ANCIENT ROOTS MANY BRANCHES

The quest to understand the individual and human conditions has led to a reevaluation of health care practices from indigenous cultures around the world.

This book searches for such models of therapy and healing which have stood the test of time, and how these can be integrated effectively in our lives.

ANCIENT ROOTS MANY BRANCHES

Energetics of Healing Across Cultures & Through Time

DARLENA L'ORANGE
GARY DOLOWICH

New Age Books

ISBN: 81-7822-126-8

First Indian Edition: Delhi, 2006

Disclaimer:
This guide is not meant to represent definitive guidelines for the treatment of illness or injury. As with any injury or health concern competent professional treatment is recommended.

Published by
NEW AGE BOOKS
A-44 Naraina Phase-I
New Delhi-110 028 (INDIA)
Email: nab@vsnl.in
Website: www.newagebooksindia.com

For Sale in South Asia Only

Printed in India
at Brijbasi Art Press Ltd.
A-81, Sector-V, Noida-201301

I live my life in growing orbits
which move out over the things of the world.
Perhaps I can never achieve the last,
but that will be my attempt.
I am circling around God
around the ancient tower,
and I have been circling for a thousand years,
and I still don't know if I am a falcon,
or a storm,
or a great song.

RAINER MARIA RILKE

Dedications

My contribution to this book is Dedicated to
Sena, Jordana, Ariel & Elisa

DR. GARY

Dedicated to Terry Theocharides, Teresita Perez &
Jazmin Tyler Cubilla — our first granddaughter
born May 15, 2000

May your grandchildren and their grandchildren . . .
and their grandchildren still find
our beautiful blue planet a delightful place to dwell.

DARLENA

In Memory of

Donna Dolowich, a dear sister, whose warmth and generosity of spirit made her a true Taoist.

Earl LaOrange, a kind-hearted, big brother, whose love of music, nature, Native American ways and work with the Shoshone and Bannock tribes helped light my own path. You will be sorely missed by all of us.

Ackey Harris, our dear friend, always a joy - forever in our hearts.

Acknowledgments

Dr. Gary:

Thanks to Darlena for asking me to participate in the creation of this book. It has been a joy to work together.

I am grateful to many teachers along the way, in particular, Fritz Smith, J. R. Worsley, Rabbi Zalman Schachter, and my buddy Wayne Souza, whose insights on Jungian psychology have been formative.

A host of friends have supported my journey; I especially want to acknowledge Len Beyea, Gary Klapman, Phil Wagner and Jim Zeno. Many thanks to Gary Hillerson, who provided the technical support that allowed my ideas to find expression.

To Dorit and fellow faculty at the Academy for Five Element Acupuncture, I am thankful for the opportunity to teach this wonderful system of medicine.

My gratitude extends to Mary Huse, Charlie Singer and all my colleagues at Jade Mountain Health Centre, together we learn about healthcare as a spiritual practice. And to my patients who, daily, are my greatest teachers.

Thanks to my daughter, Jordana, whose skill in language has been a great help in editing.

And, finally, to my wife and partner, Sena, whose support and love has made this work a reality.

Darlena:

Baba Hari Dass, thank you for your crystal clarity and being a constant source of light and inspiration in my life. Ma Renu, thank you for your wise compassion, loving guidance and dedication to the betterment of so many lives.

Dr. Gary Dolowich, my 5 Element guide, thank you for your deep wisdom and insights into the world of archetypes and energetics. So many of your teachings are reflected in my work. Without you, this book could not have materialized.

Michael Tierra, my herbal and 8-principle acupuncture teacher (in the Miriam Lee tradition), thank you for your eclectic vision of planetary herbal energetics and profound love of our earth's green inhabitants.

UCSC Professors Triloki Pandy and Diane Gifford-Gonalez - your thought-provoking lectures were instrumental in forming my world view - thank you.

Lesley Tierra, my dear friend with whom I share so many paths, we have laughed often and enjoyed countless fascinating adventures (including Egyptian "sound and light" shows!) - I'm certain we'll share many more.

Savarna McCabe, thank you for your warm caring heart, our friendship, innumerable therapeutic giggle sessions and your help in naming this book.

Ellen Holm, Mary Huse, and Charles Singer - Earth, Fire & Water, our wild, witty, wonderful 5-Element companions - it's a pleasure and delight to work with you!

Vanessa Stafford, thank you for your artistic sensitivity in creating the lovely artwork that graces the following pages.

Cathy Hoselton, your excellent editing skills were invaluable - thank you for your patience and guidance in bringing this work to fruition.

Roger and Peggy Mastrude, your tender love and dedication to each other, and gentle, compassionate ways warm and enrich the lives of those you touch - thank you for touching ours.

Special friends & family, thank you for your support and encouragement - you bring so much meaning to my life: Barbara Bender; Martha Benedict; Madhu & Swarup Brodkey; Roberta Bristol; Lara, Kili, Jazmin & Vivi Cubilla; Reva & Amitabha Damir; Mary Fenton; Lito, Pablo & Patricia Galbani; Margot & Dario Grasso; Susan Hansen; Prema Harris; Janaki Hattis; Claudia Kenyon; Dena, Pauls & Kai Krasts; the entire Lansdale clan & Emily, our goddaughter; Joan, Desiree, Monte, Karla, Karly & Ashlyn Rose LaOrange; Rajiv & Sanjivani Martel; Savarna & Devendra McCabe-Wiley; Rachel McKay; Maureen Moore; Ann Murphy; Julito, Nora & Juli Perez; Lona, Lonnie, Lanny, Penny, Tessa, Jessica & Chris Saloga; Debbie & Mohan Siegel; Vicki Swaynie; Senta Tierra; Shasta & Arnold Tierra-Tayam; Harry, Mary and Nico Theocharides; Barbara Trovato; Lupe Vega; Lorraine Washington.

Contents

Foreword

The introduction of Energy into the Western view of health and healing has been one of the formative events in our culture over the past 30 years. Not only have concepts and models of Energy fueled the acceptance and growth of alternative and complementary medicine, but they have added to the ferment of our times fostering changes of our basic values, life style, and self responsibility. From the influences of the East we have seen yoga, martial arts, Tai Chi, Qi Gong, and meditation emerging into the main stream; from cultures around the world we have seen the introduction of herbs, shamanistic practices, and alternative ways of viewing the individual; from East and West we have seen the introduction of major systems of healing such as Traditional Chinese Medicine, Ayurvedic Medicine and Homeopathy.

Central to these non-Western, non-scientific viewpoints, whether they have come from China, India, Tibet, South America, Europe or our own Native American Indians, is the concept of Energy, in one form or another, and a fundamental understanding of Energy as a basic factor in our health, well being and satisfaction in life. As one looks at the world of alternative medicine it is apparent that Energy is the basic theme that runs throughout these approaches to health, and it is a theme little known in Western scientific medicine. Time proven ideas from other cultures have been pivotal in the grass roots revolution that has been and is occurring in our culture, and in the increasing acceptance and prominence of alternative/complementary medicine in our personal health care.

The impact of non-Western thinking and alternative ways of viewing the individual and the human condition has led to the reevaluation of health care practices from indigenous cultures around the world. It has stimulated the search for models of therapy and for specific treatments and herbs which have stood the test of time, and which have provided glimpses of healings and cures seemingly impossible from the Western viewpoint. This book, ***Ancient Roots, Many Branches,*** is a reflection of that excitement and research as it specifically describes and organizes divergent cultural ideas and therapies into frameworks of healing.

No one health care system has all the answers. Whereas Western Allopathic medicine is brilliant and critically important for all of us, it does not preclude the importance - the necessity - of learning from time proven non-scientific traditions. I commend the authors for stretching their collective beliefs to encompass other cultures and traditions, and to select and organize ideas and therapies into a meaningful form for the Western culture. This book is another step in our expanding understanding of health, healing and wholeness. ***Ancient Roots, Many Branches*** is an important publication for the culture, the health care practitioner, the student, and, perhaps most important, for the patient or individual searching for personal health.

Sincerely,

Fritz Frederick Smith, M.D., author of *Inner Bridges*

Introduction

BY GARY DOLOWICH, M.D., B.AC.

Health and illness have always been inseparable in human life. Like the Chinese concept of *yin* and *yang*, it is impossible to conceive of one without the other. Wanting a life free of illness would be comparable to expecting summer without winter, or day without night. The American poet Wendell Berry said it like this:

When I rise up,
let me rise up joyful
like a bird.
When I fall,
let me fall without regret
like a leaf.

Notice that he doesn't say, "*if* I fall," it is rather, "*when* I fall." The implication is that illness is an inevitable part of the wholeness of human experience, a challenge each of us must eventually face. The choice is whether we go "kicking and screaming" or manage to find a more dignified response that balances acceptance with some active intervention.

Over the ages it has always been an aspect of cultures to deal with illness, and people have come up with solutions to this fundamental human problem in ways that reflect their unique cultural expression, combined with centuries of creative experimentation. Drawing upon an intimate relationship with a particular environment, treatments have evolved that range from herbs and foods to acupuncture needles. Before the advent of Western biomedicine, traditional healers tended to both individual health and to the wellbeing of the community. This was a work as vital to the life of the tribe as that of the hunter or warrior. It was the role of the shaman to create the sacred space where appropriate remedies could be brought in, so that healing could occur.

In this book, Darlena draws upon diverse medical traditions from ancient cultures. She takes us on a journey from India to Egypt and China to roots of Western thinking in Greece, and on to Native traditions from the Americas. Like a rich banquet, she blends therapies that have survived the test of time. The treatments presented here are not seen as an alternative to replace the achievements of Western medicine, but rather as a complement to expand the range of conditions that we can address effectively. In the wisdom of these healing practices we find teachings that are as relevant today as they were thousands of years ago.

Most remarkable, as we explore therapies developed in faraway lands, is the striking similarity in the solutions that are discovered. Although the methods always reflect particular cultural styles and environments, we find a consistency in approaches, and sometimes even the identical remedy being prescribed across the planet. Some of this can be explained through communication via caravans and trade routes, but there can be no doubt that many of these treatments have developed independently. Uncovering this "archetypal" dimension to healing brings a certain satisfaction. From the point of view of Jungian psychology, it confirms the concept of the "collective unconscious" - that there are patterns for our lives that people share because they are a fundamental aspect of what it means to be human. Birth, death, falling in love, the qualities of the Warrior that allow us to overcome difficulties - these are images that can be found in dreams, art, and stories all over the world - and can be considered archetypes. In responding to the perennial human predicament of illness, people from diverse traditions have come up with answers that are so similar because they originate from this archetypal level and reflect universal principles of healing. According to Richard Wilhelm who, in translating the ***I Ching,*** brought ancient Chinese wisdom to the Western world, "the truth can be reached from any direction, provided one digs deep enough."

As we examine the range of modalities available to us, it is useful to distinguish between symptomatic and wholistic treatments. Addressing the symptom can be quite appropriate in acute situations and with physical level problems. This is the realm where Western biomedicine excels and we also find many herbal prescriptions that are directed primarily at specific complaints. There can be no quarrel with this approach when it is successful, and we are all grateful to discover effective remedies that can remove annoying discomforts. In the case of life threatening situations, dealing with the immediate situation is essential, as we must first put out a fire in our house before searching for the cause in the electrical wiring.

We face the limitation of symptomatic treatments, however, in the case of chronic illnesses, where this type of medicine merely suppresses a manifestation of the problem and leaves the deeper cause untreated. We know this to be the case when the condition keeps reoccurring or, because the root is not addressed, suppression forces the disturbance to a deeper level. Here is the appropriate arena for wholistic medicine, which does not separate the symptom from the person in whom it is occurring. This approach works under the assumption that the illness is a meaningful occurrence and, in fact, has something to teach us about how we live our lives. The unremitting nature of the problem creates a demand to be heard and raises the question, "what is the message behind the symptom?" The chronic condition then becomes not just "meaningless suffering," but a part of one's life journey. In this view, illness occurs when we no longer are expressing our truth, and actually becomes an opportunity to come back into "the stream of life."

There obviously needs to be a balance between therapies that focus on the symptom and those that look at the larger picture. In Chinese medicine this distinction is known as "treating the branches or treating the roots." In my own life, it was the desire to address a deeper more meaningful level that brought me to the study of the traditional medicine of China. So many of the cases that were part of the general practice of Western medicine left me frustrated with tools that merely suppressed the presenting complaint and left the source of the problem untreated. Conditions such as headaches, irritable bowel syndrome, back pain, depression, and asthma were clearly asking for an approach that included another level. Chinese medicine allows us to uncover the imbalance beneath the condition because it directs treatment to the *energy* which underlies life. It shares this approach with traditional healing systems around the world that have understood there to be a vital force (the Chinese called it *ch'i*) that is the basis for existence. This spiritual influence moves within the physical form - when it flows harmoniously, there is health; when there is a block in the energy, illness arises. It is the goal of *energy medicine* to diagnose and treat this deeper level, thereby addressing the pattern underlying the symptoms.

Despite the best efforts of science, the vital energy retains an element of mystery. This is actually an advantage in understanding the wholeness of life experience, which cannot be grasped solely through the analytical mind. Throughout this book, we will be taking an anthropological view of how people, across cultures, have approached this elusive concept of energy. Traditionally, symbols are used for this purpose, often arranged in a particular numerical pattern that brings meaning to life's events and order out of chaos. Based on the idea that we are an extension of the natural world, these models for understanding nature are then applied to the human condition. And so we find that traditional medical systems have evolved, built on symbols, and based on a particular numerology, for working with *ch'i*. Our journey through these models will take us from *one* (the essential unity of all things), to *two* (*yin-yang* in Chinese philosophy and hot-cold in the Americas), to *three* (the doshas in the Ayurvedic tradition of India), to *four* (the humors in Greek thought and the directions in Native American understanding), to *five* (elements in acupuncture). In the later chapters of this book, we will see how these models can be applied to individual conditions.

When the deeper roots of illness are examined, we find that conditions tend to involve three levels of human experience: *body*, *mind*, and *spirit*. Any chronic disease will in time be expressed on all three, though there certainly may be an emphasis on one level or another. The approach taken in energy medicine allows us to avoid the unhelpful notion that our mental state is the *cause* of physical symptoms, especially when they cannot be measured in the laboratory. This assumption operates in both the concept of psychosomatic illness and in alternative medicine as well, derived from the Western model of cause and effect and the Descartian view that separates the mind from the body. Holding illness in this way creates a double burden for us - not only do we have the condition to contend with, but we are somehow to blame for it. Implied in this thinking is the idea that, if we did everything right, we wouldn't get sick. In the face of the unexplainable tragedies in human life, such as childhood leukemia, this way to approach disease simply does not work. We need, rather, to navigate a middle course that allows us to be "responsible *to* the illness, not *for* the illness." Instead of splitting the person into parts, the model of energy medicine holds to the basic unity of the *body*, *mind*, and *spirit*, while addressing the underlying imbalance that lies at the root of manifestations that may occur on all levels. It provides us with unifying symbols that support genuine healing. As a paradigm, it allows acceptance of what can't be changed, while encouraging us to work creatively to achieve the most favorable outcome.

A case from my practice to illustrate these principles involves a woman who developed adult onset asthma and was treated with bronchodilators and steroid inhalers. The Western trained physicians involved in her case never reflected on a possible meaning to the illness, even though this patient was diagnosed late in life (which is unusual for allergic asthma). Despite the latest chemical treatments to suppress the condition, her problem was not clearing and, indeed, her ability to get a deep breath was becoming more compromised. In addition, she was feeling increasingly depressed and described a general loss of purpose. An in depth history revealed that this woman had suffered a terrible tragedy: she lost a child in a car accident. The asthma, it turns out, began exactly on the one-year anniversary of this event. In acupuncture, the energy pathway of the Lung is associated, in addition to the physical organ of the lungs, with the emotion of grief and, on the deepest level, with the function of receiving life energy from the heavens. This woman had experienced an almost unbearable loss that impacted on this specific energy pattern and eventually manifested on all levels, including the disease we call asthma. To merely suppress the symptoms on the body level would clearly not be sufficient. Rather than implying that the grief is the cause of her physical condition, in Chinese medicine we can look at all the expressions of the body, mind and spirit as a reflection of an underlying energetic disturbance. Treatment included a range of therapies: herbs, psychotherapy, ch'i gong exercises, as well as acupuncture to treat the Lung meridian. Western pharmaceutical agents to support her breathing were continued during the initiation of these complementary approaches. Ultimately, the pain of losing a child is something that we can never cure but, as the deeper pattern was treated in a compassionate manner, the woman could gradually return to the stream of her life. I knew that healing had indeed taken place when she eventually became a volunteer at the local hospice in order to help other parents who had suffered similar tragedies. As for her asthma, the symptoms gradually subsided as the deeper root of the problem was addressed, and in time she was weaned off the inhalers.

Generally there are two strategies in approaching imbalances through energy medicine. The first would be to provide the factor that brings things towards center, that balances the disturbance. This is seen, for example, in treating a hot condition by prescribing cooling herbs. Similarly, if someone is too active and excited, unable to sleep or shut off their mind, interventions that offer quiet and rest would provide a balancing influence that can lead towards health. The second principle in healing on the energetic level takes the opposite approach, based on the concept that "like cures like." In this case, an imbalance is treated through a remedy that produces a similar effect, thereby bringing the disturbance to the surface in order to allow its release. We find this operating in psychotherapy, for example, when we encourage a person to express a buried emotion and find that this has a healing effect. Homeopathy is built on this idea and uses minute doses of remedies that produce similar symptoms (such as coffee to alleviate insomnia) to help the body resolve a disturbance on a deep level. Listening to blues music when we are depressed and finding that this indeed lifts our mood is an everyday example of this principle of healing. In the remedies described in this book, we will find both approaches operating.

There is a third possibility in dealing with illness that needs to be acknowledged: the problem may not be susceptible to our interventions. Traditional medicine has always allowed for this category and has understood that illness could be "sent by the gods," in which case it was not our place to eradicate it. The humility that allows us to accept our human limitations, and bow to forces that are beyond our control, was built into the worldview of traditional cultures. Here the task presented by illness is a spiritual one. This is where faith comes in, the intuition that, regardless of the outcome, there is a deeper meaning and purpose that we can trust. As the Native American tradition has said, "sometimes I go about pitying myself, and all the while I am being carried by a great wind across the sky."

In coming to terms with illness, we find ourselves on a journey of growth and exploration. Fundamental is the self-discovery that is the inevitable outcome if we choose to dig deeper to uncover the roots of the condition. This book can serve as a resource for such a journey - providing ideas and materials that have been useful across cultures and throughout the ages as people have dealt with this very human challenge. Sometimes the solution, if we are fortunate, is a simple remedy that neutralizes an ailment. In other cases, the situation requires a more fundamental change in lifestyle or attitude. Often healing may then require a sacrifice - be it of a job, a relationship, a point of view, or some destructive habit. Always, in dealing with the archetypal problem of illness, there is the opportunity for finding new meaning and appreciation for our lives. And, as Jung has said, "meaning makes a great many things endurable, perhaps everything."

1

Natural Healing Traditions of the Ancients

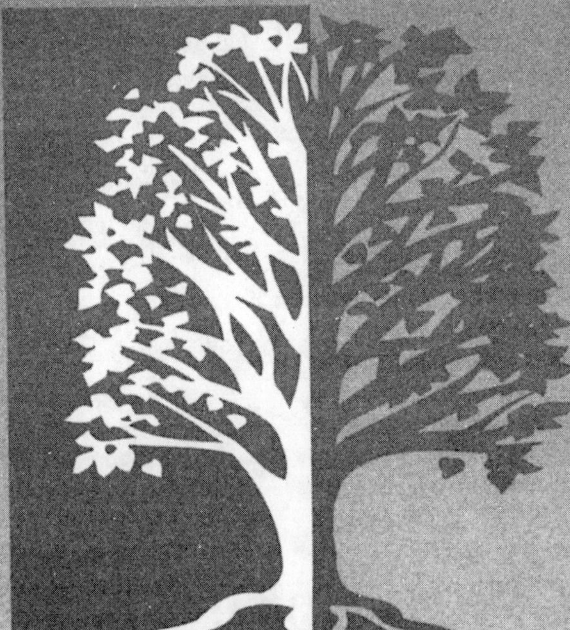

A Path of Wholeness

Western Biomedicine meets Traditional Healing

BY GARY DOLOWICH, M.D., B.AC.

An eye is meant to see things.
The soul is here for its own joy.
Mysteries are not to be solved:
The eye goes blind when it only wants to see why.
RUMI

After twenty years of integrating the traditional methods of acupuncture and herbs, along with the bodywork system of Zero Balancing, into my practice of Western biomedicine, I've come to realize that it is simply a matter of selecting the appropriate tool for the condition to be treated. Common sense dictates the conditions where the techniques of conventional scientific medicine excel: surgery, acute emergencies, high technology interventions, and diseases that can be measured in the laboratory. It is the chronic problems, situations that involve the mind as well as the body, diseases that are labeled "functional" because no precise etiology exists or tests prove negative, that are suitable for traditional medicine. Even if there are positive X-ray findings, as for example in osteoarthritis, whenever biomedicine can only suppress the symptoms, more natural therapies may offer a more effective treatment that addresses a deeper level. By most estimates, at least 75% of the patients seen today in general practice would benefit by incorporating traditional healing methods into their treatments.

What is needed, from both the patient and practitioner, is a mind big enough to hold a range of possibilities. It is far too easy to allow a biased viewpoint determine the way we approach a condition, and lead to inappropriate, or even harmful, treatments. I remember a case that occurred when I first began incorporating Chinese acupuncture into my medical practice. In my enthusiasm for Five Element theory, I began to interpret a patient's report that he was urinating six times during the night as a *Water* imbalance to be treated with needles and herbs. Only as an afterthought did it occur to me that I ought to check his urine for sugar. When the test turned positive, and subsequent measurement of blood sugar proved the onset of acute diabetes that responded to life-saving therapy with insulin, I received an important lesson in keeping my balance. In approaching traditional medicine from other lands, we clearly must build upon a foundation in our own culture's understanding of life. It would be a tremendous loss to disregard the gifts of our Western heritage and seek the answers entirely from without.

Fundamentally, science deals with what can be measured, with things that can be known for certain. Diseases that can be approached in this physical way often respond quite nicely to Western biomedical treatment. Where a definite etiology exists, for example when a bacteria that is the cause of pneumonia can be grown in the laboratory and an antibiotic can be shown to suppress its growth, the tools of conventional medicine are unsurpassed. Science also offers one way to know about other systems of medicine. There is, for example, an impressive body of literature documenting the clinical efficacy of Chinese medicine. It has long been known that acupuncture can influence physiological measurements, such as blood pressure and cardiac output. Electroencephalograph recordings clearly show the ability of acupuncture to influence brain wave responses to electric shock. Recently, in response to overwhelming evidence, a panel at the National Institute of Health concluded that acupuncture is beneficial in treating nausea due to chemotherapy and most forms of pain.

These studies are certainly useful and serve as a bridge for introducing traditional medicine into the West. The problem with the research, however, is that it tends to force these systems into the Western paradigm, ignoring, or worse, deriding aspects that don't fit the model. Most disturbing is the insistence that rigorously conducted scientific tests are the only way to evaluate unconventional methods of healing. The editors of the Journal of the American Medical Association, spokesmen for orthodox medicine, even go so far as to insist that:

> *until solid evidence is available that demonstrates the safety, efficacy, and effectiveness of specific alternative medicine interventions, uncritical acceptance of untested and unproven alternative medicine therapies must stop.*

This is quite a pronouncement in light of the fact that over four billion people (some 80% of the world's population) currently rely on herbal medicine for some aspect of primary health care. In the United States alone it is estimated that 40% of adults use some form of unconventional therapy.

Much of herbal medicine is indeed amenable to scientific study, and there is an increasing interest in isolating the chemical components responsible for their effects. However, when practiced in a wholistic way, traditional medicine does not separate the disease from the patient or the treatment from the practitioner, and it then becomes impossible to isolate single variables to "prove" their efficacy. In fact, any method that is truly wholistic will approach ten patients with migraine headaches with ten entirely different treatments. It is a real concern that, in order to fit the rigid criterion for modern scientific research, medical therapies based on energetic models will increasingly be studied as symptomatic, cookbook formulas. Each disease category then receives the identical prescription and the patient, once again, is treated as a broken machine rather than as a unique individual. In an effort to conform to accepted research designs, the real value (and potential contribution to health care in the West) of these traditional medical systems will be lost.

Rational thought can excel within its appropriate arena, but reason sets the boundaries far too narrowly for us, and a great deal of life falls outside its realm. When we explore the issues that lie at the root of illness, we are often led to aspects of life that elude the methods of science. Traditional medicine, built on centuries of observation and developed in cultures where there is an intimate connection to nature, offers an approach that embraces the wholeness of the human experience. In seeking to understand the energetic pattern beneath the symptoms, we focus on the process rather than content and are led to a deeper level of our being that includes the emotions and the spirit. However, *ch'i*, the vital force which is the fundamental principle behind many of these traditional systems, like life itself, remains a Mystery. Perhaps there will be a time in the future when science will develop instruments that are sensitive enough to measure it, but for now *ch'i* cannot be known through these tools. To try to interpret energy medicine solely in terms of current Western models mistranslates it miserably.

The unnecessary conflict between biomedical and traditional approaches to healing is not unlike the struggle between science and spirituality in Western history. The over-emphasis on "correct" religious belief during the Middle Ages led to an equally one-sided belief in science with the coming of the Renaissance. Yet, it seems to me that some things naturally fall within the province of science and can be known through its methods, while other areas of life are best explored through poetry, spiritual practices, and by trusting one's heart. Life is sufficiently complex and mysterious to allow for both approaches. As Jung points out in his essay, "Yoga and the West":

> *There are no grounds whatsoever for any conflict between these two things. Both are necessary, for knowledge alone, like faith alone, is always insufficient.*

Of course, very few patients come for treatment with questions about scientific validity. Their concern is likely to be much more pragmatic: finding the approach that will alleviate their condition. For the health care provider it also ought to be a matter of applying the most effective therapeutic intervention. The practitioner is not being asked to master these wide ranging fields, only to have the open-mindedness that allows referring elsewhere when appropriate. It is a missed opportunity when the patient is advised prematurely that they must "live with the problem."

In so many ways we find the scientific and energetic medical models to be useful in just the areas where the other is lacking. For this reason, I would avoid using the oppositional term "alternative medicine" and support the more inclusive phrase "complementary medicine." We can see how this can work in chronic conditions such as hypertension, where Western medicine is able to prescribe medications to successfully lower blood pressure, preventing serious complications. Because the disease is labeled *idiopathic* (which means we don't know the cause), it is not surprising that the root of the problem remains untreated. When this is the case, herbs and acupuncture are appropriate ways to address the problem on a deeper level, with the goal of reducing or eliminating the reliance on drugs. The experience in China, where practitioners of Western and traditional methods work side by side, has been quite illuminating in this respect. In treating certain cancers, for example, chemotherapy and radiation are used to eradicate the tumor while acupuncture, herbs, and internal exercises are prescribed to lessen side-effects of treatment and to support the immune system and the patient on the whole.

Another arena where traditional methods can blend quite easily with scientific technique is in the treatment of infertility. In many cases, high tech interventions can place the fertilized egg in the woman's uterus, but fail to achieve the desired goal. What is often not addressed is the human factor in pregnancy - receptivity, openness, and the ability to nurture - qualities that are basic to this natural process and often lost in our fast-paced, modern world. The sterile atmosphere and focus on results often creates an anxiety that works in just the opposite direction. Five Element acupuncture, through encouraging us to think metaphorically, offers the insight that the woman must indeed *be* the Earth for the potential new life to take hold inside her. In my experience, treatments that reinforce such positive images, both through visualizations and acupuncture therapy, can complement scientific techniques and lead to a more favorable outcome. In addition, a more balanced, wholistic approach may benefit a person's life in ways that extend beyond the immediate concern, as in this example, where a woman may come back in touch with her feminine side. It is clear that the complementary use of traditional and biomedical therapies holds great promise and is, as yet, largely unexplored.

For those engaged in the practice of Western medicine, it can be frustrating not to have a model for treating the whole person, or for working on improved well-being; health is merely defined as the absence of disease. This is particularly evident in general physical exams where, in the case of basically healthy clients, there is very little the physician can offer besides ordering expensive tests to rule out pathology. In the arena of preventive medicine, traditional methods offer a positive vision of wellness, based on living in harmony with nature. When diagnosis addresses subtle energetic imbalances, there is the possibility of improving conditions before they become manifest in organic disease. Since it is at this stage where interventions in life-style, such as diet, exercise, and herbs are likely to be most effective, there is typically a strong emphasis on the prevention of illness in energetic approaches to healing.

All systems of medicine share a common concern, the care of the patient, and ask a similar quality from the practitioner, a "mind of caring." Professor Worsley, my acupuncture teacher in England, has compared the world of medicine to an orchestra, where each system is a section that has a particular function. It is only through working together that we can approach the healing process in a way that treats the whole human being in *body, mind, and spirit*. There is a beautiful symphony to be played, one which can support the healing of the individual and, in the bigger picture, the healing of this planet. It will require a full range of skill and experience from many traditions for this to take place.

In studying healing systems from around the world we are led on a path that takes us away from the complexities of modern life and back to the simple rhythms of nature. The rewards extend far beyond the learning of new medical techniques to suppress symptoms. It is a journey that holds the potential for a deeper healing, as we examine the patterns of life and come to know the energies of our own inner being. It is only as we become more whole in ourselves that we are in a position to assist others, and to address the real issues underlying the problems of our world. Indeed, the true role of traditional medicine in the West is "to help society, in general, to rediscover its natural roots."

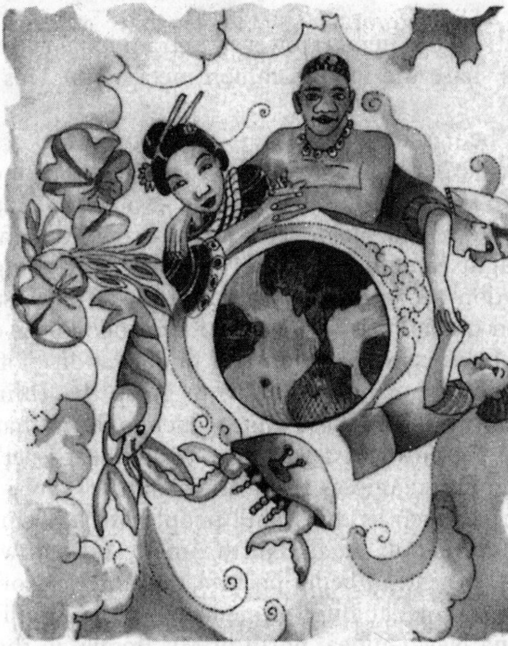

Patterns of Life

What pattern connects the crab to the lobster
and the orchid to the primrose
and all four of them to me?
And me to you?

GREGORY BATESON

If an anthropologist walked into your home or room, what patterns would they find that define YOU... who you are... the way you think... your unique take on the world? In order to truly understand a person or culture, anthropologists may first attempt to distinguish the four or five major symbols that dominate a particular person or culture's world view. For example, in your room would someone find a Grateful Dead or Beatles' poster, or perhaps a copy of Monet's *Water Lilies* - maybe all three? Do you have books and magazines on health, sports, the stock market or computers? Perhaps you have a crucifix on the wall, a Buddha statue on the shelf or a copy of the Koran or Bible on your night stand. In our widely diverse and complex culture, the great melting pot, in any given city block we might find all of the above items. However, in traditional cultures, most inhabitants share the same common metaphors. This is how it works...

Human beings are web weavers and pattern makers - we are trying to make sense of a world we do not understand. In trying to make sense out of our experiences we create art, music, religion and other ideologies. We literally construct a world out of our thoughts, and, like UCSC Professor Shelly Errington says, "The imitation becomes our world and the world disappears." The human tendency is to concretize symbolic forms originally created to help expand our limited understanding of the universe and provide a means for us to grasp the Infinite. The "real" world gets lost in those finite, concrete forms that we have created. To get an idea of what this really means, let's look at some intriguing examples from other cultures, very different than our own, such as the Kaluli people of New Guinea and the Zuni/Hopi people of the North American Southwest.

Let's say, instead of being born in the Americas or Europe, you are the son or daughter of members of the Kaluli tribe living in Papua New Guinea, north of Mt. Bosavi, in the tropical rain forest. Let's look at just two basic symbols or patterns that dominate your Kaluli view of the world and how they influence your life and take on reality - *birds,* and *landscape.* As a Kaluli, from an early age you would spend much time learning the descriptions and nesting habits of the forest avifauna, as well as their calls. The Kaluli compare themselves to birds; spirits are birds and birds are spirits. Because of the dense forest habitat, you would recognize the birds primarily through their "voices." Bird voices are believed to be spirit communications from deceased men and women - your ancestors.

Kaluli memories are tied intrinsically to the landscape; their lush forest home is a large topographical memory bank. For example, as a Kaluli person, you might identify a certain tree with a place you once ate honey with a friend, or a particular stream might be associated with memories of fishing with a dearly loved but deceased grandfather. Time is nonexistent in your culture, in the typical Western sense, and in much the same way that certain dates serve as memory nodes for us (i.e., I graduated in 1975, or my daughter was born in 1980), places in the forest are memory nodes for the Kaluli.

Now, let me whisk you away to the arid, North American southwestern lands of the Zuni/Hopi people and look at two important themes that help form their view of life - *corn* and *rain*. Eagle instructed the Hopi ancestors to propagate human life by growing corn, and, according to tradition, corn is your main source of nourishment. As a member of the Hopi tribe, there would be 35 words in your vocabulary which mean "corn." Many Hopi rites of passage center around the corn theme. Corn would even be a factor in selection of your future mate since courtship actually takes place while the girls are grinding corn. Special blue corn tortillas would be served at your wedding and in one special ceremony, your newborn baby would be introduced to corn and told that it is the food given to it by the ancients.

A prime requisite for the growth of corn is rain. Most ceremonies in Zuni/Hopi culture center around fertility, with rain being a central focus. If someone close to you passes on, as a Hopi/Zuni you believe they become a Kachina spirit who resides over the mountains in spirit form as a cloud. You would look forward to visits from your cloud ancestors who bring life-giving rain with them to nourish the corn crops.

Interesting, but what does all of this have to do with healing? Sometimes, it is extremely difficult to see beyond the patterns we have created. Here's a good example that may bring all of this closer to home. Walking with a friend in nearby Niseen-Marks forest the other day, Jeannie expressed concern for her brother Craig who works as a machinist in nearby San Jose. Craig experiences extreme pain from arthritic knees and, over the years, he's come up with some rather interesting home remedies based on his particular view as a machinist. Most recently, perhaps half in jest, Craig applied a spray used for rusty hinges to his knee *(not recommended)*. It didn't seem to help. While this true story may seem extreme or bizarre to some people, it is perfectly logical if you spend eight hours a day working on machines. The view that the human body is a machine, after all, forms the basis for the model used by our modern biomedical system. Just think of all our cultural references to the body as a machine - the heart is a pump, the joints are hinges, the brain is a computer. The truth is that each of us is constantly making decisions, some good, some maybe not so good, based on the unique patterns that govern the way we perceive our world. And, the way we see the world depends largely on how the family and the culture in which we grew up views the world.

Earth, our home, from time immemorial has been inhabited

by ingenious patternmakers, weavers of realities, makers of myths, creators of cultures, civilizations and vast empires. They are our ancestors. In the upcoming pages we will be looking at healing systems and cures from around the world. While volumes can and have been written about each of these great cultures and their unique healing systems, our delicate shrinking globe cries out for synthesis - not separation. The intent of this book is not to romanticize one system as being superior but to open new vistas of thought by suggesting each system has much wisdom to offer while we explore the patterns found in each. A lovely poem by a Zen monk named Kukai, who lived between 774 and 835 A.D., calls us to open, grow and expand our views:

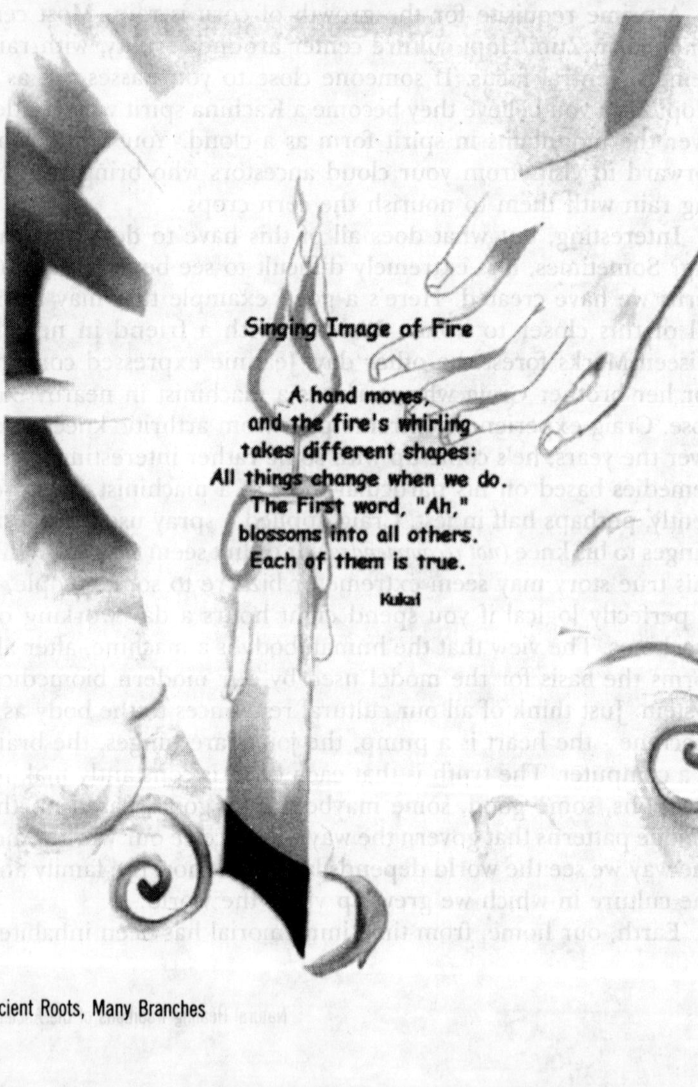

Singing Image of Fire

A hand moves,
and the fire's whirling
takes different shapes:
All things change when we do.
The First word, "Ah,"
blossoms into all others.
Each of them is true.

Kukai

Harnessing the Power of Earth's Age-Old Medical Traditions

From the beginning of time our ancient ancestors not only survived, but thrived and multiplied in our earth's vastly diversified ecosystems - from icy tundra to tropical islands. Shaman, curanderos, witch doctors, mid-wives, monks, mendicants, herbalists, physicians, homeopaths, chiropractors, acupuncturists, nutritionists, psychologists, scientists, nurses and doctors - health care providers of all types from all continents - have contributed to the rich legacy of earth's healing practices from our planet's herbal pharmacopoeia to pharmaceutical drugs. This chapter is dedicated to all true healers, those of a compassionate heart, from all cultures and through all times. It is dedicated to each and every one of us who, in big or small ways, contribute care giving to ourselves and others.

Entering the new millennium we are witnesses of a remarkable resurgence of interest in tried and true healing practices that have survived the tests of time. If only in a small way, we hope to bring some of the wisdom of many of these traditions to life in the following pages. Everyday complaints will be discussed, along with many different techniques, foods and herbal formulas for easing discomfort. Depending upon our individual constitutions, some methods will work better than others for each of us. Often you will find that you already possess the cure for minor ailments right on your spice rack, in the kitchen cupboard, or growing in your own backyard!

Before getting started, I can't resist taking you on a brief, whirlwind adventure. To get a sense of the richness of our world's remarkable healing legacy, we'll take only one simple substance, silver, just to see how it has been used for healing in various cultures throughout time.

Bacterial infections have long plagued humankind, however, our ancestors demonstrated incredible ingenuity in the numerous ways they overcame microbial invaders - from herbs to minerals to antibiotics. Silver is one of those substances that has enjoyed a long and distinguished history of usage in the healing arts.

In ancient Greece, over 3,000 years ago, wine and water urns were lined with silver to kill bacteria. Romans applied poultices of silver 2,000 years ago to aid in the healing of sores, cuts and burns. About 1,500 years ago doctors advised patients to eat with silver utensils if they wanted to maintain their health. In Europe, 400 years ago, the bubonic plague decimated 25 percent of the population; however, very few wealthy persons succumbed to the black death. Their children maintained good health by sucking on silver spoons (that's where our expression, *"Born with a silver spoon in his mouth,"* comes from!). From that time on, silverware became a highly-valued household item.

Since refrigeration was not a convenience enjoyed by settlers of the American West, silver dollars were placed in fresh milk to keep it from spoiling during warm spells. In 1884, Dr. K.S. Crede, a German obstetrician, discovered that a mild silver solution significantly reduced eye infections if placed in the eyes of newborns. Use of silver nitrate is required by law in most countries to this day. In the early 1900's, Dr. Henry Crookes successfully used silver in the treatment of tuberculosis, gonorrhea and other diseases. In 1916, the medical journal *Transactions of the American Association of Obstetricians and Gynecologists* reported that silver enhanced immunity by building the number of white blood cells as well as by killing bacterial and viral invaders.

During the 1960's, the healing properties of silver were praised when studies demonstrated its effectiveness in combating infections such as syphilis, malaria and candidiasis. In 1970 Dr. Carl Moyer, at the Washington University Department of Surgery, demonstrated that an ultra-fine, low-dose form of silver solution in the treatment of burn victims was far superior to the use of antibiotics. Burned skin developed an immunity to the drugs while a mild silver solution simply killed the bacteria quickly and efficiently, facilitating healing of the burned tissue. Clinical researchers at the VA Hospital in Syracuse, New York confirmed Dr. Moyer's research by conducting their own tests.

During this same time frame, and perhaps even hundreds of years earlier, Ayurvedic sages in India had discovered the therapeutic value of various metals and gemstones. In the land of Gandhi, silver is prized for its cooling properties that help balance pitta (heat symptoms); and its ability to increase stamina and strength, thus balancing vata (air/ether elements). It was and is still used to ease chronic fever, heartburn, inflammatory conditions of the intestines and profuse menstrual bleeding. Ayurvedic practitioners utilize silver as a disinfectant, an antiseptic and as an antibacterial agent. To increase strength and endurance, people in India drink warm milk that has been heated in a container made of high quality silver.

But, please wait, before you run out to purchase silverware! In the upcoming pages you will be introduced to many extraordinary healing substances that might be more appropriate for your constitution or particular condition! Be sure to take the brief tests in Chapters 9, 10, 11 and 12 to learn more about the energetics of healing substances. In the upcoming pages you will be reading a lot about *energetics*. When we talk about *energetic healing systems,* we are referring to models that are very distinct from our own cultural image of the body as a machine. All of the other systems view the human body as a microcosm of the universe, as part of, and, as an extension of nature. Basically, there is the bipolar model which categorizes people, diseases and healing substances as hot/cold or yin/yang. In East Indian Ayurveda we find a five element system that categorizes in terms of a model of three - Vata, Pitta and Kapha Dosha. In ancient Greece, Rome and Arabia a four element model was used while North, Central and South American Natives utilized bipolar and four and five element models. In Asian medicine the healing system is divided into bipolar as well as five elemental categories.

Are you ready for a brief, but fascinating, historical tour of the origins of healing in various cultures? Please notice how the ancient roots of all healing traditions are firmly planted in a system of energetics based on observations of nature as described above. Throughout the history of humankind, those **ancient roots** have sprouted in to the **many branches** of healing arts practiced in our world today.

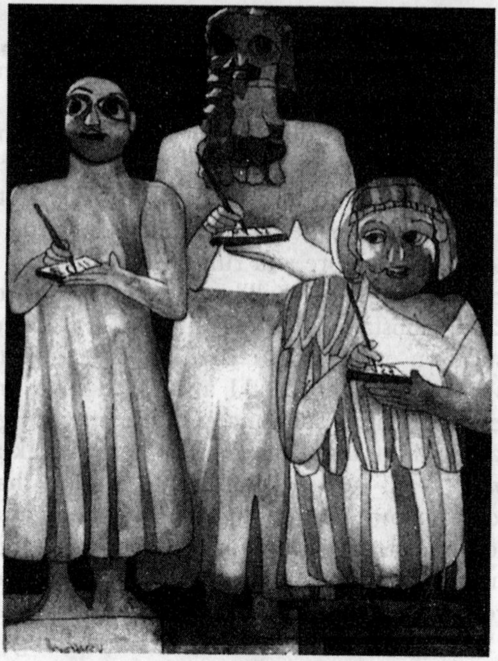

Medicine in Mesopotamia

Some of the earliest written evidence of the practice of medicine comes to us from the ancient civilizations of Assyria and Babylon in the form of cuneiform writing that has been preserved on baked clay tablets dating from as early as 3500 BCE. Hammurabi ruled Babylon around 1940 BCE. From this ancient civilization some of humankind's very first codes were written on an eight foot long pillar, or stele, known as the Laws of Hammurabi. The responsibilities of a physician are outlined along with other laws regarding economic regulations and social conditions. At this early date the medical profession was already highly scrutinized with penalties for failure clearly stated. The unsuccessful surgeon could lose his hand as a punishment for surgical incompetence.

Herbalism was formally practiced by this time in human history; the evidence comes to us once again from Assyria. Over 250 healing herbs are described on clay tablets dating from around 2500 BCE. It is unknown, at this time, if these ancient peoples were using a system of healing energetics or if the roots of bipolar and four or five element humoral thinking first began to sprout in ancient Egypt.

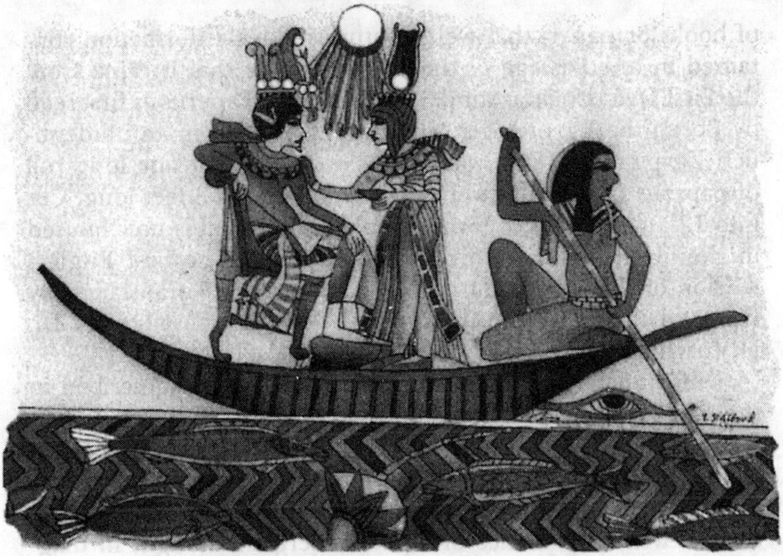

Secrets of Healing from the Land of the Pyramids

It is the power of truth that endures!

PTAHHOTEP, 2400 BCE

In every culture, some type of medicine develops early on. The use of malachite as an eye paint and salve can be traced back nearly 7,000 years to the Badarian Culture that thrived on the banks of the Nile in Upper Egypt from approximately 4800 to 4200 BCE. A circumcision operation is clearly represented on the wall of a Sixth Dynasty tomb (c. 2625 to 2475 BCE); and embalmed bodies exhumed from ancient graves dating from around 4000 BCE show traces of the operation. The skill of an early dentist is illustrated by a mandible found in a tomb of the Fourth Dynasty (2900 to 2750 BCE); the alveolar process under the first molar was pierced to drain an abscess.

While there are fragments of seven or more medical papyri that date back to 2000 BCE, most of them reflect knowledge going back as far 2700 BCE. The Ebers Papyrus, often called the oldest medical "book" in the world, was written around 1600 BCE; however, it is believed the text was copied from a series of books or papyri that were centuries older. Information contained in one passage of the Papyrus states that it came from the First Dynasty, or around 3400 BCE. The Papyrus as first seen by Ebers, the Egyptologist who purchased it from an unidentified Egyptian in 1862, was not a book at all but one long roll of papyrus measuring twelve inches wide and 68 feet long. Cut into 12 inch lengths to form a book, the original is now housed in the library of the University of Leipzig. The first English version of this document comes to us as a 1927 translation by Dr. Cyril P. Bryan from the original German translation by Dr. H. Joachim.

Unfortunately, many of the herbs and diseases described in the Papyri seem to be lost to antiquity and have not yet been translated. In reading through Bryan's translation of this ancient document, it's truly amazing to find scattered references to "heat or cold" in treating diseases, which could make this the earliest written evidence of bipolar energetic thought in diagnosing and treating illness. Any natural healer familiar with Asian medical arts will clearly understand the truth that rings out across centuries from one part of the text on the heart and circulatory system, "When anger arises in the Heart, behold it is a seething-up of the parts of the Intestine and the Liver." In Chapter XVII, *Diseases of the Ear, Nose and Mouth*, we find the following advice regarding cases of "Ear-that-Discharges-foul-smelling-Matter": The physician is told to "Treat it with cooling remedies, not warm ones." *(From a Chinese Traditional Medical perspective this is sound advice since we use bitter, cooling, antibacterial/anti viral herbs to treat middle ear infections).*

While many of the 877 prescriptions contained in the Papyrus may sound outlandish by today's standards; some of the cures are still with us through eons of time, for example, application of raw meat to a black eye; or, electrical stimulation to ease the pain of muscle strains. Yes, the ancient Egyptians were quite aware of the pain relieving affects of electrical current. Scribonius Larigus, in 45 CE, wrote about the Egyptian cure for gout pain: An electric eel was placed under the foot of the patient, then, "the patient stands on a wet beach, covered as long as possible with water, until the foot is asleep to the level of the knee." (While full grown eels can give charges up to 200 volts, the Egyptians undoubtedly used younger creatures for this cure). Inoculations? - the first known inoculation against smallpox was Egyptian in origin. The dried scab from a smallpox victim was ground into a fine powder and blown up the nostrils of the immunees with a hollow papyrus reed. Antibiotics? - In many of the prescriptions for preparing poultices to dress burns, blisters and wounds we find "rotting bread" - or moldy bread - the Egyptians were familiar with the antibacterial properties of molds more than 4,000 years ago. Suffering from a crocodile bite? You will be given the ancient Egyptian remedy for this, as well as other maladies, in the form of some very interesting and rather exotic formulas in the upcoming chapters.

A much shorter but slightly older (by about 100 years) papyrus called the Smith Papyrus could be called a surgical treatise, the spirit of which is far more "scientific" than the Ebers. It gives 48 case studies with the ailments listed in order of the body parts, starting from the head. Unfortunately, it stops a little below the shoulders because the rest of the manuscript was lost or the work of the scribe was interrupted. The author of the Smith Papyrus systematically organized his work on each case in the following way: 1) Title, 2) Examination, 3) Diagnosis, 4) Treatment (unless the case was considered fatal and untreatable) and 5) Glosses, or definitions of terms found in the text that might be considered obscure. This is truly remarkable when you think that the author lived at least two thousand years before Hippocrates. The Smith Papyrus contains some of the earliest surviving evidence of the inductive thought process in the evolution of the human mind.

Imhotep, the grand vizier of King Zoser (founder of the Third Dynasty, who ruled around 2980 BCE), is often cited as the father of Egyptian medicine; in later times he was worshipped as a hero and god of medicine - the prototype of Aesclepius. One of the rites associated with his worship (as well as that of the later Greek god of medicine, Aesclepius) was known as incubation or temple sleep. Patients would sleep in the temple and the god would appear in a dream, giving them the appropriate remedy for their malady. Imhotep was not only an astronomer and physician, but possibly the architect who designed the first large pyramid at Sakkara.

Not unlike health care professionals today, Egyptian physicians were already specializing in their trade as early as 2700 BCE. From his tombstone, we are told that Iry, head physician to Pharaoh Pepi II, who ruled during the Sixth Dynasty (2625-

2475), bore the titles of "Palace Eye Physician," "Palace Stomach Bowel Physician" and "Guardian of the Anus."

From the Egyptian papyri we learn that herbal medicine and surgery were extensively practiced in ancient Egypt. Hundreds of different substances, including mineral, plant and animal byproducts are listed to treat various ailments ranging from diseases of the eyes, teeth, nose, tongue, skin, head, extremities and bowels, to diseases of women with special tips regarding wrinkle control, cosmetics and formulas to prevent balding and graying of the hair. In reading over these ancient manuscripts you can't help but feel connected to these people who lived over 5,000 years ago grappling with many of our same, everyday concerns and complaints.

(Note: For additional information on Egyptian medicine and herbalism, see recommended reading in the Resources Section at the end of the book.)

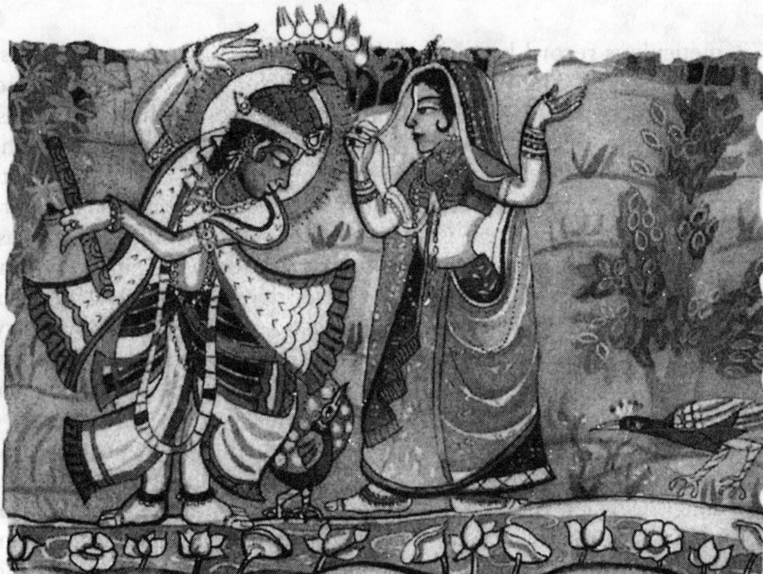

4000 Year Medical Tradition of the East Indian Yogi's

Whenever I have read any part of the Vedas,
I have felt that some unearthly
and unknown light illuminated me.
In the great teaching of the Vedas,
there is no touch of the sectarianism.
It is of ages, climes, and nationalities and
is the royal road for the attainment
of the Great Knowledge.
When I am at it, I feel that I am under
the spangled heavens of a summer night.

HENRY DAVID THOREAU

The Vedic world view was introduced to India approximately 2000 BCE by the hunting/gathering Aryan peoples. As the Aryans migrated in to India from the northwest, the agricultural Dravidian people were pushed southward. Hunter/gatherers found no practicality in carting around recorded volumes of Vedic lore (as compared to the meticulous record keeping of their agriculturally oriented Chinese counterparts). The Vedas were transmitted orally, in the form of verse, from teacher to disciple over thousands of years. While it is impossible to give an exact date, it is estimated that sometime around the 6th century BCE Sushruta, the East Indian father of surgery, wrote detailed procedures for complicated surgeries like removal of urinary stones, cataract removal, Caesarean section, tonsillectomy, even plastic and brain surgery. In the *Sushruta Samhita* (the word *Samhita* means "collection of writings"), we find a description for over 120 pieces of surgical equipment, as well as in depth knowledge of embryology, anatomy, physiology, digestion, metabolism, genetics and immunity. This comprehensive medical text also includes an herbal pharmacopoeia which lists over 750 medicinal plants.

It would seem logical that the world might not be as friendly a place for a hunting/gathering people, resulting in an Aryan patriarchal world view that was somewhat less earth-centered than the Chinese agriculturalists' view. However, earthly existence is uncertain under the best of circumstances and both the medieval Chinese and Aryan people made elaborate sacrifices to placate or solicit the aid of elemental deities, as well as regular offerings to propitiate the spirits of dead ancestors.

According to K. L. Bhishagratna, in his translation of the *Sushruta Samhita*, Sushruta gained valuable insight into comparative anatomy by dissecting many of these quartered animal sacrifices. India has never invaded any country during the last 10,000 years of history, but skilled surgeons were kept busy healing the wounds of Aryan warriors injured while protecting the settlements. If a warrior suffered from a lance or arrow wound which severed the intestine, black ants became living sutures to hold the two pieces together - once they had firmly attached themselves, the ants' bodies were then cut off, leaving only the heads. In fact, our modern word "suture" is derived from Sushruta's name. It was Sushruta who first talks of grafting of skin in mending an earlobe. In the Rigveda we find mention that legs were amputated and fitted with prostheses made of iron. Foreshadowing modern germ theory, Sushruta recommends that sick rooms be fumigated with the burning vapors of a number of herbs including white mustard, Nimva leaves and resinous gums from Shala trees. Even with this level of surgical sophistication, therapeutic massage, as well as dietary and herbal therapy were the treatments of choice. Surgery was considered mutilation, not doctoring, and was resorted to only if the vital energy of the patient was not strong enough to enable a cure.

Two other important names in early Hindu medicine include that of Caraka and Vagbhata. Exact dates for both of these men is uncertain. Caraka, who lived in the millennium before Christ, wrote a medical treatise known as the *Caraka Samhita*; which is regarded as a classic text of Hindu medicine. The *Astranga Sangraba*, written by Vagbhata sometime between 200 BCE and 700 CE, encompasses medicine, surgery and midwifery.

Like the Chinese, Vedic seers perceived a close relationship between humankind and the universe - the same Cosmic Energy (*ch'i* for the Chinese; *prana* for the East Indians) flowed through all of creation. Five basic elements were also central to the Vedic world view. According to Ayurveda, ether, air, fire, water and earth elements resulted from the union of male and female energy - *Purusha* and *Prakriti* (also referred to as *Shiva* and *Shakti*) - which, in turn, gave birth to the whole of creation.

There were no atoms yet,
let alone stars or galaxies:
All was empty.
We tend to think of it as a
serene, hushed nothingness,
an insubstantial, uneventful void,
but it was in fact seething with
all the pent-up energy of the
primordial explosion.

TRINH XUAN THUAN

Birth of the Universe: The Big Bang and After

Very similar to modern Big Bang Theory, Ayurveda, as it is being taught today, tells us that the universe was born in one instant. From that first subtle vibration of union of *Purusha* (male) and *Prakriti* (female) came the Ether element; as Ether began to stir, the Air element was created. Friction produced by the movement of Air generated heat, forming light particles or waves - the Fire element manifested from this light. Intense heat caused ethereal elements to dissolve and liquefy, creating the Water element. The Water element solidified to form molecules of the Earth element.

East Indian Ayurveda teaches us that the five basic elements are present in all matter, in varying degrees. Since humankind is a microcosm of nature, these five basic elements also exist within each individual. Our individual characteristics and differences are dictated by the relative quantities of each element. And, similar to Traditional

Chinese Medicine, when taken together, these five elements form one complete whole - self-contained, self-renewing, and self-regulating.

The five basic elements of Ayurveda are building blocks of creation. Ether *(Akasha)* is unmanifest, clear, light and subtle - giving dimension to the creation; Air *(Vayu)* is rough, clear, light and cold in quality and is responsible for movement; Fire *(Tajas)* is dry, rough, light, clear, hot and pungent - providing heat; Water *(Ap)* is oily, sweet and slightly salty, cold and soft and produces fluidity; Earth *(Prithivi)* is dense, heavy, rough, hard and gives firmness or structure.

In an individual, the Ether element manifests as "spaces" in the nose, respiratory tract, abdomen, thorax, tissues and cells. The Air element is Ether or space in motion and manifests in a human body as heart pulsations, muscular movements, the expansion and contraction of the lungs during respiration, etc. The central nervous system

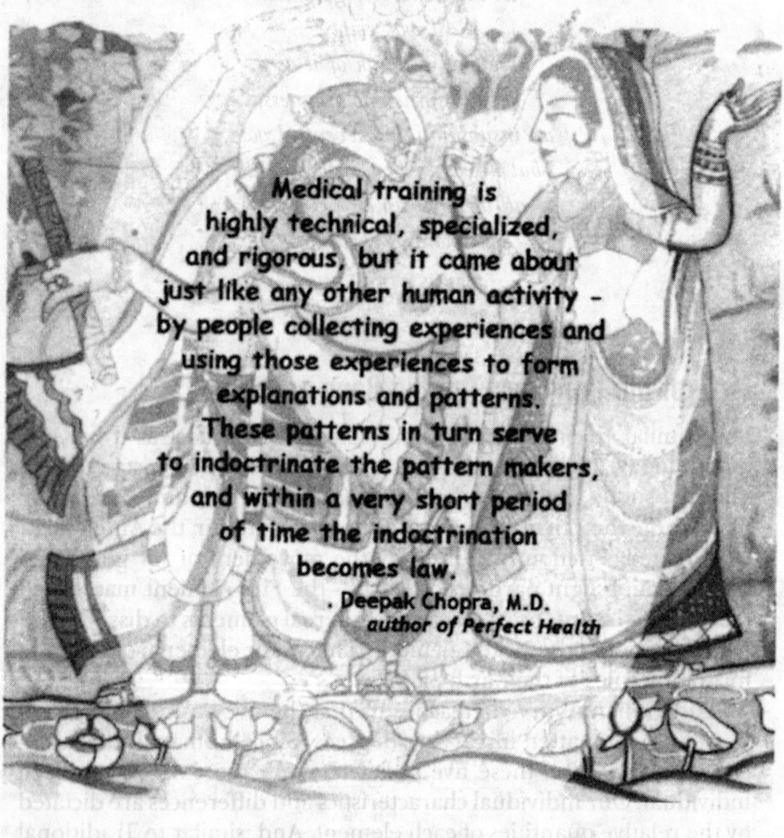

is governed by the Air element. Fire is the third element and is responsible for metabolism, enzyme production, body temperature, intellect and vision. The Water element manifests in the secretion of bodily fluids such as saliva, digestive juices and mucous. Essential to life, water is found in the plasma and cytoplasm. In the human frame, the Earth element is responsible for the creation of solid structures such as bones, cartilage, muscles, skin and hair.

The five elements, according to Ayurveda, manifest in the human body as three basic principles known as Tridosha. *Vata dosha* is produced by the combination of Ether and Air elements; *Pitta dosha* is the combination of Fire and Water elements, while Water and Earth elements combine to form *Kapha dosha*. Disharmony or illness is the result of an imbalance in the doshas. Excess *kapha* can produce diseases associated with excess mucous such as bronchitis, sinusitis, or pneumonia. Excess *pitta*, or heat, can manifest as stomach or duodonal ulcers, inflamed skin irritations, allergies, etc. Arthritis, dry skin, and disorders of the nervous system are all examples of *vata* imbalances.

(Note: Fill out the questionnaire in Chapter 10 to determine your unique Tridosha balance based on physical and psychological characteristics. When working with the various healing substances you will find in the upcoming chapters, it will be very helpful to know if your tendency is to suffer from kapha (heavy, damp, cold); pitta (hot) or vata (dry, cold) imbalances in order to choose herbs and foods best suited to alleviate your discomfort. For additional information on this age-old healing system, see recommended reading in the Resources Section at the end of the book.)

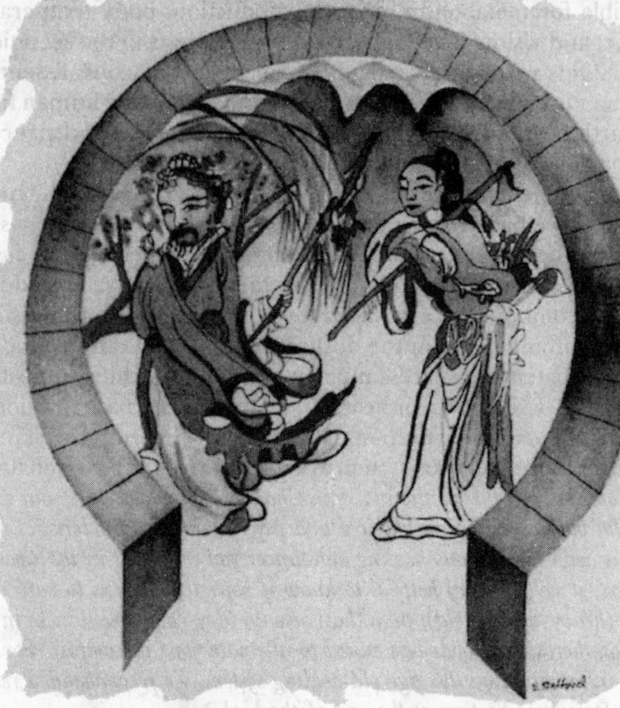

Traditional Medical Wisdom from China

BY GARY DOLOWICH, M.D., B.AC.

It's like a tear in the hands of a Western Man,
it'll tell you 'bout salt, carbon and water.
But a tear to a Chinese Man,
it'll tell you 'bout sadness and sorrow -
and the love of a man and a woman.

- JEFFERSON STARSHIP, FROM THE SONG, *"RIDE THE TIGER"*

Chinese medicine is said to have been practiced for over five thousand years and its origin lies in the earliest stratum of Chinese history. According to tradition, acupuncture was invented by Huang Di, the Yellow Emperor (2600 BCE); herbs were discovered by Shen Nong (3400 BCE) - mythical sages that symbolize a timeless wisdom. The medical system that evolved in China cannot be separated from its two indigenous spiritual traditions which continue to be meaningful for people today. In Taoism we have a mystical path for living simply, free of attachments, in harmony with the rhythms of nature. Confucianism is more about life in the world - correct relationships and responsible actions. These two philosophies themselves embody the teaching of *yin* and *yang*, and the ideal balance is to be Confucian in one's public life while a Taoist in private.

As it developed through centuries of empirical observation, Chinese medicine always kept its roots in these ancient traditions. Health is seen as a result of following nature's laws. Illness arises when we violate the natural order of things. Unlike the emphasis in Western biomedicine, which focuses on ruling out pathology, the traditional medicine of China holds a positive vision of wellness that encourages a relationship with both the laws of the natural world and the "inner law of our being."

In Chinese medicine we have a prototype for a wholistic approach to healing. Committed to uncovering the energetic pattern that underlies the symptoms, its very framework directs us to a deeper level in our quest for health. Therapeutic interventions are also wholistic, in that they extend beyond acupuncture needles and herbs to include diet, exercise, meditation techniques, and attention to lifestyle. The emphasis is on prevention and the techniques of diagnosis are subtle enough to uncover problems before they manifest in organic disease. In the ***Yellow Emperor's Classic of Internal Medicine*** the earliest written source of this tradition, we find such a prescription for preventative health care:

"The sages did not treat those who were already ill,
they instructed those who were not yet ill.
To administer medicines to diseases which have already developed
is comparable to the behavior of those persons
who begin to dig a well after they have become thirsty.
Would this action not be too late?"

In ancient times practitioners were paid only as long as the client stayed healthy; if the patient became ill, then the doctor had to support the family. This economic structure strongly encouraged prevention and regular treatments to address imbalances at the earliest possible stage.

As we explore the positive attributes of Chinese medicine as it has been traditionally practiced, it is important to note that a wholistic approach is not the property of any one system, but can be used by anyone who takes the time to uncover the deeper roots of an illness. A caring, concerned Western doctor can certainly practice preventatively and in a way that treats the whole person. Unfortunately, this is just not very likely when the average visit under *managed care* is now seven minutes. It is also true that Chinese medicine is often applied in a symptomatic, cookbook fashion where acupuncture points are used to merely suppress symptoms and no effort is made to relate the presenting problem to the person's life. The crucial factor is whether the practitioner is fully *present* and allows sufficient time to discover the source of the imbalance.

The fundamental concept in Chinese medicine is *ch'i*, or life energy. *Ch'i* is defined as "the breath of heaven" and is the spirit which animates life. Our bodily form comes from the earth, but the essence of life is much more than this and can be better described as a "meeting of heaven and earth." An image which depicts this interrelationship is the bamboo flute, which has a physical structure but does not produce sound (its reason for being) until the breath moves through it. The ancient Chinese understood the value of integrating the form and the formless, and this view, presented in the ***Yellow Emperor's Classic***, still has meaning today. Life can be understood as a flow of vital energies within a concrete and tangible environment.

Energy flows unceasingly through the Yin and Yang Meridians.
Energy is immaterial, the body is material; together they form man.
SU WEN, *CHAPTER 6*

Ch'i is the foundation for Chinese Medicine. Symptoms can be understood as a manifestation of an imbalance in this internal energy. Diagnosis is aimed at assessing the *ch'i* and uncovering blocks in its movement. Clues from the patient's color, sound, emotion and odor help uncover the state of their vital force. Chinese pulse diagnosis is a highly refined system that allows the practitioner to directly palpate twelve distinct energies that flow in the meridians. These pathways are ancient descriptions of the flow of the *ch'i* within the body, and can be understood as the anatomy of our energy body. The acupuncture points themselves are precise locations along these meridians where we can contact and treat this deep energy.

As discussed in the introductory chapters, there are some interesting Western biomedical studies which now demonstrate the effectiveness of acupuncture and Chinese herbs. Studies with laboratory animals consistently document the ability of needles to elevate pain thresholds, and the successful use of acupuncture to treat animals at veterinary schools shows that there is more than suggestion going on here. Imaging techniques can record changes in the visual cortex when points are stimulated that are known to affect sight. Research using double-blind methodology, reported in the Journal of the American Medical Association, demonstrated the effectiveness of acupuncture in correcting breech presentation and the benefit of Chinese herbs in the treatment of Irritable Bowel Syndrome. In the endorphins, morphine-like compounds that naturally occur in the brain, science has found a biochemical mediator for the effects of acupuncture. Giving a drug which blocks the action of this chemical, prevents the measurable effects of acupuncture treatment. It should be pointed out that though these studies may be useful in proving the efficacy of Chinese medicine, they fail to elucidate the *ch'i* that is the basis for its action. The *vital force*, like life itself, ultimately remains a mystery and lies beyond the range of our instruments. Here it is best to follow the advice of the Sioux medicine man who advises that we "marvel and accept and imitate, but leave mystery to mystery."

In order to navigate this world of energy we need a map for the journey. One such construct from China is the model of *yin* and *yang*. According to ancient wisdom, this system of polar complements enables us to discern the workings of heaven and earth. All things are said to have a *yin* and *yang* aspect, which allows there to be comparisons. Thus we can contrast dark and light, cold and hot, water and fire, rest and movement, falling and rising, feminine and masculine - each pair representing a *yin/yang* relationship. Neither is seen as more valuable than the other and, in fact, *yin* and *yang* are inseparable, each mutually creates the other. The concept of beauty defines the category of ugliness, the idea of winning requires there to be losing. At the extreme, *yin* and *yang* transform into each other, just as the moon, when full, begins to wane. In the ***I Ching***, the oldest source of this teaching and a book that has been called "the soul of Chinese medicine," *yin* and *yang* becomes the foundation for a philosophy that can describe the nature of change, lead to freedom from attachment, and help the individual find a spiritual center.

Everything on earth is subject to change.
Prosperity is followed by decline: This is the eternal law on earth.

This conviction might induce melancholy, but it should not;
it ought only to keep us from falling into illusion
when good fortune comes to us.
As long as a person's inner nature remains
stronger and richer than external fate,
fortune will not desert him.

The system of Chinese medicine known as Eight Principles uses *yin/yang* theory as a way to diagnose and treat the *ch'i*. The practitioner seeks to understand the person in terms of this model and defines their condition as deficient or excessive, cold or hot, internal or external. Steps are then taken to restore balance and harmony. An example, based on this approach, would be a person who presents with hypertension, anxiety, insomnia, restlessness, and feelings of heat in the body - symptoms that can be diagnosed as an excessive *yang* condition. Treatment would include acupuncture points and herbs aimed at quieting and sedating the hyper energy. This pattern can be contrasted with the typical menopausal syndrome when the ovaries stop producing female hormones, a situation that can be interpreted as a depletion in fluids *(yin)*. The symptoms of hot flashes, irritability and insomnia are indeed similar to the first case. The cause, however, lies in the lack of hormones and what appears to be an abundance of *yang* in the body is really only a *relative* excess that is actually due to a deficiency in *yin*. This distinction is crucial if we are to direct treatment to the root of the problem. Here the more effective intervention would be to select the acupuncture points and herbs that build and nourish the *yin* side, and in this way bring things back into balance.

The teachings of *yin* and *yang* reveal a cardinal principle of Chinese medicine - that of moderation. It encourages us to embrace our wholeness and accept the rhythms of nature. Whenever there is a one-sidedness, it upsets the natural order and can lead to illness. Thus health derives from a flow between rest and activity, play and work, relationship and solitude. A vital part of the practitioner's task is to use this model to counsel the client, in order to help them find the unique harmony that is true for their lives. Even illness and health are ultimately part of the dance of *yin/yang*, as is life and death, energy and matter. As the Chinese philosopher Chuang Tsu has said,

The person who wants to have right without wrong,
order without disorder,

Does not understand the principles of heaven and earth.
He does not know how things hang together.
Can a person cling only to heaven and know nothing of earth?
They are correlative: to know one is to know the other.
To refuse one is to refuse both.

Another traditional system for understanding the flow of life energy is the Law of the Five Elements. This circular arrangement describes a fundamental interconnection in which Wood creates Fire (in the way wood feeds the flame); Fire, in turn, creates Earth (as ashes fall to the soil); Earth creates Metal (in the minerals and mountains that arise out of the earth); Metal then creates Water (as seen in the rivers and waterfalls that come down from the mountains); and, finally, Water creates Wood (as the source of living and growing things). This cycle of creation is known as the *Shen*, or Mother-Child relationship.

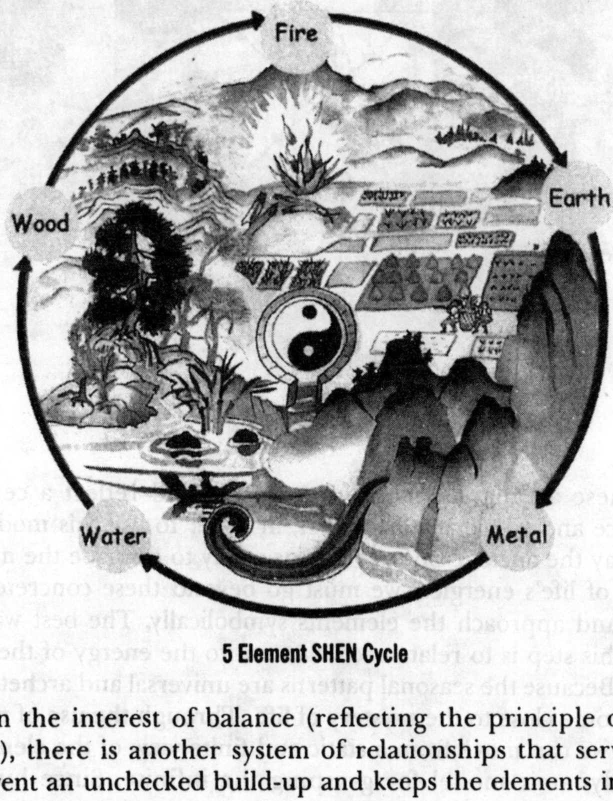

5 Element SHEN Cycle

In the interest of balance (reflecting the principle of *yin/yang*), there is another system of relationships that serves to prevent an unchecked build-up and keeps the elements in control. This is known as the *K'o* cycle. It describes the fact that Wood controls the Earth (the way trees keep a hillside from eroding); Earth, in turn, controls Water (as the banks keep a river running in its course); Water controls Fire (in that water puts out a blaze); Fire then controls Metal (as seen in the way fire can melt metal); and, finally, Metal controls Wood (in that an axe can fell a tree).

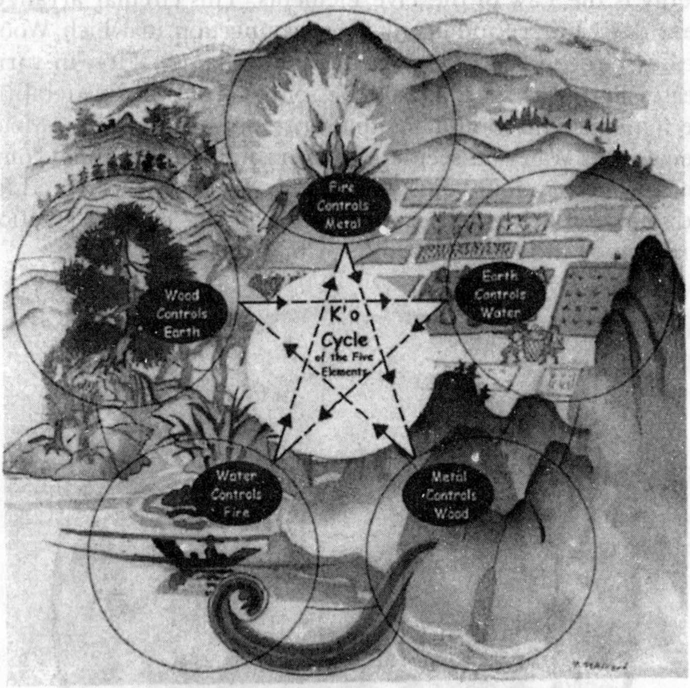

5 Element K'o Cycle

These arrangements are intriguing, and reflect a certain balance and wholeness. However, in order to use this model in the way the ancient Chinese did, as a way to describe the movement of life's energies, we must go beyond these concrete images and approach the elements symbolically. The best way to take this step is to relate each element to the energy of the seasons. Because the seasonal patterns are universal and archetypal, they come close to the mystery of life. Through the use of metaphor, we can move from a static and finite view of the elements to a dynamic model for grasping the infinite. Since human beings are seen in ancient tradition as a microcosm reflecting the same patterns as the larger macrocosm, this understanding can be extended to human behavior - and it then becomes the basis for a system of medicine.

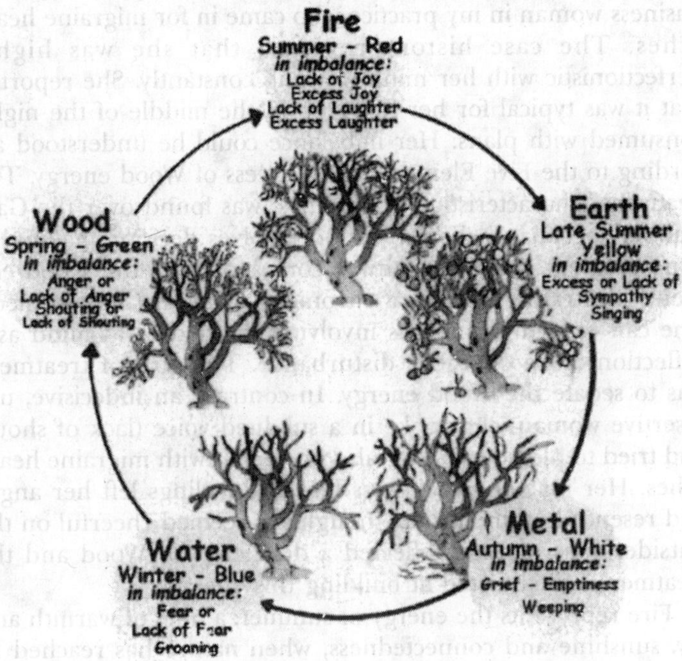

5 Element Movement

The Five Element model essentially describes the alternations of the energy with the seasonal rhythm of the year. Thus, the Wood element corresponds to the energy of spring, a time in nature of birth, growth and creation. It has an upward movement, as seen in a tree reaching up to the heavens and unfolding according to the plan inherent in its seed. For humans, Wood is a symbol of growth. It is a way to describe the energy that allows for new beginnings, decision-making, and vision; the force that provides the focus and direction for creation to occur. Evaluating a person according to the Wood element asks whether, like the tree, they are unfolding according to the inner law of their being. When this does not occur, there is inevitably frustration, anger, and often a shouting voice; these signs become diagnostic information as to the state of a person's Wood energy.

As with each of the elements, we find that this energy can be out of balance in either an excessive or deficient way (bipolar dysfunctions that reflect *yin* and *yang*). For example, I treated a business woman in my practice who came in for migraine headaches. The case history revealed that she was highly perfectionistic with her mind working constantly. She reported that it was typical for her to be up in the middle of the night, consumed with plans. Her imbalance could be understood according to the Five Elements as an excess of Wood energy. The headache, characteristic of migraines, was found over the Gallbladder meridian, whose function involves decision-making. It is no accident that this pathway corresponds to the Wood element, illustrating how, in a chronic imbalance, Chinese medicine can explain symptoms involving the body and mind as a reflection of an energetic disturbance. The goal of treatment was to sedate the Wood energy. In contrast, an indecisive, unassertive woman who spoke in a subdued voice (lack of shout) and tried to please everyone also presented with migraine headaches. Her inability to express her true feelings left her angry and resentful on the inside, though she seemed cheerful on the outside. This pattern reflected a deficiency of Wood and the treatment was directed at building this energy.

Fire represents the energy of summer, a time of warmth and joy, sunshine and connectedness, when nature has reached its zenith. For humans, the Fire element is expressed in relationships, sensuality, communication, and the full manifestation of our nature. The spirit of this element is often best captured in poetry and music:

An orange on the table, your dress on the rug
- and you in my bed,
Sweet present of the present
- cool of night, warmth of my life.

To understand the state of a person's Fire element, we can ask whether they experience heart-felt connection, joy, and love in their life. As is so often the case in our high-pressured, technological world, there is little time for these simple pleasures and we often see the consequences in the treatment room, expressed as a lack of Fire. This may manifest on a physical level with freezing cold hands and feet, an inability to get warm, and low blood pressure. On an emotional level, it may show up as a lack of joy. One of the tools used in Chinese medicine for treating deficient Fire is moxibustion. This technique of burning the herb mugwort on a needle or directly on an acupuncture point brings warmth directly into the meridian system.

The other side of an imbalance in Fire may be expressed on the physical level in the symptoms of hypertension, anxiety, rapid heart rate, and hot flushes - all signs of overactive Fire. In the emotional realm, we might expect an excess of joy and, indeed, a person who is always partying, incessantly laughing, and cannot refrain from being engaged with others may appear to be abundant in this element. Frequently, when we dig deeper, we discover that these compulsions may actually be compensating for a deficiency of Fire on the inside, which is the driving force behind their external behavior. Often, when an element is out of balance, there is such a mixture of excessive and deficient symptoms. Clearly, health lies in finding "the middle-way." We find that, according to the principle that *yin* and *yang* mutually create each other, extremes may turn into their opposite, as they prove to be "two sides of the same coin."

The Earth element symbolizes nourishment and stability. It is the energy of the late summer and represents, as an expression of that season, the harvest. For humans, this energy can be evaluated by asking whether we feel nurtured, are grounded, and can bring things to harvest in our lives. Eating disorders reflect the state of the Earth element, and compulsive overeating may be an attempt to bring in from the outside what is lacking on the inside. Once the problem is understood as stemming from an energetic disturbance, it is obvious why the external physical level solution can never be enough. Conditions such as anorexia are seen to represent the other side of the same imbalance. On the emotional level, Earth is the mother element and is related to sympathy.

I treated an older woman living in a mobile park who repeatedly would ignore her own needs in order to take care of others, and eventually developed gastritis. In Chinese medicine, the stomach, since it is involved with bringing in food, is associated with Earth. A person who is overly sympathetic, mothering everyone, trying to please and fix every situation, may be expressing an imbalance in the Earth element. Applying the *K'o* cycle relationship of the Five Elements, it is Wood that brings the Earth into balance (just as trees prevents the hillside from eroding). Some healthy anger (I HAVE A LIFE TOO!) could enable this person to set limits on their excessive behavior. The goal of treatment, through both counseling and acupuncture, was to strengthen the Wood energy and thereby restore a healthier balance.

Metal is the energy of the autumn and corresponds to the spirit. It is a time in nature of letting go (as the leaves fall from the trees) and in this season there is a sense of great peace and of finding the quality of things. For humans, it is required for self-esteem and, in the extreme, when a person is out of touch with this element, there can be the deepest grief and despair. The Metal element connects us to meaning and purpose, provides quality rather than quantity - without it there is an emptiness inside. It is not surprising that our modern world, cut off from traditions and meaningful rituals, suffers from a lack of spirit. Though the essence of Metal has little to do with material possessions, people typically attempt to compensate for a deficiency in this energy by seeking money and jewels (concrete aspects of the element). Those who endlessly search for spiritual truths, traveling in search of a guru, may be again seeking on the outside what they are lacking (and can ultimately only find) on the inside. One of the healthiest expressions of the Metal element I've come across was the statement by an impoverished but very spiritual Hispanic woman who, when asked whether her life had meaning, replied simply: "God did not make junk."

The Water element corresponds to the energy of the winter, a time of stillness and going back to the depths. In nature it is the season for allowing the reservoirs to fill up, an opportunity for cleansing as the winter rains bring fluidity and freshness. Water symbolizes the seed that can unfold with the coming year. For humans, it represents the deep reserves that can only be replenished by rest and is the potential for our life. The emotional aspect of the Water element is fear, which makes sense when one considers the fear of drowning or the feeling that would be engendered by a scarcity in the storehouse during the wintertime.

I recall the case of a carpenter who, despite long term bodywork therapy, suffered from chronic back pain. Of interest was the fact that his symptoms were especially severe in the winter months. His fear at not being able to earn a living was quite apparent and, since the meridians of the Water element run through the back, his situation fit the Five Element model. He failed to respond to physical level treatments simply because the problem did not have a structural cause. Rather, it was an energetic disturbance of depleted reserves, and held the deeper message that he needed to rest during this time of year. Like so many in our culture, he ignored the sensations in his body as he was swept into a frenzy of activity during the Christmas season, a pattern clearly not in harmony with nature. The advice found in the ***Yellow Emperor's Classic*** for staying healthy in the winter would apply here: get plenty of rest and stay in bed until the sun is well up in the sky. It was only when he began to integrate this counsel into his life that his back pain subsided.

The Law of the Five Elements is based on patterns of nature that are as true for us today as they were for the ancient Chinese thousands of years ago. It can therefore provide an archetypal understanding that brings order to the myriad manifestations of life. It is both a guide for harmonious living, as well as a medical model for restoring health and balance. A more in depth study of the Five Element patterns can be found in my upcoming book - ***The Five Elements of Chinese Medicine: Archetypal Acupuncture for the Western World.***

Within each of the elements we find two organs, except for the Fire element which has four. This creates the Twelve Officials, another model used to organize the wholeness of human experience.

Unlike the reductionist approach of biomedicine, which studies the smallest measurable variable in order to conform to double-blind experiments, Chinese medicine always seeks the broadest possible understanding. This system is no exception, and the Twelve Officials expands our view of anatomy and physiology. In addition to the corresponding physical organ, each official includes a meridian that is the path of a specific energy within the body, as well as a dynamic functional activity that takes place on all levels.

Within the Metal element, for example, we find the Colon and Lung officials. On the physical level, we know that the colon is responsible for letting go of undigestible food and waste products from digestion. When we refer to the Colon function in Chinese medicine, however, we are speaking of letting go of all aspects that no longer serve us. Thus, on the mental level we need to let go of negative thinking, toxic experiences, and all the old programs that keep us stuck in destructive patterns.

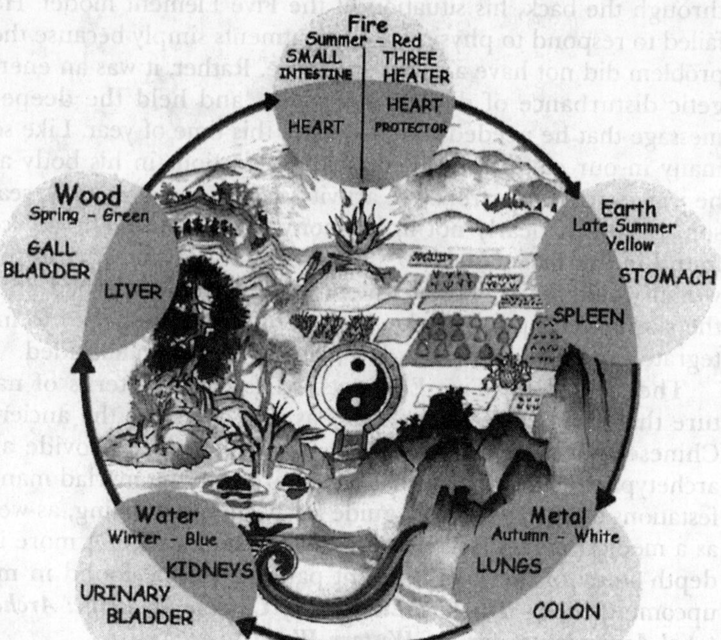

5 Element Officials

On the emotional level, it is important not to hold on to anger, grief, and fear. In Chinese medicine, these emotions are all considered normal, and can be appropriate expressions; they are not unhealthy as long as the Colon official is able to release them in due time. In the spirit realm, it is essential to stay uncluttered in order to be in touch with a higher awareness, as in the teaching from the ancient classics, "keep empty and you will be filled." We can see how the Colon official is essential for a healthy Metal element, since holding on to negativity would inevitably damage self-esteem, cutting us off from quality and meaning. The Colon is coupled, in Chinese medicine, with the Lungs, the official responsible for "receiving pure *ch'i* from the heavens." Again, this is more than a physical function and refers to our ability to receive and take in on all levels of experience. The Colon and Lung must work together in the dance of letting go and then receiving new inspiration. Understanding these relationships helps make sense of the fact that so many spiritual traditions emphasize both cleansing rituals and breathing practices as a way to cultivate the spirit.

In the ancient description of the organs first found in the ***Yellow Emperor's Classic***, the functions of the body are compared to the organization of the Empire. Each of these "officials" is likened to one of the "ministers" that carried out a specific task and together allowed for the proper balance of the whole. The Heart, in this view, was seen as the Emperor or Supreme Controller, the part of ourselves that holds the center, providing a sense of calmness and order in our lives. It is no accident that the Heart meridian is treated in Chinese medicine for anxiety, panic, and insomnia - symptoms that would result from not having an emperor on the throne. In this system the Lung would be considered the Prime Minister who counsels on spiritual matters; the Stomach is known as "the Official of the Public Granaries." Each of the officials can be understood as arising out of its particular element. For example, the Liver is called "the Military Leader who Excels in Strategic Planning;" the Gall Bladder is "the Official of Upright Judgment and Decision-making." It is obvious that these two functions belong to the Wood element and allow for vision, focus, and action that makes growth possible. Again we can take the Western view of the liver, a biochemical factory that provides a *plan* for molecules involved in the metabolic function of the body, and see how Chinese medicine expands it to a more wholistic perspective, looking at planning on all levels.

The ancient model of the officials closely resembles the concept of the archetypes found in modern depth psychology. These primal images can also be understood as inner energetic potentials which must find expression in our lives, and work in a balanced way, for there to be health. In the Jungian view, we are hard wired for these instinctive aspects (an idea that corresponds to the meridians). They become activated as our life unfolds in order to allow for a full range of function. Fairy tales, myths, and stories serve to help us get in touch with the qualities of these energies, such as the power of the Warrior, the joy of the Lover, or the compassion of the Queen. Sometimes we become aware of these possibilities through another person, such as the guru, who embodies the wisdom of the Sage. In time, life experience will typically teach that others cannot hold these archetypes for us, ultimately they must be found within. In a very real way, the archetypal model of Jungian psychology is another description of the same internal world of *ch'i* that is the foundation for Chinese medicine.

One of the most useful ways to understand both the archetypes and the concepts of Chinese medicine is as symbols that allow us to describe what is basically a mystery, the energies of life. The acupuncture points themselves can be seen as archetypes, images within the body that can be accessed for balance and health. Points such as "the Meeting of One Hundred Ancestors", "the Spirit Storehouse", "the Great Eliminator", or "the Inner Frontier Gate" all reflect energies that are part of our potential as human beings. It is the genius of Chinese medicine to be able to assess the state of the life energy through careful observation including the twelve pulses, to formulate a diagnosis in terms of archetypal models, and then to intervene creatively by treating a specific energy that can restore balance. Since it is a system based on images that are fundamental to the human condition, it has withstood the test of time and remains applicable across cultures.

Later in tnis book we will explore how these concepts can be applied to specific conditions and provide insights into the deeper meaning of symptomatic manifestations. In truth, the traditional medicine of China opens up an entirely new way of understanding the *body*, *mind*, and *spirit*. To interpret it solely in terms of the scientific model not only mistranslates it miserably but, in the words of Joseph Campbell, misses "an opportunity for the West to regain contact with a forgotten side of life, and with the whole history and heritage of mankind's life in the spirit."

(Note: Based on Five Element Theory, numerous charts can be found in Chapter 12. Fill out the questionnaire that is available to help you determine your unique Five Element balance based on physical and psychological characteristics. When working with the various healing substances you will find in the upcoming chapters, it will be very helpful to know if your tendency is to suffer from Wood, Fire, Earth, Metal or Water imbalances in order to choose herbs and foods best suited to alleviate your discomfort. For additional information on this healing system, see recommended reading in the Resources Section at the end of the book.)

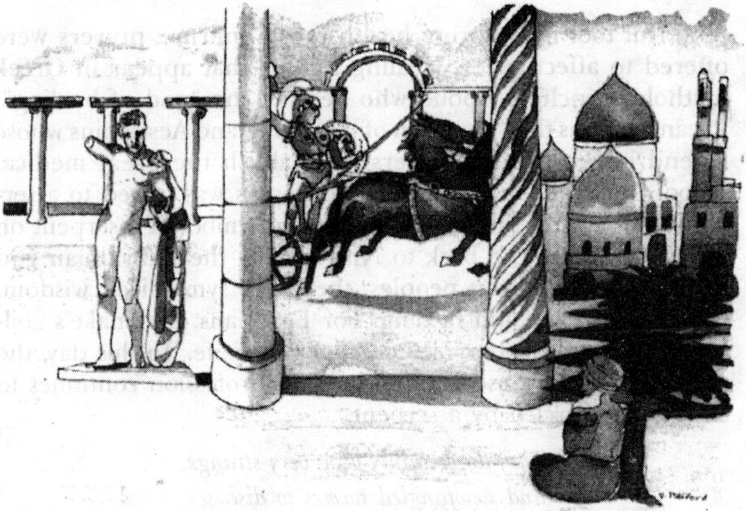

The Greeks, Romans, Arabians and the Roots of Western Medicine

Men do not think they know a thing till they have grasped the "why" of it.

ARISTOTLE, ***PHYSICS***

The writings of Homer (9th century BCE) tell us a great deal about the practice of medicine in ancient Greece. It is not known if Homer was one man, or if the works credited to him were written by different hands. It is interesting, however, that throughout his writings, accounts of medical practices vary. For example, the *Iliad* tells us that physicians were considered, "professionals and servants of the public," and that the practice of medicine was a "noble art". Good hygiene and good health were equated in the thought of Greek physicians; wounds were first cleaned, then treated with medicinal herbs, compresses and bandages as deemed necessary. A song of healing was sung while treatment was underway, thus, early Greek medicine contained elements of both magical and empirical thought treating body, mind and spirit.

However, in Homer's *Odyssey*, we find a different trend - society's changing view now considered magic to be the most powerful tool in restoring health to the infirm - prayers were offered to affect cures. Healing figures that appear in Greek mythology include Apollo who became the "god of healing"; Paean who was the "physician of the gods"; and Aesclepius whose legend inspired his followers to establish the great medical school in Cyrene (c. 429 BCE). Aesclepius was linked to a serpent (symbolic of the healing arts). The symbol of a serpent on a staff can be traced back to Ningishzida, the Babylonian god of healing. To ancient peoples, the snake symbolized wisdom, fertility, longevity and healing. For Egyptians, the snake's ability to shed its skin represented renewal of life. To this day, the symbol of healing used by the medical profession continues to be a staff encircled by a serpent.

They do certainly give very strange,
and newfangled names to diseases.

PLATO (429 - 347 BCE)

Hippocrates of Kos (460 to 377 BCE), the father of Western medicine, established ethical standards for medical practitioners defining professional relationships with patients based on truth, compassion and morality. This inspired the Hippocratic oath taken by M.D.'s today. Fundamental to the Hippocratic School of thought was that nature inherently possesses the power to cure itself. Hippocrates stated, "Leave your drugs in the chemist's pot if you can heal the patient with food." For him, the art of healing consisted of providing a positive environment for the patient along with an appropriate diet and exercise. In one of the 79 books attributed to him, *On Airs, Waters, Places,* Hippocrates states that, based on observation of the changing seasons, climate and locale, the physician should be able to determine the state of a patient's health without ever questioning him. For Hippocrates, all disease could be explained in terms of natural causes and no disease was thought to be 'sacred', or of a supernatural nature.

Whoever wishes to investigate medicine should proceed thus:
In the first place, consider the seasons of the year
and what effect each of them produces.

HIPPOCRATES

Hippocrates adopted his views regarding humoral theory from Empedocles, a Sicilian philosopher who lived c.500 to 430

BCE. Similar to Ayurvedic and Chinese medical thought, the basic tenet of the Doctrine of Four Humors is that everything on earth is created from four elements: Air, Fire, Water and Earth. The cause of disease, linked to an imbalance in one of the elements, is due to an excess or deficiency in dryness, warmth, coldness, or dampness. The four elements were linked to four body types (sanguine, choleric, melancholic and phlegmatic) and four humors in the body (blood, yellow bile, black bile and phlegm). Similar to Chinese and East Ayurvedic Medicine, the Four Humor system of thought assigned qualities, seasons, personality traits, and, as the system evolved, zodiac signs to each of the four elements.

The Greek philosophers did not hold a uniform view of the four elements. Empedocles referred to them as "roots" while Plato called them "simple components". Aristotle, similar to Chinese Five Element thought, believed that the elements represented dynamic qualities of Nature that could transform into each other as well as generate each other.

Earth and Fire are opposites also due to the opposition
of the respective qualities with which they are revealed to our senses:
Fire is hot, Earth is cold.
Besides the fundamental opposition of hot and cold,
there is another one, i.e. that of dry and wet:
hence the four possible combinations of hot-dry (Fire), hot-wet (Air),
cold-dry (Earth) and cold-wet (Water) . . .
the elements can mix with each other and can even
transform into one another . . .
thus Earth, which is cold and dry, can generate Water
if wetness replaces dryness.

ARISTOTLE

This age-old medical tradition, once practiced throughout the Mediterranean, slowly passed out of existence with a few exceptions. Known as Unani Medicine (in the Arabic language, "Unani" means Greek), an Islamic form of the Four Humor medical thought system still survives and is being practiced in India today. Remnants of the Four Humor system can also be found in Central and South American indigenous healing traditions. *(Note: For charts and information on the Western Four Humor tradition, please see Chapter 9).*

One of the most famous names in Greek, Roman and Arabian (or Islamic) medicine is that of Galen. Born at Pergamum in Asia Minor, 131 CE, Galen was appointed as surgeon to the gladiators there; he later lived in Rome, writing over 125 medical texts on anatomy, physiology and practical medicine which stressed four element humoral theory. His works codified all existing medical knowledge and were used as the standard medical texts throughout Europe and the Arab world until the Renaissance. In the 1500's Galen's theories would be planted in the New World by Spanish physicians. These ideas would be adopted by Native Aztec and Mayan healers and a new hybrid system of healing would be born.

By 750 CE the Arabs had conquered over half of the known world. Avicenna, one of the great physicians of the Islamic world, followed the teachings of Hippocrates in theory and those of Galen in practice. Avicenna, called the "prince of physicians" by contemporaries, wrote his *Canon of Medicine* around 1000 CE. Translated into Latin in the 12th century, this work greatly influenced Western medical thought up through the Renaissance. In reading through a history of Islamic medicine, one cannot help but be impressed by the advances made in care giving - actual palaces were converted in to hospitals to treat the infirm. The luxurious grounds, buildings and costs of care were maintained by donations or endowments from the wealthy.

In 1248 CE one of world's largest and most elaborate hospitals was constructed in Cairo, Egypt. According to Husain F. Nagamia, M.D., Clinical Assistant Professor of Surgery, University of South Florida Medical School in Tampa, Florida, the Mansuri Hospital in Cairo could house 8000 patients. There were separate wards for men and women, lecture halls, a library, pharmacy, a chapel for Christian patients and a mosque for Muslim patients. The Waqf document states that no one could be turned away regardless of their race, religion or citizenship, and there was no limit on the length of their stay: *"The hospital shall keep all patients, men and women until they are completely recovered. All costs are to be borne by the hospital whether the people come from afar or near, whether they are residents or foreigners, strong or weak, low or high, rich or poor, employed or unemployed, blind or sighted, physically or mentally ill, learned or illiterate. There are no conditions of consideration and payment; none is objected to or even indirectly hinted at for non-payment. The entire service is through the magnificence of Allah, the generous one."*

From around 300 BCE we have two herbals written by the Greek philosopher Theophrastus, *Enquiry into Plants* and *Growth of Plants*, describing over 500 herbs based on his own observations and the botanical writings of Aristotle. A Roman naturalist, Pliny the Elder (77 CE) wrote *Natural History*, 37 volumes of plant lore which included information on the medicinal use of plants as well as the Doctrine of Signatures. During the first century CE, Dioscorides, a Greek physician, wrote what would be the most influential Western herbal of all time. *De Materia Medica* became the standard reference work for the next 1500 years; it describes over 600 herbs, many of which are still used today. The books of Pliny and Dioscorides were translated into Arabic by the two famous Islamic physicians Avicenna and Rhazes.

Moses Maimonides, the most renowned Jewish physician of the Middle Ages, lived in Egypt during the 12th century. As personal doctor to the Sultan, he developed many of his medical ideas as a way to advise patients among the royal court. His teachings, written in Arabic, drew upon Greek and Mid-Eastern medicine, while integrating basic concepts from Judaism. Maimonides is also widely regarded as one of the most important scholars of the Hebrew scriptures and his commentaries on the Bible are quoted to this day. Practicing medicine amidst the excessive indulgences of the sultans of Cairo, he stressed the value of moderation. For Maimonides, the first aim of the art of medicine is to instruct individuals on how to follow a healthy lifestyle. His statement, "the ability of a physician to prevent illness is a greater proof of his skill than his ability to cure someone who is already ill," is strikingly similar to the advice of the Yellow Emperor in ancient China (see page 25). Steeped as he was in a rich spiritual tradition, his approach to the human condition was based on the understanding that, fundamentally, we are born in the Spirit. Maimonides considered life sacred and the soul, the breath of life, to be man's divine endowment. The guiding principle which pervades his work is the need to balance *body, mind and Spirit*, an idea that certainly parallels Chinese wisdom. As is true throughout traditional medicine, he made distinctions between hot and cold states, for example, advising smaller meals during warm weather and increasing the quantity of food when the air becomes colder. Of all his contributions to medicine, probably the one that most endures is his deep compassion for human suffering and appreciation of the role of the doctor. Maimonides "Prayer for the Physician" can be found today on the wall in many a doctor's office (including my own). - *Dr. Gary*

Exalted God - Before I begin the holy work
of healing the creations of your hands,
I place my entreaty before the throne of your glory
that you grant strength of spirit and fortitude
to faithfully execute my work.
Let not desire for wealth or benefit blind me from seeing truth.
Deem me worthy of seeing in the sufferer who seeks my advice
- a person - neither rich nor poor.
Friend or foe, good man or bad, of a man in distress,
show me only the man.

MAIMONIDES, EXCERPT FROM ***PRAYER FOR THE PHYSICIAN***

Herbalism in Europe went through a great setback during the Dark Ages, now referred to as the Early Middle Ages and Middle Ages (approximately 420 to 1500 CE). The Christian Church taught that disease was sent by God as punishment for sin, so little was done to relieve suffering. It is said that women giving birth actually welcomed the pain (thinking it was a penalty sent from God for the original sin) and viewed it as a time to atone for their transgressions. As late as the sixteenth century, persons living in Germany and Scotland were condemned to death by fire if they used pain-relieving herbs or medicines. However, luckily, monks continued to painstakingly translate herbal works throughout this period.

It was during the 9th century that the first apothecaries were opened in Baghdad and by the 13th century London became a major trading center for spices and herbs. With the Renaissance, herbalism blossomed once again and the best selling herbal of all time was written by Nicholas Culpeper in 1653; *The English Physician and Complete Herbals*, still in print today, contains descriptions of 398 herbs. However, with the advent of "reason and experimentation," the golden age of herbalism came to a halt. Village "healing women" were disposed of as witches; folk healers were declared heretics and women were forbidden to study. The use of healing herbs became equated to the occult or magic and herbalism was dropped from medical training.

Bridging East and West

As a crazy Christian kid growing up on a tiny farm in Kansas, I was always intrigued with "why I thought what I thought". It seemed logical that if I spoke another language and lived somewhere else, other than the Kansas prairies, I'd be thinking totally different things! It was questions like this that ultimately lead me into the fields of Herbalism, Anthropology and the Asian healing arts. Now I'm only more intrigued with many more questions than answers. However, what became apparent to me is the significant difference in the way we modern Westerners think when compared to individuals living in more traditional, nature-oriented cultures. Most Asian and Native American traditions view life in relationship to nature's constantly changing cycles - the cycles of the moon; the cycles of the seasons; the cycles of the heavens as our incredible universe spins through space. In comparison to the cyclical thought systems of nature-oriented cultures who tend to view distinctions, like black and white, as complementary pairs that work in harmony; we linear Western thinkers most often see things in terms of polar opposites that clash with each other. Since Zoroaster, and Aristotle after him, we have been contrasting everything under the sun this way - black/white, hot/cold, male/female, us/them, good/bad. In this process of comparison, we frequently split our universe into an inferior/superior dichotomy - something is either *good* or it is *bad*.

History is replete with examples demonstrating our Western tendency to view nature as inferior to reason; female as inferior to male; them as inferior to us; black as inferior to white (just think of the enslavement of the African people or the holocaust). Unfortunately, nature and native peoples became something to be conquered and dominated; their landscapes were not sacred to us, but yet another object to be owned and exploited. What now remains of many traditional cultures are merely remnants of a once-proud past - their lifestyles, belief systems and self-esteem have been largely destroyed by Western expansionism and colonization. While it may not be pleasant, I think it's extremely important that we come to grips with the effects the acts of our ancestors had on other cultures. As a teenager studying American History back in Kansas, I know I was not told that the government of California had actually paid $10 for each Native American scalp (man, woman or child) brought in by the settlers. Were you aware of these genocidal acts? While it is impossible to go back in time, we need to be aware, to fully evaluate the impact we are currently having on the precious few remaining native cultures, natural resources and virgin forests on this incredible planet.

Not everything that can be counted counts,
and not everything that counts can be counted.

ALBERT EINSTEIN

Realities are created by our thoughts. Since Descartes, Darwin and the scientific revolution, our Western minds have been preoccupied with measuring, categorizing, calculating, quantifying, comparing, cataloging and collecting. With the advent of Newtonian physics, the universe became conceptualized as a gigantic clockworks - a machine. In the spirit of this machine metaphor, we Westerners constantly attempt to break things down in to their smallest components - we are not interested in the whole, but are intrigued by the individual parts of which it consists. We separate ourselves from nature just as we separate our bodies from our minds. Our Western minds seek to discover the *cause* of phenomena while nature-oriented thought systems seek an understanding of the *relationships of things* in the web of phenomena. It seems important to understand our cultural tendencies so that they can be moderated by a more wholistic view - the other half of the equation. Each system of thought constitutes one half of the whole; and they can complement one another perfectly.

Science cannot solve the ultimate mystery of Nature.
And it is because in the last analysis we,
ourselves, are part of the mystery
we are trying to solve.

MAX PLANCK

Now it's time to move on to the Americas! So many of the Native American tribes and cultures have shared a similar view of a cyclical universe with their Asian counterparts. According to many traditional Asian and Native American cosmologies, everything - in the heavens and on earth - is intricately interwoven into the web of phenomena. Knowledge, within that framework, consists in our ability to understand the patterns in the weaving.

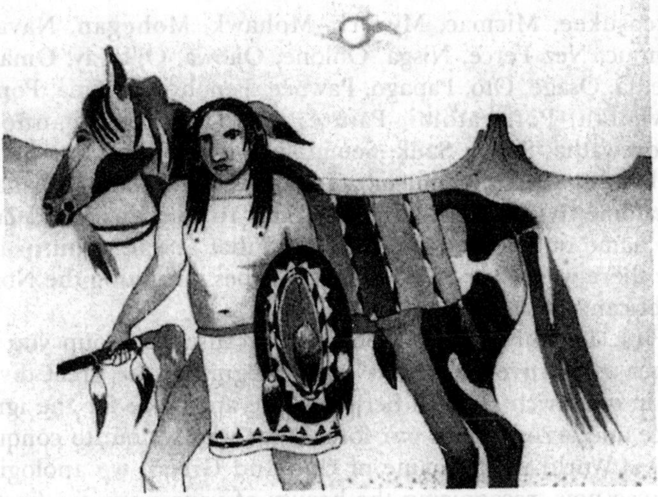

Healing Traditions of the North American Natives

This we know - the earth does not belong to man,
man belongs to the earth.
All things are connected like the blood that unites one family.
Whatever befalls the earth befalls the sons of the earth.
Man did not weave the web of life; he is merely a strand of it.
Whatever he does to the web, he does to himself.
One thing we know.
Our God is also your God.
The Earth is precious to Him.
And to harm the Earth is to heap contempt on its Creator.

CHIEF SEATTLE, 1854

In tribute to the rich and complex cultures of the original North Americans: Abenaki, Absarokee, Algonquin, Alabama, Anasazi, Anishinabe, Apache, Arikara, Athapaskan, Bannock, Blackfeet, Caddo, Catawba, Cherokee, Cheyenne, Chickasaw, Chinook, Chippewa, Choctaw, Chumash, Comanche, Costanoan, Cree, Creek, Crow, Dakota, Delaware, Eskimos, First Nations, Flathead, Hawaiin, Hidatsa, Hopi, Houma, Huron, Ioway Nation, Iroquois, Karuk, Kaw, Kiowa, Kwakiutl, Malecite, Maya,

Miccosukee, Micmac, Miwork, Mohawk, Mohegan, Navajo, Nipmuc, Nez Perce, Nisga, Ohlone, Ojibwa, Ojibway, Omaha, Oneida, Osage, Oto, Papago, Pawnee, Penobscott, Pima, Ponca, Powhatan, Potawatomi, Paiute, Quapaw, Rappahannock, Sagoyewatha, Salish, Sauk, Seminole, Seneca, Shoshoni, Sioux, Skokomish, Taino (Timucua), Tonkawa, Tsimshian, Wabanaki, Watatome, Winnebago, Wyandot, Yahi, Yuma, Yup'ik, and Zuni - to name only a few. It is estimated that at one point in history there were over 3,000 different tribes inhabiting the North American continent.

First, it's important to apologize because we group you together as "Native Americans" not recognizing the great diversity in your rich cultural heritages; we apologize for the ignorance and arrogance of our forefathers who set out to conquer a New World in the name of God and Greed; we apologize, because now, recognizing the beauty of your ways, we (in the ways of our ancestors) *collect* your sacred objects, your sacred ceremonies and your healing herbs. We cannot undo the injustices of the past; but we can join together, through mutual understanding and respect, to create a more balanced world. Native American traditions ought not vanish into a remote past. May the visions and wisdom of their Ancestors, the stories of their proud heritage and the healing ceremonies of their Forefathers that joined the Heavens and the Earth live on so we can all move forward to create a brighter future for the generations to come.

First, they say, there was only the
Creator, Taiowa.
All else was endless space.
There was no beginning and no end,
no time, no shape, no life.
Just an immeasurable void that had its
beginning and end, time, shape and life
in the mind
of Taiowa the Creator.
Then he, the infinite, conceived the finite . . .
BEGINNING FROM THE HOPI STORY OF CREATION

While the fascinating field of Cultural Anthropology emphasizes the detailed study of the unique differences between cultures, the work of Carl Jung and Joseph Campbell brings to light similarities in the thought patterns of all people through all time.

Delving deeply into the mythic symbols of traditional peoples, archetypes emerge - these are the images we all share; common experiences, thoughts and feelings that bind us together in this human experience called life. Those *ancient root* ideas of our ancestors, archetypes which form the very matrix of the human mind, gave birth to *many branches* of thought, which manifested in concrete form as our earth's greatly diverse cultures and civilizations. However, if one digs deeply enough, no matter how distinct a cultures's religious or healing practices, or their customs, costumes and cuisine, these root images are bound to emerge. Creation myths from around the world, when compared, have amazing similarities as do approaches found for dealing with illness. The Hopi Creation myth above is a good example of such an archetypal thought form as are images of the Sage, the Warrior, the Lover, the Father, the Mother and the Trickster. *(Note: In Chapters 3, 4, 5, 6 and 7, Dr. Gary will discuss these images in relation to the Chinese Five Element healing system, when we talk about life's stages and preventive medicine).*

The circle is another one of those archetypal images. Many Native North American tribes use what is known as a medicine wheel in their healing and spiritual practices. You'll notice a correlation can be drawn between the Native American Medicine Wheel, European Four Humor, East Indian Ayurvedic and Chinese Five Element Systems of thought. While the medicine wheel system of symbols varies between tribes, each of the four directions symbolizes an animal totem, a wind or season, a personality type, spiritual qualities and energies as well as diseases and herbal medicines. For example, the East, frequently symbolized by a hawk or eagle, represents spring, mental clarity, enlightenment and wisdom; the Southerly direction, represented by a coyote or mouse, is associated with summer, growth, compassion and maturation; the energy of the West, symbolized by a grizzly bear or elk, represents autumn, strength, responsibility and introspection; while the North, symbolized by the white buffalo, is associated with winter and the qualities of purity, patience, balance and renewal.

Life goes on in a circle, a medicine wheel.
We humans are one part of the circle, but not the only part.
The minerals, plants, the people of the water,
the winged ones, the four-leggeds, the spirit keepers,
the powers of the directions, the times and the seasons

are also part of this great circle.
We are their relatives, and they are ours.

SUN BEAR, CHIPPEWA MEDICINE MAN & MEDICINE CHIEF,
TRIBE MEDICINE SOCIETY

Sometime in the remote past, hunter gatherers living in Western Canada and the Great Plains areas constructed wheel patterns out of stones. While no one knows what they were called at that time, most archaeologists and historians believe that these "medicine wheels" served as ceremonial calendars. The famous Bighorn Medicine Wheel in Wyoming accurately charts the heavens, marking the position of the sun and other stars that appear at dawn on the summer solstice. A number of tribes from the area claim this particular Medicine Wheel as their own including the Cheyenne, Crow, Shoshoni and Sioux.

It was sometime during the late 1500's that the legendary Iroquois chief Agonawila, later known as Hiawatha, united the feuding Native American nations with an alliance that ushered in a period of peace which lasted for more than 150 years. This alliance later became known as the Confederation of Nations; it recognized the brotherhood of the Native American people. While over three hundred different Native dialects were spoken at the time, similarities in belief systems and traditions enabled the tribes to unite. The medicine wheel became an important symbol of this healing transformation.

Medicine wheels were placed at the entrance of every teepee. Each one was uniquely decorated with colors and symbols designed to describe the occupants. According to Native tradition, members of the tribes were ordered to work on improving themselves or leave the tribe. This is how it works. A circle is drawn and then divided by a cross to represent the four directions: North, East, South and West. Somewhat similar to Western and Asian astrology, it is believed that the date of a person's birth can influence their behavior or character. Based on the individual's time of birth they are associated with a special moon as well as a certain color, mineral, power animal, plant, clan, element and healing herb which will help maintain their balance. The person's placement on the medicine wheel helps serve as a guide or map for their life in relationship to the universal plan. Since the medicine wheel reflects the unique strengths and weaknesses of each individual, it offers them a path to follow for personal growth. For example, in one Native American Medicine Wheel system (as it is being taught today) a person born between February 19 and March 20 belongs to the Frog Clan which is associated with the Water element; their healing herb is plantain; the moon phase under which they are born is called Big Wind's Moon; their power animal is the cougar and special mineral is turquoise. Rather elusive and shy Cougar People are natural healers (like other members of the Frog Clan); they are frequently called upon to give advice and to help settle arguments.

Most frequently Native American healers receive a calling to become a shaman, medicine man or woman; though sometimes these traditions are handed down to a son, daughter or another worthy family member. Many receive their calling after experiencing some type of serious illness themselves, after which they may experience a period of introspection culminating in a strong need to help others. This universal pattern, the archetype of the wounded healer, can be seen to operate for many individuals in our modern world who are drawn to the healing professions. The responsibility of being a shaman is tremendous and the person must maintain a strong relationship with the world of spirit. Medicine men and women are the moral leaders of the tribe and render many types of healing services to their community. Most medicine people have an in depth knowledge of the healing herbs found in their area.

Their (Native American) *diseases, indeed, are exceedingly few;*
nor do they often occur, by reason of their continual exercise,
and (till of late, universal) temperance. But if any are sick,
or bit by a serpent, or torn by a wild beast, the fathers
immediately tell their children what remedy to apply.
And it is rare that the patient suffers long;
those medicines being quick,
as well as generally infallible.

JOHN WESLEY, *PRIMITIVE PHYSIC*, *1747*

Native Americans were adept at treating wounds and it is quite possible that many Native tribes preceded Europeans in their use of a syringe and application of boiled water to dress injuries. The Michigan Natives cleaned wounds with a syringe made by filling a bladder with boiled herbal decoctions and attaching a quill to the bladder. People of the Ojibwa and Potawatomi tribes are said to have used a similar device. The Ojibwa people would suture torn tissues with a needle and deer's sinews while other Native North Americans used human hair, vegetable fibers (especially basswood) and deer tendons as suture material.

Massage was an important therapeutic device employed by many tribes including, but not limited to, the Pawnee, Pima, Maricopa, Yuma, Zuni and Navaho. It was used to correct breech presentation of a fetus; and to relieve the pains of labor, rheumatism and other disorders. To treat painful colic spasms, Pawnee people would massage the abdomen with an ointment made of powdered black rattlepod seeds *(Baptisia Bracteata* Ell.*)* and buffalo fat.

According to one physician, Dr. Eric Stone, "their skill in the care of wounds, fractures and dislocations equaled and in some respects exceeded that of their white contemporary." Native Americans devised form-fitting splints to treat fractures. Rawhide or wet clay padding as well as poultices were applied. The flat elastic ribs of the giant cactus became splints in the hands of a Pima healer while Ojibwa medicine people used thin cedar splints. First, the broken limb was washed with warm water and grease applied; after that came a poultice made from wild ginger and spikenard; the broken arm or leg was covered with a cloth before being bound to the splint.

It has been said that Native American practices involving childbirth were much more compassionate than those of their European counterparts whose Christian belief system dictated that the mother should feel the pain of labor to pay for original sin. Native American healers practiced what is known as "Crede's method of expelling the placenta" one hundred years prior to the publication of Crede's procedure. While European mothers were burned alive for using pain-relieving herbal medicine during labor, Native Americans drew upon any number of herbal remedies to ease delivery pain. Boiled roots of the cotton plant were used by the Alabama-Koasastis tribe to ease labor while the Zuni people utilized corn smut. Studies have confirmed that both of these substances contain phytochemicals that promote and ease labor pains. A few weeks prior to the expected delivery date, Cherokee and Penobscott women ingested frequent doses of a tea made from the leaves of partridge berry *(Mitchella repens)* to speed labor. Blue cohosh root was utilized by a number of tribes to ease delivery including the Ojibwas,

Menominees, Potawatomis, and Meskwakis. To stop postpartum bleeding, Hopi women drank a tea made from the entire buckwheat plant. Anikara women drank black western chokecherry juice to stop bleeding after childbirth. In the upcoming chapters you will learn many effective herbal remedies based on the ageless wisdom of Native American healers.

Native North Americans frequently employed similar healing techniques to those used by practitioners of Traditional Asian Medicine, including bleeding, cupping and moxa. (Don't let this scare you - when done in a gentle, caring manner, the procedures are not painful but quite effective in relieving discomfort. According to my personal experiences, an injection by a hypodermic needle can be much more painful!). For example, in Chinese Medicine we apply tiny cones known as "moxa" to a tender point on the body; the cone is set on fire and removed when the patient feels the heat. In a similar way, Virginia Natives made moxa cones from the soft wood found in knots of Hickory or Oak trees and burned them on painful areas of the patient's body. To help alleviate discomfort, Apache and Algonquin medicine men and women pierced points of persistent pain on the patient's body with a sharp object such as a splinter of glass, a needle from a cactus plant, or the fang of a rattlesnake from which the poison had been removed. Though far less elaborate than the Asian system, could this have been the North American Native version of acupuncture?

Similar to the East Indian Aryan hunting and gathering people, carting around volumes of written lore simply was not practical for most Native American tribes. Songs or stories about the healing properties of herbs as well as tribal traditions ensured that important knowledge would be passed on to future generations. Native American medicine people continue to recognize the incredible healing potential a story can offer and frequently use tales as a part of their healing art. Let's look at a myth that comes to us from Tchin, a Native American storyteller and artist *(Blackfoot and Narragansett)* from Norfolk, Virginia. This lovely tale (shortened for inclusion in this book) explains how the autumn season came to be created. It attunes listeners to the energy of autumn and can aid them in accessing and processing deeply buried emotions:

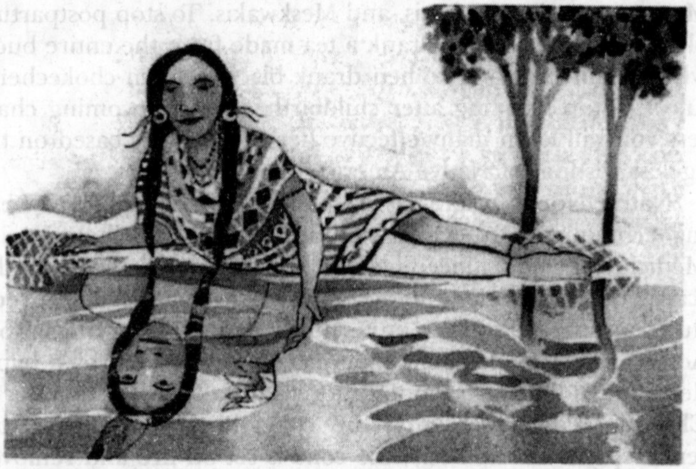

White Dove and Running Deer met at the annual Hoop Dance. As was the custom of their clans, once a year when the full moon rose high over the third notch in the mountain crest, eligible young people came together to be introduced by the elders. Here they learned the customs of their clans regarding taboos and marriage. Since young men and women were always chaperoned when they came together, this was their one opportunity each year to meet, dance and converse.

While most of the young people at the Hoop Dance changed partners frequently, parents, relatives and friends noticed how White Dove and Running Deer stayed together throughout the festivities. In soft whispers, White Dove explained how she spent her days working in her mother's field while Running Deer told of life in a nearby village and how his uncle taught him to play the flute.

The next day, after the Hoop Dance, Running Deer sat down by stream not far from the field and played a lovely haunting melody; the wind spirit carried the sweet sounds to White Dove. She understood his message and wanted to send him a sign. White Dove first asked permission of a nearby maple tree, then plucked the most perfect leaf she could find and placed it gently upon the swirling waters of the stream. The leaf message came to rest at Running Deer's feet; his heart leapt with joy; he picked up the leaf and returned to his village. Day after day, week after week, month after month, Running Deer played his flute only for the ears of White Dove. Day after day, week after week, month after month the maiden asked permission from the maple tree; then plucked a leaf and gently placed it in the swirling waters of the stream. In this way their love grew strong and deep though never a word was spoken.

One day Running Deer's uncle said it was time for him to stop playing the flute and learn how to hunt so he would be able to provide for a wife and family. This news made Running Deer extremely happy since he knew exactly who he wanted to marry.

Day after day, White Dove continued working in her mother's field but the wind no longer carried the sweet message from Running Deer's flute. At first she thought he probably had more important things to do - perhaps help the elders. She waited patiently, working in the field, always listening for the sounds of a flute, but slowly the days turned into weeks, and the weeks turned into months. One day a thought came to her, "Maybe he is playing the flute for a maiden from another clan." With this thought she felt a terrible pain in her heart. and she fell to the ground. Her parents called the medicine people, but even the medicine people could not mend a broken heart.

One day, Running Deer returned to his village, now strong and muscular from months of hunting; he joyfully ran down to the stream and played his flute for White Dove; he waited for the leaf . . . but it did not come. As he slowly returned to the village he ran into White Dove's brother on the path. They spoke of many things and finally Running Deer got up the courage to shyly ask about the boy's sister. Tears welled up in his eyes. In great sorrow he pointed west, to a rock in the distance and said, "My sister is over there." A stabbing pain ripped through Running Deer's heart and he fell to the ground. "Take me to where they placed your sister," he cried.

Together they walked in silence . . . when they finally reached White Dove's rock, Running Deer hesitated, and then began to play his flute - a song so lovely a hush fell upon the land and all of nature came to a halt . . . Up until then, from the beginnings of time, the trees had never lost their leaves, but a miracle happened . . . slowly . . . one by one . . . the leaves on the trees turned to red and gold and gently drifted down around Running Deer . . . each one carrying White Dove's message of love. No one ever saw Running Deer again . . . however . . . if you go out in the autumn, you will see how the trees and all of nature remember the everlasting union of White Dove and Running Deer.

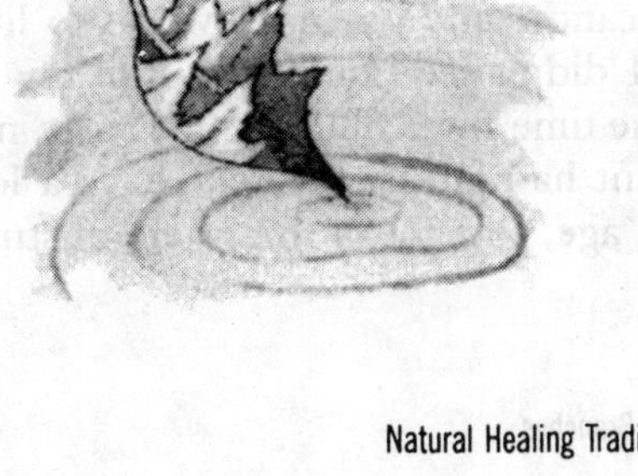

The central theme of this tale - that of grief or loss - in root form, is symbolized in a similar way by many diverse cultures around the globe. In the Western/European Four Humor tradition, grief and melancholy are linked to the cold, dry Fall season. In Ayurvedic medicine *Vata dosha* is associated with cold/ dryness, the colon, letting go, the fall season and the autumn of one's life. In the Chinese Five Element model, autumn is associated with cold/ dryness, grief, sadness, the Lung and Colon meridians (inspiration and letting go) and the westerly direction. And, as we have seen in this story, in many Native American traditions the westerly direction is associated with autumn, introspection and grief.

Have you noticed how feelings of sadness and depression tend to surface in the darker months of fall and winter? The emotion of grief or sadness is one that our modern American culture finds very difficult to acknowledge, much less express. We rarely take time to experience and process the profound grief that inevitably visits each and every one of us with the loss of a loved one - friend, lover, husband/wife, mother/father, brother/sister, aunt/uncle, pet - each loss requiring a unique healing of mind and spirit. We might take a day or two off from work, but then we expect, and are expected, to carry on as if everything is normal. All too frequently we simply turn to antidepressants. In ancient China, the sages recognized the enormous amount of healing that must take place after such a loss; the "official" mourning period was three years. In the clinical practice of Asian medicine, all too frequently we see patients who have suffered such a loss afflicted with chronic conditions associated with the Lung or Colon meridians (such as bronchitis, pneumonia, asthma, sinusitis, colitis or depression). Once the root cause of the imbalance is addressed and the deep energetic blockage created by buried grief is removed, the patient then begins to move back into the flow of their life.

On a personal note, by age nineteen I had lost most of my close family members. When I was four years old my brother left for college out of state; my mother was diagnosed with terminal breast cancer and given six weeks to live; my father left my mother (I didn't see him again until my sister's funeral at age 17). By the time I was nineteen my sister, my mother, a close uncle and aunt had all passed on. That's a lot to deal with at such an early age, so a lot of the grief got stuffed away. (Interestingly, right in line with the Chinese system of thought, I came down with pneumonia and then chronic bronchitis for about ten years). One of the best ways to deal with grief borrows an image from nature. Let me share it with you: "Notice how the emotion of grief comes on in great waves - don't fight with it, don't try to force it down. Simply allow the waves of grief to wash over you. It's the struggle to avoid feeling the pain that makes it so much worse. As time passes, slowly the waves become more gentle and, one day, the sun breaks through again as you recall the precious moments once shared with loved ones."

What is life? It is the flash of a firefly in the night.
It is the breath of a buffalo in the wintertime.
It is the little shadow which runs across the grass
and loses itself in the sunset.

CROWFOOT, 1821 - 1890
(HIS LAST WORDS)

One of the great merits of indigenous healing traditions, whether African, Native American or Australian Aboriginal, is that they address fundamental questions frequently asked by a person who wants to understand their disease process. Those questions are, "Why?" and more specifically, "Why me?" Traditional healing systems, by their very nature, are attuned to the spiritual beliefs of the culture in which they evolved and are thus ideally suited to help the individual answer those questions. In our modern world, where cultures are colliding, perhaps the more helpful approach is to assist the patient in exploring the root of the illness and addressing the question, "What is this condition asking of me?"

In its mechanistic approach to fixing the body-machine, Western biomedicine too often neglects delicate issues regarding the psychological and sociological responses of individuals and their families to illness. Western biomedicine strives to, and surpasses, other systems in its ability to explain the malfunctioning in biological processes called "disease"; but does not adequately recognize and honor sensitive cultural differences and resultant differing healing needs in our country's rich ethnic mosaic from which its patients are drawn. For real healing to take place a partnership must exist between the physician and the patient. Medical Anthropologists Kleinman & Sung state,

"What is needed in modern health care systems, in both developing and developed societies, is systematic recognition and treatment of psychosocial and cultural features of illness." These authors go even further to assert that modern biomedical clinical care "must fail" because most cases require treatment of these other aspects of illness, not just treatment of the diseased body-machine. Unfortunately, specialists have replaced general practitioners and the once intimate relationship between helper and helped has shifted to an impersonal one between strangers. In this system, the tendency is to view patients not so much as persons, but rather as a "diseased heart, lung or kidney". Many modern health practitioners have lost knowledge of their patients as real people.

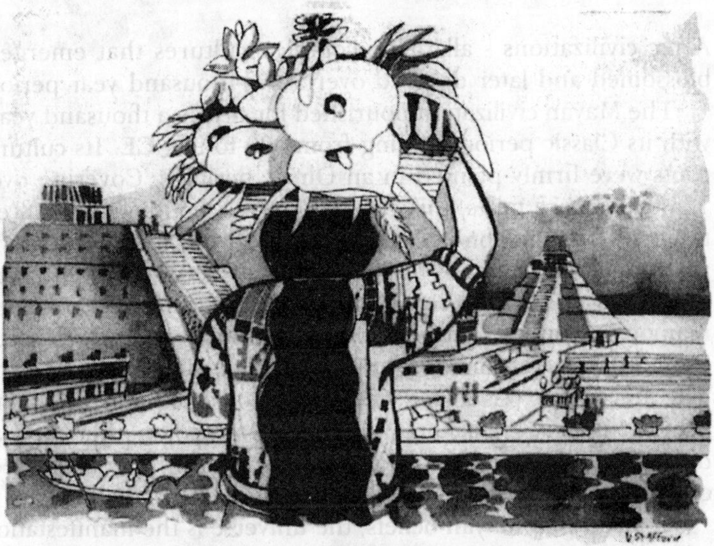

Myths, Legends & Health Care Practices from the Land of the Mayas & Aztecs

"The roots of all living things are
tied together. When a mighty tree is felled,
a star falls from the sky;
before you cut down a mahogany you should ask
permission of the keeper of the forest,
and you should ask permission of
the keeper of the star."

CHAN K'IN OF NAHA, MAYA

Are you ready for an adventure - a real anthropological challenge? Although difficult, it can broaden our understanding of life to see how we human beings create concrete realities with our thoughts. The best way to do that is to try to project ourselves into a completely different reality: we are going to become Aztec healers around 1500 CE. But first it's important to get an idea about how we would view the world, based on the beliefs of our ancestors. Let's set the stage.

In Mesoamerica, as early as 800 BCE, hunter gatherers banded together to form the Olmec culture. After the Olmecs came the Teotihuacan empire, the Mayan, the Toltec, and the

Aztec civilizations - all richly complex cultures that emerged, blossomed and later decayed over a two-thousand year period.

The Mayan civilization flourished for nearly a thousand years with its Classic period ranging from 300 to 900 CE. Its cultural roots were firmly planted in an Olmec heritage. Covering over 125,000 square miles, this vast empire was populated by an estimated three million citizens at the height of its development. An agriculturally based society, Mayan farmers cultivated maize as their principal crop along with beans, squash, sweet potatoes, manioc, cotton and cacao. It was a complex society with social status being determined by birth, and/or possibly by occupation. The aristocracy was formed by a ruler, or chief, and the members of his clan; craftsmen and artisans formed another class, as did the scholars and the peasants. The Mayan State was theocratic in nature with priests holding positions of power.

According to Mayan beliefs, the universe is the manifestation of one supreme divinity, Hunab K'u, who functions through dynamic dualism - hot/cold, light/dark, masculine/feminine, heavens/earth, spirit/matter. This single god, responsible for all of creation, is sometimes symbolized by a feathered serpent called Quetzalcoatl. The feathers represent the heavens and the spirit, while the snake represents the earth or material manifestations of matter. Somewhat akin to Asian philosophy, the Maya believe that all of creation is animated by an invisible life force - plants, animals, clouds, stars, minerals, humans; a concept not unlike that found in East India *(prana)* or in China *(ch'i)*.

Similar to the ancient Greek four elements, Ayurvedic and Chinese five element model, and Native American thought system, the Maya people divided their universe into five directions. Each direction had many associations and was assigned a specific color, time, plant and god. As is common in many North American Native traditions, the center constituted the fifth direction (up-down dimension), and the Maya assigned the green ceiba tree (*yaxche*, "green tree") to the center. The pantheon of Maya deities gets quite complex because each deity is divided into four different aspects and given a different name when assigned to each one of the four directions.

The Mayans founded their belief system upon rhythmic cycles of creation and destruction, much like we find among the Hindus. The cosmic struggle of four brother demigods to rule the world was fundamental to the Mayan creation myth and belief system. Their history was divided into five periods called "Suns"; one of the brother gods would rule during a Sun and then creation was destroyed and the brothers would struggle to gain control. According to one version of the creation myth, Tezcatlipoca Rojo ruled the time period corresponding to the First Sun (13 Mayan centuries, or 676 years). He was god of the east and the color red; the First Sun came to an end when Tezcatlipoca became angry and sent jaguars to eat the people. However, the other three brother gods helped Mayan ancestors hide in caves to avoid the destruction. Next came Quetzalcoatl, god of the south and color yellow, who ruled during the Second Sun for seven Mayan centuries, or 364 years. He decided to destroy the world with wind; but the other three brothers changed the people into monkeys so they could cling to the trees. Tezcatlipoca Negro, god of the west and color black ruled for six Mayan centuries, or 312 years. He destroyed the world by fire, but the other three brothers came to the rescue, changing the people into birds so they could fly away. Huitzilopochtli, god of the north and color white, ruled for 13 Mayan centuries, or 676 years. He destroyed the world with a flood but his three brothers changed the people into fish so they could save themselves by swimming away. You see a very complicated belief system emerging in which the gods gave life but, in a capricious sort of way, were also capable of whisking it away in an instant.

Finally, at long last, the four feuding brothers reached an agreement. They divided the Mayan century of 52 years into four periods of 13 years each. They would take turns - each would rule for 13 years. We are currently living in the Mayan period of the Fifth Sun. Modern experts on Maya chronology believe that the Fifth Sun began on August 12, 3113 BCE. Based on Maya prophecies, they say this Fifth Sun is supposed to come to an end when the world is destroyed by earthquakes on December 24, 2011 CE.

Cultural Perspectives on Time

Could Someone Please Tell Me What Year It Is?

Most Westerners believe it is now the year 2000;
in reality, there are many different views on this subject!
According to the ancient Babylonians it should be 2749;
the Buddhist calendar says it will be 2544;

it's the Year of the Dragon according to Chinese calendars;
1716 according to the Coptic calendar;
the 1st Egyptian calendar indicates it should be 6238;
208 according to the calendar of the French Revolution;
the Jewish calendar says it will be 5760;
5119 in the current Maya great cycle;
1420 according to the Muslim calendar;
1378 according to the Persian calendar;
and, by the old Roman calendar it will be 2763.

DAVID EWING DUNCAN, EXCERPT FROM *CALENDAR*

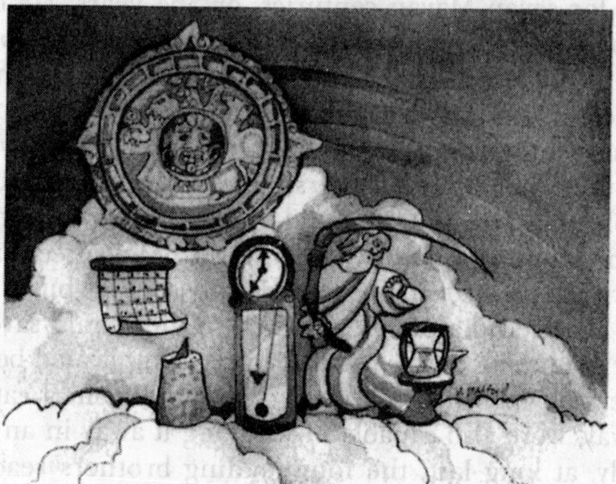

Master engineers, architects, astronomers and mathematicians, the Mayans developed their mathematical system (based on the value of 20 rather than 10) to such a degree that it surpassed that of the Greeks and Romans. Fascinated with time, all important events of their lives were calculated in accordance with celestial cycles and, similar to the Chinese tradition, living rulers repeated the rituals of their ancestors. Time was circular for the Mayan people - and a person, by completing the circle, could return to the same place in time and space. History was perpetually repeating itself.

This Mayan obsession with time led to the sophistication of a mathematical system which gave them the ability to plot the movements of the planets, sun and moon with such remarkable accuracy. The Maya developed five inter-related calendars: 1) The Sacred Year calendar consisting of 260 days (13 months of

20 days each); 2) the Solar Calendar consisting of 365 days (18 months of 20 days and one month of 5 days); 3) the Moon Calendar of 29 days; 4) the Calendar of Venus consisting of 584 days; and, 5) the Calendar of Mars consisting of 780 days. Just to demonstrate the accuracy of the Mayan astronomical calculations, let's consider the Venus Calendar (keeping in mind that all calendars were equally accurate). The Maya knew the Venus cycle was 583.92 days instead of 584. To compensate for the discrepancy, they dropped four days every sixty-one Venus years.

Every 18,980 days, or 52 years (representing a Mayan Century), all of the calendars "lined up" and started with "Day One" again. The Mayan people believed that if their world was going to come to an end, it would happen at this time. Every 52 years, the priests prepared the people for the end of the world: All activities halted; fires were extinguished; and the people gathered to pray. If "Day One" passed without incident, they had another 52 years!

(Note: Descendants of the great Maya civilization still occupy vast regions of Guatemala and eastern Mexico today. Their children speak Mayan languages. Despite heavy pressures to change, they have managed to cling tenaciously to many of their age-old traditions mixing native beliefs and practices with Christianity. Unfortunately the Maya system of hieroglyphic writing did not survive the conquest. The invading Spaniards destroyed thousands of ornate and exquisitely decorated native books called codices - only four remain today. Here are the words of Bishop Diego de Landa who presided over the 16th century purge, "We found a large number of books in these characters and, as they contained nothing in which there were not to be seen superstition and lies of the devil, we burned them all, which they regretted to an amazing degree, and which caused them much affliction.")

Life of an Aztec Healer

The existence of writing in state-level societies allows knowledge to accumulate, be passed on, and achieve an increasing level of sophistication.

The Aztecs are a crucial example because written records make theirs the best documented state-level civilization of the New World. Their medicine was ideologically coherent and sophisticated, with obvious appeal for anthropologists and medical and religious historians concerned with the nature of non-Western thought systems.

BERNARD R. ORTIZ DE MONTELLANO,
AZTEC MEDICINE, HEALTH, AND NUTRITION

It's 1500 CE and we're physicians living in Tenochtitlan, one of the three major cities of the large Aztec empire that spans from coast to coast. Chocolate beans serve as our monetary unit; rumor has it that our ruler, Motecuhzoma II drinks 50 to 60 cups of chocolate daily. Sometimes we can't help but wonder if each of his 600 wives drink that much chocolate as well! Like the Maya and ancient Egyptian civilizations, our system of writing is hieroglyphic. The citizens of our city enjoy a game played with a solid rubber ball, and we frequently have to look for our children playing at the ballcourt not far from our homes. The streets of the city are swept and watered daily by over a thousand city employees. Between 1466 and 1478 CE, our ancestors constructed aqueducts to carry fresh water to Tenochtitlan from Chapultepec (people living in London drank polluted water from the Thames River until as late as 1854). Human waste is collected and used as fertilizer to nourish the city's lush floating gardens or *chinampas*. Our beautiful city is laid out along canals like Venice, Italy; but instead of gondolas, Aztec boatmen make their way through the canals with poled canoes. Hygiene and personal cleanliness are of great importance to us and fragrant herbs are used to create soaps, dentifrices, breath sweeteners and deodorants.

As health care providers we enjoy visits to the royal botanical gardens and zoo in Huaztepec, established by Motecuhzoma I in 1453. We work at a nearby hospital with other nurses, surgeons and medical staff where patients do not pay for medical treatment. Herbs are cultivated for medical research and we give remedies to patients without charge as long as they report back on the results of their cure. Sweat baths, massage and manipulation are the treatments we most frequently recommend for persons who have been injured in a fall. We apply splints to immobilize broken bones and traction and counter traction to reduce sprains and fractures. As surgeons, if a broken bone doesn't mend, we open the fracture and insert a resinous stick in the hollow to hold the two bones together; the laceration is then sutured with hair and a healing poultice applied. (This technique, of inserting an intramedullar nail, was not used in Western medicine until the 20th century). We perform plastic surgery with obsidian scalpels that have edges much thinner than those of surgical steel (the sharper the blade, the less damage is done to tissues). If a nose is cut off in battle, we sew it back in place with hair and apply salted bee honey to prevent infection; in case the nose fragment was lost, we can even make a prosthesis. (Note: It is believed that Native North, Central and South American people were familiar with the use of herbal anesthetics hundreds of years prior to Carl Koller's experiments with cocaine in 1884. The Aztecs utilized a number of herbs with narcotic-like effects including one called *yauhtli [Tagetes lucida]* to relieve pain).

Some illnesses are not caused by accident or war. We have come to understand them to be punishments sent by one of the many nature spirits or demigods that has been offended. Many of these "internal" disorders were classified by our ancestors before us and they are treated effectively with herbs and healing rituals. For example, the rain god Tlaloc might send a cold disease that we refer to as *coacihuiztli* (symptoms include fever, colic, phlegm) to one of our patients. We use an herb called *iztauhyatl (Artemisia mexicana)* to induce sweating and help remove excess mucus. When in doubt about a particular disease or remedy, we can always go to the library at the university to look through some of our elaborate Aztec codices on healing. Very frequently we prescribe a single herb to treat a specific ailment. *When Aztec lands were conquered, Spanish physicians praised the efficacy of native treatments while criticizing what they perceived to be an overly simplistic healing system. Of course, they didn't take the time to understand the wealth of knowledge the Aztecs accumulated over the centuries. In Europe, during the 1500's, the tendency was to create herbal formulas using a great quantity of herbs.)*

Fundamentally, our belief system is somewhat similar to that of the Mayas, we believe in one Creative Force, but daily life requires placating a very complex pantheon of deities and nature spirits. Even though past civilizations were disrupted when bands of hunter gatherers came in from the North, for the most part, they settled in, adopting the lifestyles and belief systems of our semi-agricultural ancestors already living off the land. They brought new demigods with them which were readily incorporated into our own belief system. *(When the Aztecs were conquered by Hernan Cortes, his conquistadors and the Catholic missionaries, they found it fairly easy to accept the new patron saints in much the same way)*. Traditions have been handed down orally from the beginning of time and this will continue with our descendants, in the same way, into the unknown future.

As physicians, we're constantly called upon to mend the wounds of valiant warriors who must seek new victims for sacrifice to the sun god. If he is not fed, our universe will come to an end. Similar to the Maya people, we believe that after the destruction of the Fourth Sun, the gods met at Teotihuacan to recreate the sun, giving new life to the world. Two of them fought for the privilege; the wealthy one claimed the prize because of his possessions, however he was cowardly and balked three times just as he was about to jump into the fire. Nanahuatzin, the small pimply-faced god, did not hesitate and jumped heroically into the flame to become the sun. Feeling ashamed, Tecciztecatl, the wealthy god followed, but the other gods intervened and punished his cowardice by converting him into the moon. Once transformed into the sun, Nanhuatzin was weak and stationary - unable to move. In order that he might gain the strength necessary to create the world, the other gods drew blood to nourish him so that he could continue his life-giving journey across the heavens. Unfortunately, the self-sacrifice of the gods was not sufficient. Since that time, human blood must be fed to the sun on a daily basis. It's not that he is blood thirsty, quite the contrary, he is simply weak and requires nourishment to give him strength to make his voyage across the sky. Our society is continually engaged in ritualistic warfare; prisoners must be taken alive so they can be offered to the sun, otherwise, all of creation will perish. The key duty imposed upon the Aztec people is to maintain the existence of the universe and to do this we must supply energy to the sun through human sacrifice.

Though extremely difficult to try to project ourselves into another time and culture, at least now we might begin to comprehend why these sacrifices were required - from the viewpoint of the sacrificer. But what about the sacrificial victim? Aztec citizens accepted the necessity of this practice because they understood their fate after life depended on their manner of death - not on their earthly behavior. For example, persons chosen to die by the rain god Tlaloc might be hit by lightening, drown or succumb to *wet* and *cold* diseases associated with him such as paralysis, gout, rheumatism, dropsy or leprosy; these people went to Tlalocan, described as a place of joy and abundance. Persons who died from an accident or ordinary death went to the place of the dead called Mictlan; the hazardous voyage took four years filled with trials and ultimately ended up in oblivion. The most auspicious death was that of the warrior in battle or as the sacrificial victim. These "fortunate" souls won the privilege of accompanying the sun on its travels from sunrise to noon; after four years they would be reborn as butterflies or hummingbirds.

Our Aztec society is a moderate one - priests and elders have taught us that the forces of duality must be maintained in balance for order and health to prevail. While there may be brief moments of joy or laughter in this life, they quickly pass. It is essential to maintain equilibrium, states of anger or sexual excesses could make us vulnerable to illness. Diseases can also result from violating rituals or offending a particular god. Since childhood we were instructed that life on earth is ephemeral; humankind is destined to feel physical pain, thirst and hunger. Our proper attitude towards life must be one of stoicism and forbearance and we should faithfully perform our duties. Sex is one of those duties; our duty to populate the earth. However, as young men we were instructed to refrain from any sexual activity for as long as possible since it would result in the serious depletion of our *tonalli*. Tonalli, a vital force that enters our bodies through the crown of the head, links us to the gods and the universe. It is a force that creates warmth, growth, bravery and vigor. Men have more tonalli than women; and to be a very influential noble you must have very strong tonalli. As persons age, their tonalli grows stronger, therefore we treat our elderly with great respect.

Our world changed forever when Hernan Cortez took control of our city in 1521; we thought he and his men were gods and we treated them as such. By the time we learned they were not, it was too late. We did not understand their lust for our gold; for us, it was simply "excrement of the sun god." We did not understand their type of warfare. War, for us, was ritualistic, we fought to take victims alive for sacrifice to the gods so the universe would not perish; the Spanish fought to kill us on the battlefield for their god of greed. Some of the Spanish missionaries, including Bernardino de Sahagun, Bartolome de las Casas and Diego Duran, were sympathetic to our ways and would later comment that our conservative lifestyle, child-rearing practices, rules on sobriety and system of laws were far superior to Spanish colonial customs. They believed that by simply converting us to Christianity, by exchanging our Sun God for their God and replacing our demigods with their patron saints, an ideal society could emerge.

(Note: Demographers estimate that in 1519, between 20 to 25 million people lived within the boundaries of what is Mexico today. A census taken by the Spanish in the late 1500's found only a scant million Native survivors of the Spanish Conquest. Millions of Native Central Americans perished due to warfare, disease brought by the conquerors, and the New World Inquisition. The conquerors brought their own medical practices to the New World; Native Central American healers adopted some elements of the European Galenic humoral approach while continuing many folk medical practices of the time. A new folk system of healing emerged).

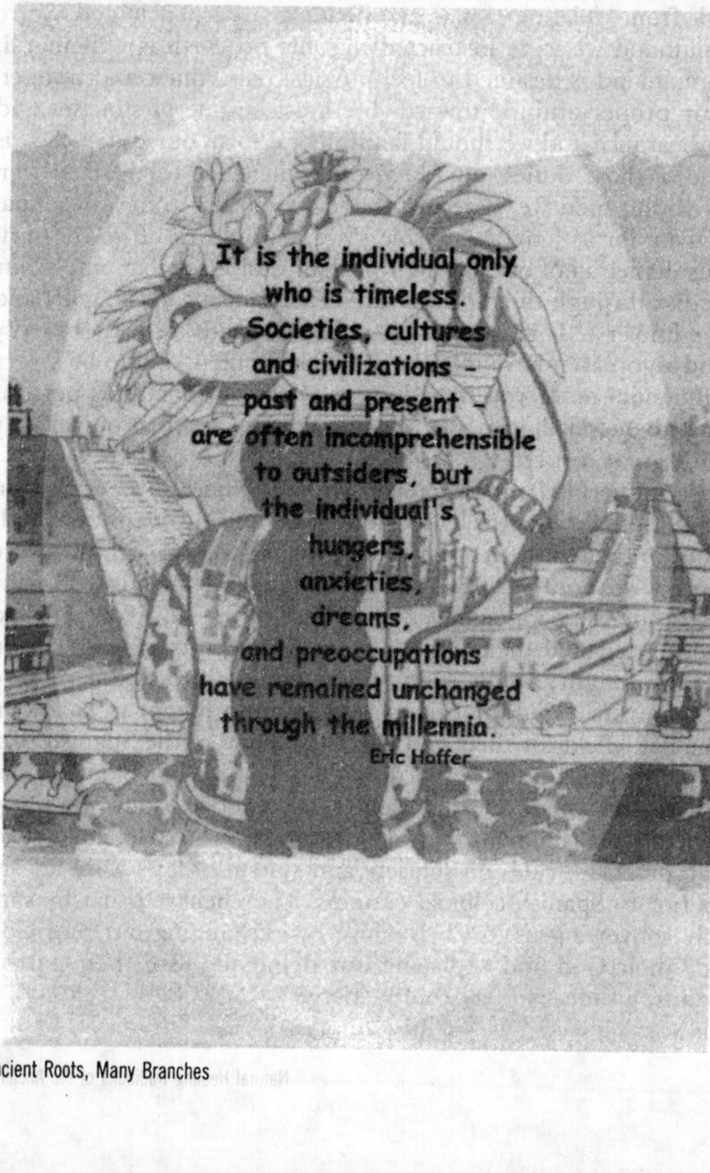

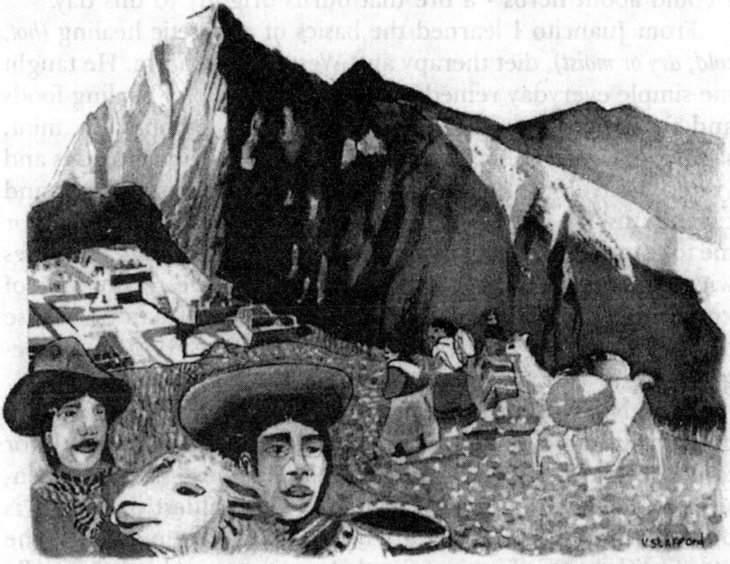

Lost Medical Arts from the Land of the Incas

Now I would like to take you on a visit to the land I call home, the land of tropical jungles and ice bergs, gauchos, magnificent waterfalls, Machu Pichu, and the hauntingly lovely flute music of the high Andes - South America. It was here that I was first introduced to healing with herbs some twenty-five years ago. I suffered from chronic bleeding duodonal ulcers for years; was hospitalized for this condition; had exhausted the plethora of Western pharmaceutical treatments, and was now facing surgical removal of part of my stomach and duodenum. At the time, I was studying music at the Universidad Nacional de Musica in Mendoza, Argentina. My clarinet professor, when hearing about the upcoming surgery, literally threw me in his car and took me to see his herbalist Juancito. What was there to lose? So I brewed up the bags of smelly blossoms, leaves, twigs and barks as directed. Amazingly, the pain subsided in four days. Suffice to say that six weeks after starting Juancito's recommended diet and herbal therapy (one that is completely contrary to all Western notions of ulcer care) the Xrays showed the ulcers had completely healed for the first time in eight years. I have never been plagued with the problem since that time; this positive experience with natural healing sparked an intense desire to learn all

I could about herbs - a fire that burns brightly to this day.

From Juancito I learned the basics of energetic healing *(hot, cold, dry or moist)*, diet therapy and Western herbalism. He taught me simple everyday remedies involving the use of healing foods and gentle herbs and spices like chamomile, lemon balm, mint, sage, garlic and rosemary. Later I became more adventurous and visited Native South American herbal healers, curanderos and curanderas. Theirs was a fascinating world that was difficult for me to comprehend. However, I witnessed some remarkable cures with strange substances and incantations. Due to my lack of knowledge at the time, I did not understand many of those cures; but I knew they worked. These are the roots of my beginnings as a practicing herbalist.

From Native South Americans we have inherited many medicines including cocaine, curare, pau de arco and quinine. Prior to the conquest of Pizarro their forefathers possessed an extensive herbal materia medica. While in our wildest dreams it is probably impossible to get a true and complete picture of the accomplishments of ancient South American peoples, let's briefly examine some of their achievements. It's important to note that new archaeological finds constantly rewrite our understanding of their lives, customs and healing practices.

The Incan civilization, the last great South American empire to emerge before the appearance of the conquistadors, was relatively short-lived (from 1430 to 1532 CE), when compared to earlier cultures such as the Chavin, Moche, Lima, Nazca, Huarpa, Tiahuanaco, Wari, Chimu and Chancay. The sprawling Incan state, called Tahuantinsuyu, translated as "Land of the Four Quarters", stretched down the long Andean mountain chain for more than 5,500 kilometers or 3,418 miles - surpassing the Ottoman Empire and Ming China as the largest nation on the globe in the 1500's. The Incan empire, more than any other, symbolizes human mastery over extreme environmental conditions. While the original Incan predecessors were montane in origin, their conquests incorporated natives from marine, jungle and desert habitats into their state. If we can conceive of a thriving civilization that flowered atop the Himalayas while encompassing a jungle more vast than the Congo, the Sahara desert and a coastal fishery brimming with more life than the Bering Sea we might begin to appreciate the triumphs of the Incan people. It should be noted that the word "Inca" actually only refers to a select group of related individuals that numbered less than 40,000; the head of the royal family ruled over an estimated ten (or more) million people who were his subjects but were not Incas. Since there was great variance in linguistics between the tribes and societies conquered by Inca legions, *Runa Simi* (a version of the Quechua language) became the official tongue.

Cuzco, known as the "navel, or sacred center, of the universe", was the capital city and heart of Tahuantinsuyu. From accounts of the Spanish invaders, the great metropolis was magnificent with a broad highway leading into the urban center. Sacsahuaman, an enormous fort exhibiting the superb masonry skills of Native builders, dominated the imperial capital; it is said that over 30,000 laborers worked simultaneously for decades to complete its construction. Sparkling fountains adorned spacious malls and precious metals glistened on the walls of temples, palaces, villas and shrines that flanked paved avenues. In Incan thought, gold was the essence of their god Inti, or the Sun. The temple, known as the Coricancha or "House of the Sun," contained images of the solar deity and other celestial luminaries that comprised the imperial pantheon. Following is a description of the the grand palace of the Incan gods in the words of Pedro de Cieza de Leon, one of the conquistadors and author of *Chronicle of Peru, 1540:*

The stone appeared to me to be of a dusky or black color, and most excellent for building purposes. The wall had many openings, and the doorways were very well carved. Round the wall, half way up, there was a band of gold, two palmos (bandwidths) wide and four dedos (fingers) in thickness. The doorways and doors were covered with plates of the same metal. Within were four houses, not very large, but with walls of the same kind and covered with plates of gold within and without. . .

In one of these houses, which was the richest, there was the figure of the sun, very large and made of gold, very ingeniously worked, and enriched with many precious stones. . .

They had also a garden, the clods of which were made of pieces of fine gold; and it was artificially sown with golden maize, the stalks, as well as

as the leaves and cobs, being of that metal . . .
Besides all this, they had more than twenty
golden sheep (llamas) with their lambs, and the
shepherds with their slings and crooks to watch them,
all made of the same metal. There was a great
quantity of jars of gold and silver, set with emeralds;
vases, pots, and all sorts of utensils, all of fine gold.

Only about 40,000 persons of Incan descent resided in Cuzco. Another 200,000 non-Incan citizens lived in the outlying suburban areas - they were the government workers, artisans and technical personnel. Work performed by conquered tribes transformed the entire imperial heartland into luxurious estates adorning lush park lands of sculpted hillsides and terraces kept verdant by irrigation canals. Agriculture in the Andes has been plagued, from time immemorial, by an enormous dilemma - where there is water, there is little land and, where there is land there is little water. Over hundreds of years, through sheer ingenuity and amazing feats of engineering, Andean cultures constructed complex canal networks covering millions of hectares. In the Western Hemisphere, to this day, abandoned Andean agricultural systems are considered to be the "largest archaeological phenomena". Steep mountainsides became terraced farms; so successful were the Incan lords at exploiting the Andean highlands that today, by comparison, there is less land in cultivation than there was in 1500.

In this South American empire people were required to pay three types of taxes to the state, these included agricultural products, textiles or pottery, and a labor tax, called *mit'a*. It was *mit'a* that enabled the Incas to construct a vast all-weather highway system through the rugged Andean mountains from Ecuador to Chile - complete with tunnels and impressive suspension bridges of rope. While it is believed that some of the routes actually date from Wari times, or 700 to 1100 CE; Incan subjects constantly improved and maintained the major thoroughfares and trunk lines which spanned at least 30,000 to 40,000 kilometers (or 18,000 to 25,000 miles).

The Incas were adept at risk management practices with food storage facilities widely distributed throughout the highlands. These well-constructed, one-room warehouses called *qollqa* were conspicuously located for high visibility and contained surplus agricultural "taxes" or commodities. In a land plagued with climactic and tectonic disasters, citizens must have felt reassured by the presence of these storage facilities that guaranteed their survival. Thousands of *qollqa* surrounded Cuzco; over 2,400 were located in Cotapachi, Bolivia. Once again, from writings of Pedro de Cieza de Leon in 1540, we might get an idea of what Pre-Hispanic Incan life was like:

As this kingdom was so vast, in each of the many provinces
there were many storehouses filled
with supplies and other needful things;
thus, in times of war, wherever the armies went
they drew upon the contents of these storehouses,
without ever touching the supplies of their confederates or
laying a finger on what they had in their settlements . . .
Then the storehouses were filled up once more
with the tributes paid the Inca.
If there came a lean year, the storehouses were opened
and the provinces were lent what they needed in the way of supplies;
then, in a year of abundance, they paid back all they had received.
No one who was lazy or tried to live
by the work of others was tolerated;
everyone had to work. Thus on certain days
each lord went to his lands and took the plow in hand and
cultivated the earth, and did other things.
Even the Incas themselves did this to set an example.
And under their system there was not want in all the kingdom, for,
if he had his health, he worked and lacked for nothing;
and if he was ill, he received what he needed from the storehouses.

Though Native life could never be romanticized as "idyllic"; five-hundred years ago the Incas managed to devise a governmental system capable of providing for the needs of all the inhabitants living in their empire in case of a disaster. To this day, such a safety net for the hungry and homeless continues to elude us here in the United States and in our world as a whole where someone dies of hunger every 3.6 seconds.

How is it that Francisco Pizarro and a handful of mercenaries (62 horsemen and 198 foot soldiers) managed to topple the largest nation in the world in 1532? This story is truly one of ruthlessness, deceit and greed. At the time Pizarro landed at Tumbez on the northern coast of Peru, two Incan brothers,

Atahuallpa and Huascar, were struggling to become emperor. Atahuallpa was informed that the Spanish were waiting to have a peaceful meeting with him in Cajamarca, and being more concerned about his brother's rebellion, headed into Cajamarca with his guard down. Pizarro and his men, aided by the military edge their horses provided, captured Atahuallpa and his retinue. Still relatively unconcerned about the Spanish threat, Atahuallpa offered Pizarro an enormous ransom in return for his freedom: a room, measuring 17 x 22 feet and 8 feet from floor to ceiling was to be filled with gold; and, the room would be filled twice with silver objects (payment amounting to approximately $50 million in today's bullion standards). While being held captive, waiting for the ransom to arrive, Atahuallpa ordered the execution of his half-brother Huascar, who had been captured. The gold and silver finally came, fulfilling Atahuallpa's part of the bargain; Pizarro repaid the ruler by executing him on July 26, 1533. Though the conquistadors met with some fierce resistance, the Spanish conquest of Tahuantinsuyu was successfully completed without major battles. Native opposition was rapidly squelched by the well-armed Castillian reinforcements who began to arrive in force once word was out about the fabulous treasures housed in Cuzco, Inti's golden city. Particularly devastating were the Old World infectious diseases brought to the New World by the conquerors. It is estimated that smallpox alone could have been responsible for the deaths of up to 2/3 of the New World population. However, greed and the religious zeal that motivated the conquerors took a terrible toll on live's and living standards of Native survivors of the battles and disease. Following are the words of Pope Paul the Third from a decree issued June 9, 1537, protesting the harsh treatment of Native people:

> *. . . Some of his ministers, who wanted to satisfy their greed,*
> *presume to affirm repeatedly that the Indians of the West*
> *and those of the South and the rest of the people*
> *of whom we have been informed in our times have to be treated*
> *like dumb animals and brought into our servitude.*
> *This is justified on the assumption that they are unfit for*
> *the Catholic faith, and on the pretext that they are incapable*
> *of receiving it, they are brought into servitude, and they*
> *are so afflicted and harassed that even the*
> *servitude to which animals are subjected is no greater*
> *than that of these people.*

The clash of cultures and the desire to dominate and suppress those who hold different views has created so much agony in our world. History has demonstrated, time and again, how the gods of conquered peoples become the devils of the conquerors. Sacred sites are ransacked and destroyed; the images of foreign gods defaced; and the conquerors own representations of the Infinite soon occupy the niches of the "pagan" gods. Too frequently, we are so caught up in our own belief system that we fail to see the inherent truth and beauty that can exist in other systems of thought. Particularly telling is one story about the Incan ruler who, when confronted by a Catholic missionary holding a staff topped with Christ on the cross, was truly puzzled upon hearing that the crucifix represented the Savior of the Spanish who had died and been resurrected into the heavens. Perceiving that the Spanish worshipped a metal representation of a dead man, Atahuallpa pointed to his god, Inti, the sun, saying that the Incan people worshipped a god who was alive and well - a god who was not human and therefore could not die - one who was clearly visible every day in the heavens.

The Incan culture was quite unique when compared to other civilizations and it is interesting to examine the root metaphors that organized the world view of these people. Similar to the Chinese and many New World cultures, inhabitants of the high Andes believed the balance of the cosmos was dependent upon the interactions of bipolar forces - interdependent and complementary pairs of opposites. Their reality was further sub-divided into four directions with their homeland,Tahuantinsuyu (translated as "Land of the Four Quarters") being laid out as an earthly representation of its celestial counterpart - the nightly heavens. The vast stream of stars known as the Milky Way, called *Mayu* or "celestial river" in the Quechua language formed the organizing principle for the Incan universe. When viewed from the southern hemisphere, the Milky Way slants left to right during six months of the year and, right to left during the other six months, creating a luminous grid that divides the heavens into four quarters called *suyu*. Andean societies tracked the movement of this celestial river of stars to predict water cycles (so important to survival in this land of capricious weather patterns) - wet and dry seasons coincide with the solstices of the Milky Way.

Astronomical occurrences in each of the four heavenly quadrants formed by *Mayu* were used to forecast what would occur in the related terrestrial quadrant during the daytime. Agricultural cycles were planned based on the movement of the sun god Inti; phases of the moon dictated planting times; movement of the other constellations and planets indicated the needs of developing crops. Even stellar voids were viewed as animal constellations that predetermined zoological cycles on earth. To this day, Native South Americans still see animals such as a fox, a toad, a partridge, a serpent and an adult and baby llama in the dark clouds, or starless spaces of the night sky.

Modern Quechua and Aymara people of these regions, in the way of their Pre-Hispanic predecessors, perceive their homeland as being alive with supernatural forces. Ill health or misfortune can be caused by earth, water or mountain in this dynamic landscape that is frequently jolted by earthquakes. The recurrent wrath of the El Nino phenomena alone is capable of completely disrupting normal marine and meteorological cycles with drought devastating the highlands while catastrophic floods wash through the deserts. *Pachamama* (mother earth) continues to be revered by Native people in this part of the world with offerings of flowers, coca leaf and chicha beer on all major agricultural occasions and, whenever alcohol is consumed, she is toasted. In the same way that excess heat, cold, moisture or dryness disrupts their landscape, Native Latin American people today, like their ancestors before them, continue to believe that good health depends upon the balance of these properties both in their external world and in their internal human bodyscape. This elemental approach to healing shows the influence of the medical view of Spanish physicians trained in the Galenic four humour tradition. It also parallels the Chinese medical model which sees the human being as a microcosm reflecting the same principles as the greater macrocosm. Like the ancient Chinese and the Java/Balinese island cultures, a mountain metaphor figures predominately as an organizing principle in their perception of the world.

Native South Americans living in the altiplano divide their world into three levels. People living on the lower slopes cultivate maize, barley, beans and peas; hardier grains like quinoa and amaranth and potatoes (over 60 varieties that come in all colors) are grown in fields located on the central slopes; highland communities devote themselves to animal husbandry, herding sheep, alpacas and llamas. The wellbeing of these people depends upon their ability to exchange supplies and services between the three resource areas of their mountainous landscape. To celebrate important events, like marriage, people and produce from all three levels of the mountain come together to symbolize unity. In a similar way, good health depends upon the body's ability to exchange fluids between its three levels or divisions (the head, trunk and legs) and to integrate the three levels of human experience (body, mind and spirit). Illness is treated or cured by "putting the body of the mountain together" which represents this unification principle.

What of the actual healing practices of the ancient Incas? Unfortunately, many of the lost healing secrets of the Incas are going to remain just that - lost secrets. This is because the Incas did not develop a formal system of writing but depended upon a verbal tradition for passing crucial information to future generations. *(The Incas possessed a very complicated device called a quipu that was utilized for multiple record-keeping purposes - from tax and census information to imperial history. Unfortunately, it has been impossible to reconstruct exactly how this device was used. The quipu is a long cord which is held horizontally; from it is suspended a number of strands of yarn of various colors and from these suspended strands hang other colored strings. Knots in the strands recorded numerical data.)* Without an official written Incan history, we are forced to rely on information that comes to us from the conquerors which is, all too frequently, biased. Despite an air of superiority, the works of one priest, Father Bernabe Cobo, have proven particularly valuable. Cobo was a botanist who described New World flora with scientific accuracy and his research placed a special emphasis on medicinal plants - many of the uses for Incan herbs mentioned in upcoming chapters come from his writings. Another way of reconstructing Incan uses of herbal medicine is to study Native healing techniques still being practiced in this part of the world today.

According to chronicles written by Spanish conquerors and missionaries, massage was frequently one of the first steps taken to cure illness in the Peruvian Andes. The ancient Incas created special healing ointments concocted from sea vegetables and valerian leaves that were applied to the body. A gum resin would be chewed and rubbed around the navel and then the masseuse would follow the course of the colon. Similar to ancient Ayurvedic healers living in East India, South American Natives, as a forerunner to modern skin clips, would apply leaf cutting ants to pinch together the edges of a cut; once attached, their heads were twisted off leaving their pincers in place. Native Peruvian healers constructed artificial limbs and knew skin-flap techniques similar to those used in plastic surgery today. Special corsets constructed of bark and laced around the patient were utilized to treat injuries that required stabilization of the body's mid-section. Deep or complicated wounds were sometimes cauterized; on other occasions wicks made from bark fibers or twisted cloth were used as drains. In Peru, abundant skeletal evidence of sophisticated skull surgery (trephination) has been found; it is believed that Andean Natives used several anesthetic drugs for such operations, such as cocaine and peyote. The mild shock from an electric eel was used by Native South Americans to treat paralysis. In the upcoming chapters you will find references to many of the herbs used by Native healers as reported by their Spanish conquerors.

In Bolivia, the Qolla Kapachayuh, or "Lords of the Medicine Bag", are herbalists who still practice their trade today. Known as Kallawaya herbalists (also spelled "Qollahuaya"), their healing tradition dates from the early Tiahuanaco cultures, or 400 CE. During the time of the Inca Empire, they were the "privileged ones" who carried the chair of the Inca ruler. From the early beginnings of Andean culture Kallawaya herbalists traveled up and down the Andes, collecting herbs and learning the pharmacopoeias of many Andean groups. It was customary for aspiring herbal healers to spend up to eight years in an apprenticeship with a practicing herbalist. This age-old tradition has been kept alive and passed down to the 120 to 130 remaining herbalists in the Kallawaya ethnic group which is mostly composed of herders and horticulturalists. Familiar with the medicinal values of more than one thousand plants, Kallawayas are renowned for their herbal healing skills throughout Argentina, Bolivia, Chile and Peru. These herbalists use a secret language among themselves called *machaj-juyai*, meaning "language of colleagues". This language, composed of some 12,000 words, is a hybrid formed from the usage of Puquina words and Quechua grammar. The Puquina language actually disappeared during the seventeenth century but lives on in a modified form when Kallawayas converse about healing rituals, medicinal plants, potions and paraphernalia.

During the 1950's and 60's in South America, herbalists were classified as *brujos*, or witches, and were forbidden to practice their art in many places. Synthetic drugs took the place of herbs. It's interesting that during the same time period about forty remedies were developed in Bolivia by pharmaceutical companies. These products came from original Kallawaya herbal recipes; however, the companies consistently omitted reference to plant constituents and reimbursed herbal suppliers only minimally. Due to unfair treatment, herbalists have refused to collaborate further with pharmaceutical companies. It is only fair that patent rights be extended to herbalists and that herbal suppliers receive equitable pay for their herbs and labors. During the 1980's and 90's the popularity of Kallawaya herbalists rebounded as the Western world became interested in the medicinal properties of healing plants. In Bolivia today, herbalists and medical doctors jointly staff health clinics in El Alto, La Paz and Oruro.

Traditional healing practices continue to survive and thrive in many areas of Latin America; in fact, worldwide, the health needs of 80 percent of our earth's population are provided by herbalists and ethnomedical practitioners. In some cases, Native practices are more practical than biomedical procedures. For example, Mayan midwives practicing in Mexico were taught by health care workers to cut a newborn infant's umbilical cord with a pair of scissors and then pack it with cotton balls that were soaked in alcohol. Scissors are difficult to sterilize and the umbilical stump remained moist resulting in an increased rate of umbilical infection and neonatal tetanus. Prior to biomedical intervention, midwives had slit the cord with a freshly cut bamboo splinter; it was then cauterized with a candle flame and dressed with a piece of burnt cloth. While it is important not to romanticize the role of ethnomedicine, it is essential to recognize that it is the only medicine available to many persons on our globe - healing herbs grow in almost all environments, they're extremely safe and effective in the hands of a trained herbalist, and cost relatively little when compared to pharmaceutical drugs. Biomedicine is extremely costly and, most frequently, available only to persons possessing wealth. What does this mean for citizens living in a city that was once part of the proud Incan empire? Of the 356,000 persons living in El Alto, Bolivia in 1990, 74 percent of the population earned less than \$60 per month while the remaining 26 percent earned \$61 to \$130 monthly.

The costs of biomedical healthcare projects in countries like Bolivia tend to be so high that they must be continually subsidized. In Montero, Bolivia, a \$5 million USAID-funded community health-worker program was abandoned because neither the U.S. or Bolivian governments could continue paying the salaries of project workers. While goods required to maintain the project could have been procured much cheaper in Bolivia or Brazil, USAID required that they be purchased from the United States.

In the minds of Native peoples, Western biomedicine is frequently associated with colonization and the white power structure that brought disease and decimation to their homelands in the first place - depriving them of their rightful resources, dignity and age-old lifestyles, cultures and traditions. As it is practiced today, Western biomedicine is a cultural institution and people living in developing countries are expected to have faith in something that is completely foreign to them. In fact, many South American Native people believe that they go to hospitals "to die" - not to get well.

As a cultural institution, biomedicine has the power to redefine (or "medicalize") concepts into the terms of its own discourse. Thus "medical imperialism", in the colloquialism of our day, now encompasses not only the conquest of new diseases but also the extension of what has been called the biomedical model over the ethnomedical world. It also implies the extension of Western cultural values to the non-West.

ROY MACLEOD, EXCERPT FROM *MEDICINE AND EMPIRE*

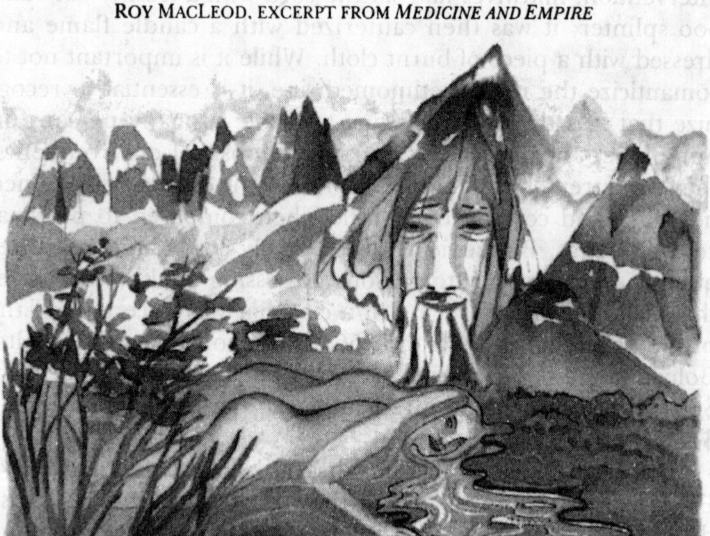

I lived and studied in Argentina for five years and became very fond of many exceptional South American people. Following is a story based on a true encounter with one remarkable old Argentine gentleman whose spirit continues to live in my heart. This story is dedicated to him and to health care providers everywhere.

One Who Left Omelas

A strange kind of trinity was forming in her mind. Students in the English Literature class were commenting on "The Ones Who Walk Away From Omelas", by Ursula K. Le Guin. The story was about a perfect city; perfect with one exception - the happiness of its inhabitants depended upon the suffering of one child who had to remain locked in a hideous cellar. The child represented the suffering, hungry and homeless masses living in developing countries; the citizens living in Omelas represented people living in the industrialized world. One student was saying that those who walk away from the city were not fulfilling their moral obligations to society. She disagreed. There are always those who talk about helping the child, but few who really ever venture out of their comfortable world to follow words with action. The ones who finally leave Omelas, walking into the darkness, are those who truly tried. They had entered that dark, dank, stinking cellar and attempted to clean, comfort and nurture the child. After many days, months or years of trying to ease the suffering, they leave the cellar; they leave Omelas and "they go towards a place even less imaginable to most of us than the city of happiness". Once . . . long ago she had an encounter with one who was leaving Omelas. The encounter was very brief, but he had mentioned where he was going, and why he was going.

Again the trinity was starting to form. She saw the worn face of a very old Argentine man; and the timeless face of the Andean mountain range as it watched over the city of Mendoza on the desert plateau below. The third face was coming into focus. Who was it? She could not quite discern the third figure in the trinity. And one again the image faded.

She had lived in Argentina from 1972 to 1977, attending the Universidad Nacional de Musica in Mendoza. Those were very difficult years for the country she called home and the people she had come to love so dearly. Peron had returned to power, died and then came the military dictatorship and missing persons. But this story is about one particular person - a very old Argentine gentleman - one who left Omelas and seemed to know where he was going.

It was a crisp autumn morning. The first frost of the season had fallen during the night. It seemed that nature's metronome was ticking faster than usual, as all living things scurried to prepare for the freezing cold nights that would follow. The craggy features of the Andean sentinels were softened this morning by the rosy colors of dawn. Morning was best because the "the old gentlemen", as the Andes were called in Mendoza, seemed more stern in the long shadows of afternoon. She hurried along the mosaic-tiled sidewalk, her breath clearly visible, rubbing hands together to create warmth. She had just left her five-year old daughter at Borboa School and now had to catch the No. 2 bus to get to orchestra practice on time. She was thinking about the long trip she had to take tomorrow - 18 hours by train to Buenos Aires to renew her resident visa.

Her pace slowed as she noticed someone ahead sitting on the ground, leaning against a tree trunk. As she neared the shivering man, she saw his feet first, no shoes, only a few rags were wrapped around them. He was holding an empty burlap bag in one hand. His clothes were threadbare.

She kneeled down and gently touched the old man's shoulder, asking, in Spanish, "Are you sick? Can I help you?"

The old man weakly turned his head and looked at her. Expecting to encounter the red, swollen eyes of intoxication, she was shocked. The old man's gaze was clear, kind and compassionate. "I am just very cold and weak, maybe you could help me back to my home," he answered.

She helped the old man to his feet; he could not have weighed over 90 pounds. They walked along slowly, in silence, arm in arm. After about four blocks he motioned to turn down an alleyway. Ahead, in a clearing in the vineyard, was an old adobe structure. She looked at him questioningly and he nodded in response. She opened the door. The small room was completely empty except for an ancient broom sitting in the corner and a cement slab. The dirt floor was swept clean. It seemed particularly bright inside; glancing up she was astonished to find the room had no roof. The old man sat down feebly on the cement slab. "He must sleep there," she thought.

"Dr. Monteverde, our family doctor, lives close by," she said, "would you like me to see if he can come?"

A gentle smile flickered across the old man's face, "Once, I was a doctor. I am O.K. Thank you for helping me."

Seeing no evidence of food in the hut, she told the old man she would return quickly. At a nearby almacen she bought a cup of steaming hot mate with milk and sugar, some fresh warm bread, cheese, and a few pieces of fruit. The old man stopped shivering as he sipped the warm mate. He slowly ate a few crumbs of bread and cheese and two or three of the purple grapes. She could tell he was feeling stronger.

"What is your name?" she asked.

"Benito Alguilar," he answered.

"Don Benito, don't you get cold at night without a roof?" she asked.

An incredible smile broke out across the old man's face, "If I have a roof, then I don't have the stars. You understand don't you?" he asked. She paused for a few moments, then nodded in agreement. She really did understand; she too, loved the stars. Nothing was more beautiful than the heavenly concerto of the stars in the penetrating blue of night.

"I see that you remember your ancient home," said Don Benito. "You know, you are made of star dust. I am made of star dust. Everything is made of star dust. Even the "old gentlemen" are made of star dust. They, too, long to return to their heavenly home - but, poor old Andes, they have such a long wait ahead of them. My wait is short, I'm 86 years old!" She looked at the strange old man. There was a special serenity about his face, and those clear brown eyes spoke of eternity. Who was he? Where were his friends and family? Why was this kind old gentleman, with the heart of a poet, all alone?

"You know," said Don Benito thoughtfully, while gnarled fingers stroked his long thin beard, "I have come to understand the universe after trying desperately to change it for so many years. The universe is perfectly balanced; there is as much negative as positive; as much black as white; as much good as evil. Whatever action one takes, the universe must react - to maintain that balance. I understand. It is good to understand, but now I'm ready to go home - to the Light Beyond the Stars where duality ceases."

She did not understand these strange thoughts and looked at him questioningly. "Don't mind me," said Don Benito, "I'm just an eccentric old man. Thank you for being so kind."

She glanced at her watch - she was already an hour late for practice. "Don Benito, I'll be back later with blankets and other supplies - please rest and try to eat a little more food." He nodded. And again that incredible smile - midday sunlight reflecting off the snow-capped Andes could not have been brighter than the light of compassion and kindness shining from his face.

She returned that afternoon with a piece of foam for a mattress; wool blankets, clothes, shoes and food. But Don Benito was not there. She left them on the cement slab.

On her way home she stopped by the church rectory to see if one of the priests could stop in to check on Don Benito while she was in Buenos Aires. Padre Juan seemed irritated by the request. He explained that they were having a very important conference and requested that she stop back by in two weeks - maybe they could help then. She told the priest that Don Benito could freeze while she was gone; but her argument fell on deaf ears. Padre Juan was anxious to get back to his meeting. She left the rectory extremely hurt and confused, vowing never to set foot in a church again.

Don Benito's image, his clear, compassionate eyes and strange words haunted her continuously during her trip to Buenos Aires. She wanted, so badly, to understand him. When she returned to Mendoza, her first stop was at Don Benito's roofless, adobe home. He was not there.

That afternoon, she was practicing her clarinet when someone knocked on the door. Dona Maria, a neighbor who had seen her leave with supplies for Don Benito, stood solemnly with the diario de los Andes in her hands. The newspaper was opened to the obituary page. A small corner article was dedicated to Doctor Benito Alguilar. He had been found under a bridge frozen to death. The article went on to explain how he had worked tirelessly in the 1930's and 40's to build the Hospital Central in order to offer free medical aid to the poor. His wife and daughter had been killed in an explosion during a political upheaval in the 1950's.

Her heart was broken. Her mother and sister had passed on when she was young. And now, Don Benito - where had he gone? She gazed sadly up at the Andes for consolation. They did not look so stern that afternoon. Perhaps they were feeling happy for their friend who had returned to his ancient home. It seemed that the wind carried a gentle message from the "old gentlemen". It softly whispered, "What WAS, IS, and shall always BE. Be silent and know peace."

* * * * *

Suddenly it all came in to focus - crystal clear. The trinity was composed of the face of the old man, the face of the Andes, and yes, it was her own face! She now understood what Don Benito had tried to explain to her twelve years earlier. "Energy is never created or destroyed." Upon transition, the energy that is "us" will return to its heavenly Source. The universe is balanced - there is nothing to change; there just IS. She was ready to leave Omelas at any time and she knew where she would be going.

(Note: It took me a few years to mellow out about "never stepping foot into another church". But I came to understand that caring and dedicated people can be found in all colors, cultures, shapes, sizes, races, religions and in all walks of life. I feel truly at peace in any religious ceremony at this point in my life, with a deep conviction that the human spirit seeks its Creator in many different and glorious ways. And the truth is, today, I'm really not ready to give up on the people living in Omelas; I think many of us are unaware of living conditions in developing countries or how our everyday choices keep other human beings, just like us, impoverished. There might be hope for our troubled globe if we all work together in a joint effort to remove that starving child from the hideous cellar - but it must be on her terms. She has a life of her own and cannot be recreated in our image).

Dis-ease on Our Planet

Never doubt that a small group of thoughtful,
committed citizens can change the world.
Indeed, it's the only thing that ever has.

MARGARET MEAD

Following are excerpts from a speech delivered by Harriet Beinfield (co-author of *Between Heaven and Earth*) at a conference for healthcare professionals in 1999. The information she presents comes from the 1998 United Nations Human Development Report:

"Worldwide, it seems the greatest underlying cause of death, disease, and suffering are the following steeply rising inequities:

The world's 225 richest people have a combined wealth equivalent to 2.5 billion of the world's poorest people, or 47% of the total world population.

Only 4% of this wealth ($47 billion) would be enough for adequate food, water, education, healthcare, and sanitation for the entire world. That translates into preventing the yearly deaths of 6 to 7 million children from malnutrition.

Imagine, 84 of the richest people own combined assets worth more than the annual incomes of the 1.2 billion people living in China.

Microsoft makes $34 million per day, the same amount sub-Saharan Africa pays in debt service.

How much do the rich countries give to the poorer ones? It is shocking to learn that the answer is **nothing**. Creditors in the rich world received more from these countries than they provided in new loans.

Yearly, Mozambique pays more on servicing debt than it spends on education and healthcare combined.

David Korten, a Stanford-trained MBA and PhD who taught at Harvard before working for several decades in Asia for the US Agency of International Development has recently written *When Corporations Rule the World* and *The Post-Corporate World*. Korten makes an analogy between the growth of global corporate entities in the social body to cancer in the personal body. Cancer, unlike a virus, is not alien but rather involves the body's own cells - threatening its survival. It develops when critical mechanisms that control cell growth become damaged, causing uncontrolled reproduction unresponsive to body needs. These selfish cells are pathological anomalies. Normally a cell functions as part of a larger organism, curtailing unbridled propagation. Ignorant of its dependence on the health of the body as a whole, cancer cells colonize more and more of the organism, expropriating nourishment and disrupting coherent function until eventually they destroy themselves by killing their host. Korten suggests that transnational corporations are defective cells in our economic system, causing individual enterprises to seek self-aggrandizement without regard to the consequences for the society that feeds them. Growth at the expense of the whole threatens the self-organizing, self-generating capacity of healthy living systems.

As some suffer, others prosper. Global pharmaceutical budgets have soared, from $22 billion in 1980 to $259 billion 15 years later. Segments of the medical industry are being swallowed up into fearfully powerful multinationals. The chemical giant known as Imperial Chemical Industries (ICI) is among the world's largest producers of chlorine and petroleum-based products, with a dismal environmental record. They were co-founders and sole financial backers of National Breast Cancer Awareness Month. They began the early detection campaign, shifting public awareness away from possible environmental causes of breast cancer and onto individual women. They own Zeneca Pharmaceuticals, makers of Tamoxifen, so they derive double benefit by marketing carcinogens and cancer treatments, while steering research dollars and public focus away from prevention. Dr. Samuel Epstein has heroically documented this "institutionalized alliance between interlocking professional and financial interests," providing evidence of how the established medical industry can harm as well as heal.

One of my college professors, political philosopher Hannah Arendt, said that it is the nature of evil to appear unremarkable and commonplace, so much so that it goes easily undetected. Whatever malevolence we witness in the US is magnified elsewhere. UNICEF estimates that due to corporate marketing of infant formula that gets mixed with contaminated water and substituted for breast milk, "Every day, between 3000 and 4000 infants die from diarrhea and acute infections because the ability to feed them adequately has been taken away from their mothers." Do these mega-corporations ever give anything back? Paul Hawken has data suggesting that US corporations now receive more in direct government subsidies than they pay in taxes. Like a malignant tumor, they suck life from the social body without conscience."

A few additional facts:

- Every 3.6 seconds someone dies of hunger; 3/4 of those deaths are of children under five years of age.
- 80 acres of rain forest are being destroyed each minute - day and night.
- In 1950 rain forests covered approximately 30% of our Earth's surface; rain forest coverage is now at 7% and rapidly declining.
- It is estimated that over 6,500 species of plants have been annihilated due to human encroachment and that each hour approximately six species become extinct.
- Indirectly, rain forest ecosystems are being destroyed due to unbridled development, which is [encouraged by the World Trade Organization and] funded by international lending institutions such as the World Bank - and the appetites of consumers living in industrialized nations, US.

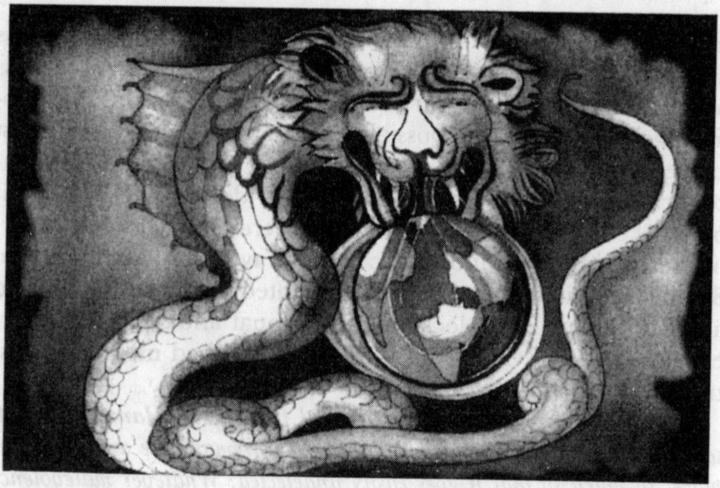

Healing the Earth and Her Children

BY GARY DOLOWICH, M.D., B.AC.

As we read through the list of injustices that exist in our modern world there are several possible reactions. The inequities are so staggering that the most common response is numbness. We've heard it all before, and anyway who can grasp what it means for six million children to die each year from malnutrition? It is hard to relate to these statistics, and yet we know that just to look into the eyes of one of these young lives lost (or their parents) would be truly overwhelming. Accompanying this reaction, and contributing to the general inertia, is a feeling of helplessness. What can the individual do in the face of the status quo? If we allow ourselves to be swept along by fears at the uncertainties of a rapidly changing world, our efforts are more likely to be directed towards personal concerns of financial security. Even when we are in touch with a more elevated, compassionate part of our self, and manage to rise above the excuses for inaction, how do we affect a meaningful change? Certainly, to look honestly at the amount of avoidable suffering in the world, the appropriate stance should be outrage. Yet, it is difficult to turn righteous anger into effective action. How do we influence the power structure, or know that new programs would not replace one oppressive situation with another? It is difficult to even identify those responsible for this tragedy, as everyone hides behind the pragmatic notion that *this is just how it is*. We can point to those who profit from the misery of others, yet if we blame individuals or corporations it can only result in a polarization that leaves everyone stuck in their position. Perhaps we don't want to carry this approach too far, as there is the vague sense that our own life-style may be dependent on the current scenario.

Applying the principles of *energy healing* to the problems we have identified may be more helpful. We would then consider the state of the planet as we would any illness, understand its problems as symptoms, and seek to uncover the *energy* that is behind the condition. Instead of *oppositional* thinking, there is the possibility of a shift in consciousness that can be the beginning of a genuine change. As we confront behavior that is destructive of human life and the earth itself, and become aware of the extent to which the suffering that is caused is the direct result of intentional actions done for profit or power, it is clear that this is what people, since ancient times, have understood as *evil*. The archetype of evil is a perennial human predicament, one that has been unavoidable throughout history, challenging philosophers and political leaders alike. Because it is so difficult to speak about, through the ages humans have created stories to better come to terms with it. In our modern age we have become too sophisticated to consider these possibilities, and it is no accident that we are the first culture not to have a myth about evil and also stand on the brink of destroying our planet. The New Age, in its efforts to cultivate only the positive side and bring in the light (for example, with crystals), shares in this massive denial of the real forces that would stifle our lives. What made leaders such as Mahatma Gandhi and Martin Luther King so effective, in fact, was their ability to identify evil in human behavior and stand up to it. Here is where their approach of *non-violence* became invaluable, as it permitted them to oppose injustices without adopting the qualities of the oppressor. Since they knew that the real problem was not the individual but the system, and even understood there to be a deeper force behind that structure, they could avoid being infected by hatred and were able to appeal to all sides. A modern day Sage, Yoda from the Star Wars epic, shares Gandhi and King's focus on confronting evil when he counsels: "don't underestimate the power of the Dark side."

As we confront life-destroying behavior, the natural tendency is to see it as existing outside ourselves. This is especially characteristic of *fundamentalisms*, which typically are unable to accept their own negative aspects and instead *project* it onto other groups. This *splitting off* of evil then can be used to justify all sorts of aggressive behavior, and is at the psychological root of moral crusades and war. The only way to avoid becoming the evil we are opposing is to accept that the darkness also exists within. When myths describe the slaying of the dragon, they are really pointing to overcoming the inner demons, such as greed and fear. Gandhi understood that this was what it meant to become a *spiritual warrior,* as witnessed in his statement that: "the only devils in the world are those running around in our own hearts. That is where the battle should be fought." Inseparable from the outer struggle with evil is an inner one. In fact, the willingness to see the darkness on the *inside* is the only way to prevent living it on the *outside*. Jung identified this archetype as part of the human *shadow*, and believed that the essence of self-growth was bringing this denied part of ourselves into awareness. He considered this process to be the cornerstone of *individuation* and crucial for the survival of the planet. In that regard, Jung said:

> *One does not become enlightened*
> *by imagining figures of light,*
> *but by making the darkness conscious.*
> *The latter procedure, however*
> *is disagreeable and therefore not popular.*

The Gnostics were an early Christian sect from North Africa. Like mystics from other traditions, they believed in direct spiritual experience, and so were persecuted as heretics by the Orthodox Church. They have received attention today largely due to the writings of Jung, who recognized in their understanding of the wholeness of the human condition, a philosophy similar to his own. These ancient thinkers identified the quality of evil, and told a myth about it. They called it *Yaldabaoth*, a being with the head of a lion and the body of a serpent. Brought into existence independently by its mother, this archetypal force was unaware of a connection to the Creator or any other unifying principle. Since it is cut off from a relationship with its Source, this energy is driven by a sense of isolation, and its characteristic stance is domination and control without regard for the misery that is inflicted on others. Existing on shaky philosophical grounds, *Yaldabaoth* is in a state of perpetual paranoia; threatened by those who are different, it responds by seeking to eliminate them.

Essentially, this is the archetype behind Western civilization's conquest of nature and colonization of the third world. It is the driving force behind oppression of those less powerful, and appears whenever another is used for gain, without concern for the consequences to that person. In the name of this false god, humans have raped the environment and destroyed countless possible futures. This is the energy that fuels the pursuit of progress and expansion at all costs, an attitude that has been the hallmark of Western history. It is the archetype that is behind ethnic cleansing, bigotry, and hatred. In fact, *Yaldabaoth* has waged a relentless attack on both the underprivileged and spiritually gifted throughout the last two thousand years - and the ancient Gnostics themselves were among its victims.

In describing *Yaldabaoth* we are speaking of an ego attitude, a value that prizes domination and power above all else. The Jungian psychologist Murray Stein, in a masterful presentation at a conference on Gnosticism, related this myth to modern depth psychology. Similar to the ancient story, the origin of the ego's sense of isolation lies in a lost connection to the Spirit or, in Jungian terms, the Self within (the Centre of the psyche). This results in a terrible sense of separateness and confronts the ego with a painful awareness of its own limitations and inadequacy. Though we may pretend that the ego is self-sufficient and totally capable, and point to the accomplishments of science and technology as evidence of our inherent brilliance, we cannot avoid the fact that there are forces at work (including illness and death) far more powerful than ourselves. Without a religious perspective, the inevitable consequence is deep-seated fear and, in an effort to compensate, unbridled greed. When a sense of relationship to the world around is missing, there is no hesitancy about using others for personal gain - and so this dynamic is played out in an attempt to exert power over others. Whenever we find abuse in family situations or personal relationships, *Yaldabaoth* is at work. In summary, we can recognize this energy on the psychological level when, having lost contact with the higher Self, the individual is taken over by material desires and all efforts become directed towards serving the ego.

As we stand on the cusp of a new millennium, all would agree that we live in a time of transformation. It is clear that to persist in an attitude of controlling others and conquering the natural world, in service of *Yaldabaoth*, portends disaster. Though we may proclaim the triumph of world capitalism, if our successes end up destroying the planet, the very foundation of life, that can hardly be deemed a victory. At this time, we must find a way to inspire the change that is being called for. This is where a symbol can function to awaken latent possibilities within the collective unconscious. It was Murray Stein's intuition that the Nazi-directed Holocaust can serve as such a symbol. The precision that characterized, what can be considered the most systematic genocide the world has seen, places it above other tragic episodes of history. The level of intense suffering, and the degree of domination and power involved, exposes the essence of *Yaldabaoth*. Even the excuse that "we were just following orders" is useful in revealing how evil can exist in a banal form, ordinary people carrying out their tasks without regard to the impact on others. To paraphrase Stein:

like a bolt of dark lightening,
the Holocaust illuminates the radical evil
that is at the heart of Western civilization's controlling attitude
over the last two thousand years.
It clearly demonstrates the fallacy in our belief in progress
– at the moral or spiritual level there has been none.

Like the crucifixion at another crossroad in the story of humankind, the Holocaust is both an historical event and a symbol of transformation. Though there were hundreds of Jewish prophets crucified by the Romans, one was selected by the forces of the unconscious and became the symbol of a new age. In the same way, the Holocaust may mark the end of one era and the beginning of a new way of being.

If we ask, what can replace the *Yaldabaothian* consciousness, it may be helpful to look towards the healing methods of traditional cultures (which is why this discussion is included in this book). The common theme among peoples whose life-styles were in harmony with nature was the sense of connectedness that pervaded their lives. Rather than dominating the world around them, they lived in relationship to it and respected the vital energy of the plants and animals in their environment. Since they had a strong sense of being part of the whole, they understood how their behavior affected others. Though certainly there existed conflict and struggle, violence was generally done in the context of survival and was never committed on the grand scale we find in recent history. Underlying all of the actions in premodern society was a connection to the Divine realm, what the Native Americans called the Great Spirit. This brought meaning and trust, as the individual knew their life to be linked to a much larger process. In place of the isolated ego that epitomizes our modern age, responding to its fear with a need to control, people in traditional cultures were able to "let it be." Some speak of this shift in consciousness as the coming of the Aquarian age. From another perspective, it is a movement from the age of Patriarchy to the return of the Goddess and the feminine principle. These are different models to describe the same necessary transformation. Clearly, the "Myth of *Yaldabaoth,*" the dominant stance of the last two thousand years, must be replaced with the "Myth of Relatedness" for humans to take the next evolutionary step in a way that affirms life.

2

The Importance of Prevention

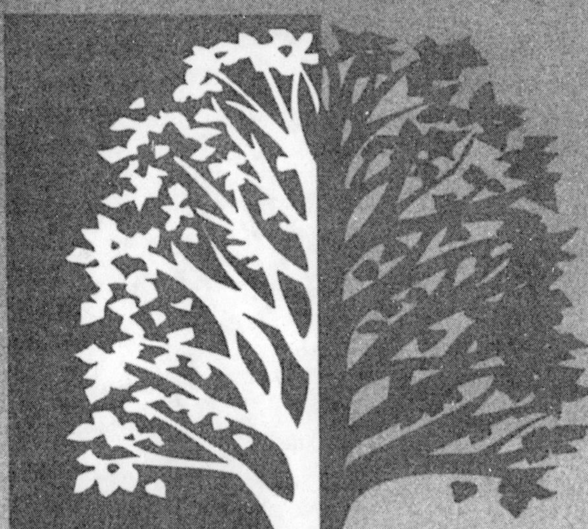

Cultivating Excellent Health Through Life's Stages

Prevent trouble before it arises.
Put things in order before they exist.
The giant pine tree grows from a tiny sprout.
The journey of a thousand miles
starts from beneath your feet.

TAO TE CHING

In honor of the spirit of the ancient Ancestors of Medicine, Imhotep, Sushruta, Caraka, Vagbhata, Huang Di, Shen Nong, and Hippocrates, the upcoming chapters on life's stages and disease prevention will focus primarily on dietary and age-old herbal recommendations to help relieve common everyday disharmonies and prevent dis-ease.

Leave your drugs in the chemist's pot
if you can heal the patient with food.

HIPPOCRATES

Prevention is by far the best medicine! Traditional healing systems provide unique insights into patterns of dis-ease that, early on, signal imbalances in our body/mind/spirit which could eventually lead to serious illness if they are not addressed. Far too frequently, when our Western medical tests finally detect a serious illness, it is already too late to reverse the disease process, so we must be content with aggressive chemical intervention, pain killers and/or surgery. The truth is that serious illnesses are preceded by many warning signals; they do not just drop in on us one day out of the blue. They quietly announce their presence every day in many ways - that persistent abdominal ache, or depression, or irritability, or stiff neck and shoulders are all trying to tell us something about the state of our health. Something is going wrong. Here in the West we view pain simply as a nuisance and immediately pop a pain killer to stop it. Pain can actually be your friend - a kindly warning signal telling you that things are not quite right in your human garden. Any serious student of East Indian Ayurvedic or Traditional Chinese Medicine cannot help but be amazed at the profound insights these medical systems offer to facilitate the early recognition of potentially serious states of imbalance that can eventually lead to life-threatening diseases.

Since Dr. Gary and I share, as common ground, a Traditional Chinese Medical view of health and healing, Chapters 3 through 7 are being presented with that medical model in mind. Dr. Gary will be sharing his unique insights as a medical doctor and practitioner of Five Element acupuncture and I (as an acupuncturist/herbalist/anthropologist) - all with a view towards prevention.

In Chapter 13, chronic disorders will be discussed in greater detail and remedies from healing traditions across cultures and through time will be presented. Since age-old traditional medical systems like Ayurveda, Western herbal and Asian medicine have their unique language, I felt it extremely important to respect the depth of thought encompassed by each and not oversimplify. All too frequently it is our Western tendency (with its love of speed, novelty and flash) to fail to recognize the value of taking the time to dig to the depths of a different perspective to truly understand the wisdom that we might completely miss otherwise. Just think of the wealth of knowledge that went up in smoke as Westerners set the Mayan and Aztec codices ablaze. To this extent, while many of the simple remedies mentioned in the upcoming chapters will be readily accessible to lay persons, I also wanted to present more complex views as accurately as possible. Practitioners of these healing systems will readily recognize the patterns of disease being described and students of different medical traditions will be able to compare the models. In the same way that basic mathematical calculations (addition, subtraction, multiplication and division) form the very foundation of advanced scientific research; energetic systems of thought are founded on simple principles that can take on great depth and complexity when applied to patterns of disease as they manifest in different body types.

Be sure to read Chapters 9 through 12 and take the tests available to help you become familiar with the "addition and subtraction" of traditional healing systems. You will not become an expert! It truly takes years and years of study and observation to begin to see the world from the unique perspective offered by Ayurvedic, Chinese and Galenic medical thought. However, even a very basic understanding of bipolar energetic thought (hot/cold designations) explored in Chapter 9 can help you make minor adjustments in your lifestyle and food selections that will ultimately lead to profound health benefits. In this book we hope to pass on to you helpful pointers in preventing disease and in treating common ailments that you currently diagnose yourself like that headache, cough, cold or flu. Hopefully the wisdom of one of the traditional systems presented will resonate with you, creating a desire to delve even deeper - in this case, please see the Resource Guide and Bibliography for recommended reading. Keep in mind that herbal therapy cannot make up for practices that conflict with good health like poor nutrition, lack of exercise, stress and overwork. It is extremely important to consult with a professional health care practitioner concerning any serious problem.

In bridging Eastern with Western thought and ancient with modern knowledge, in the upcoming chapters I would like to offer a few unique perspectives. While some modern practitioners of traditional medicine may prefer to remain "purists" to their tradition, playing an important role in maintaining the integrity of that particular healing system, others of us will attempt to synthesize and integrate the knowledge from various systems. The truth is that modern humankind is living a very different life from that of our ancient counterparts, and a natural evolution in medical thought is bound to occur as the wisdom from age-old traditions blends with scientific knowledge and technological advances.

In my own mind, and for workshops I teach on nutrition and herbs, I like to link each of the Five Elements with a specific nutrient or substance required for human life to exist. To that extent, I associate 1) Oils or FAT with the Wood element; 2) PROTEIN with the Fire element; 3) CARBOHYDRATES with the Earth element; 4) OXYGEN with the Metal element and 5) WATER and MINERALS with the Water element. Over the past fifty years, trendy diets have emphasized the importance in reducing or eliminating either fat or protein or carbohydrates to lose weight. Oxygen, water, minerals, fat, carbohydrates and protein are all essential for our existence. Without just one of these substances, we could not survive. In Chapter 13, the life-giving qualities of each of these substances in relationship to its paired element will be discussed.

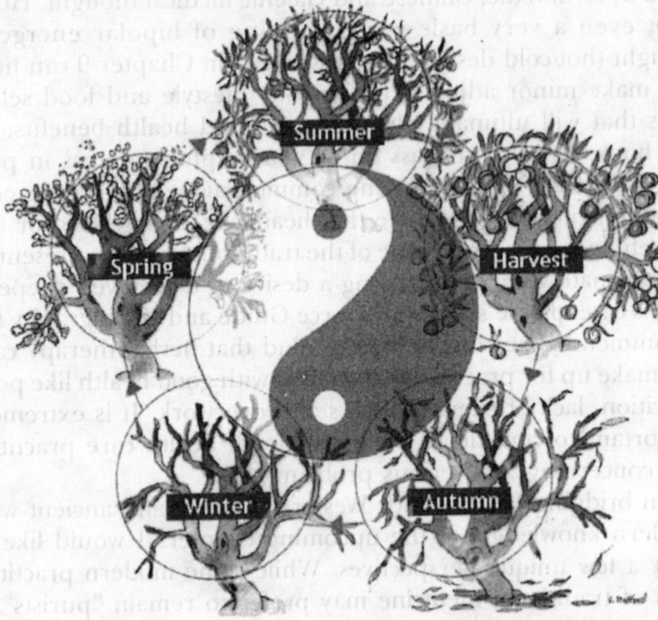

Life's Stages Viewed Through the Cycle of the Five Elements

By Gary Dolowich, M.D., B.Ac.

For every thing there is a season
and a time for every purpose under heaven:
A time to be born, and a time to die;

a time to plant, and a time to pluck up that which is planted;
A time to kill, and a time to heal;
a time to break down, and a time to build up;
A time to weep, and a time to laugh;
a time to mourn, and a time to dance;

ECCLESIASTES, CHAPTER 3:1-4

In Chapter 1 we explored the Chinese model of the Five Elements as a way to grasp the dynamic movement of life. Developed by the ancient Chinese through observation of nature's cycles, it uses the seasonal rhythm of the year to understand the stages of the vital energies. The philosophical foundation for this approach is found in the *I Ching*, a source of wisdom from the earliest stratum of civilization in China. Here, in a theory based on *yin* and *yang*, we discover that the transformation between light and dark results in "the appearance and withdrawal of the vegetative life force" that we know as the progression of the seasons.

The Five Element system describes five different energies that symbolize the predominant qualities in nature as we move through the sun's annual journey. Thus we can speak of the Wood element as the energy of the springtime, a time of birth and new growth. Fire is the symbol of summer, a time of full expansion and maturity, as the plant world reaches its fullest expression. The Earth element, the "extra" season in the Chinese model, represents a decrease from the fullness of Fire and depicts the time of harvest, the late-summer. Metal is the energy of autumn, the time of letting go and finding Spirit. And finally, in the Water element, we have the winter, a time of rest and stillness, when things return to the Source. It is the end of one cycle and, in this circular arrangement, the beginning of the next, as Water represents the seed that will unfold with the coming spring.

This model can be used to describe any cyclic movement that contains a rising and falling aspect. For example, the Five Elements can be readily applied to the pattern of a day. In this analogy, the new beginnings of the morning are represented by Wood, the fullness at noontime can be depicted by the Fire element, the afternoon with its decrease in light and fulfillment of the day relates to the Earth, the reflective time of evening when there is a quieting of activity and opportunity for quality would correspond to the Metal element, and, in the rest of night, we have Water. The Five Elements can also be used to deepen our insight into a cycle as short as one breath, which has its expansion with inhalation (Wood and Fire) and contraction in exhalation (Earth and Metal). Water, in this comparison, would correspond to the pause between the breaths. As we have seen, the elements originated as a description of the seasons of the year and can certainly be useful in understanding larger cycles of time. In the chapters to follow, we will extrapolate this system to the seasons of an entire lifetime.

Nowhere is the model of the Five Elements more relevant than in appreciating the stages of human life. It provides a map for the journey, a description of the qualitative shifts that occur as we navigate through a progression of life experiences. As we confront the various tasks for each stage, we find that an understanding of how things are in nature can enable us to respond more effectively. If, as the ancient Chinese assert, the way to stay healthy is to live in harmony with nature, then the Five Elements allow us to understand the shifting landscape. Following the elemental cycle may, in fact, help us avoid the difficulties that would inevitably arise if we were to operate according to guidelines that are not applicable to the stage we are in.

3

The Wood Stage of Life Childhood & Youth

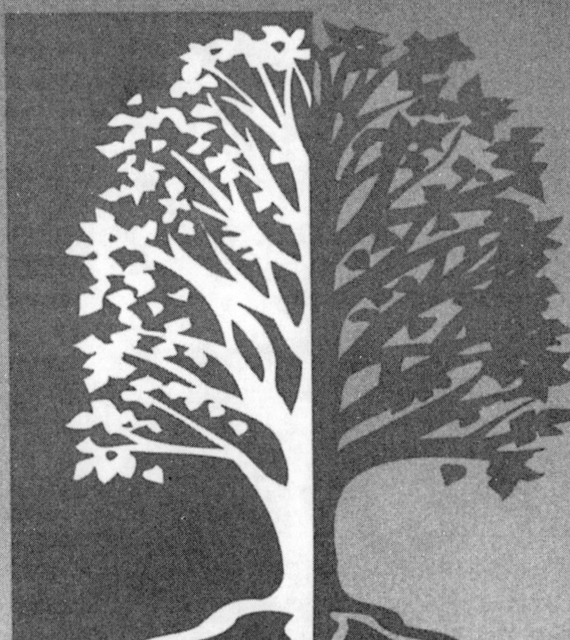

Springtime/Wood Element

By Gary Dolowich, M.D., B.Ac.

Spring comes after the fall of the leaves,
which is proof enough of the fact of resurrection.

Rumi

The spring of life, like the spring in the seasonal rhythm, brings new beginnings, expansion, and growth. The Wood element is a symbol for the energy associated with this phase of life. It is a time when nature gives birth to countless new possibilities. This pattern has an upward moving energy and, as we observe the new shoots pushing up from the ground, we sense the power contained here. The ancient Chinese called the springtime "the period of beginning and development of life." In the time of the Wood element we experience the tremendous vitality of the natural world, as the potential contained in the seed begins to manifest in the world.

In order to understand someone in this stage, the essential question to be asked is, "are they growing?" In this expansive phase of human life, the dominant themes include birth, creativity, and the free expression of one's potential. This is a time to travel different paths and explore myriad possibilities. We wouldn't expect from this energy a certainty as to the ultimate outcome. The hope would be for enough clarity to allow movement to reflect an inner truth, in the same way that the growth of an oak tree manifests the plan contained in the acorn. Of course, the issue of balance is again called for. As a young person seeks to discover their purpose in the Wood phase, the freedom to change one's direction needs to exist alongside the ability to stay focused long enough to allow a given vision to come to expression.

Behavior that would be out of place for someone in their later years, for example a person at 50 still struggling to find their identity, might be very appropriate in this phase. It is built into the way things are that an older person needs to come to terms with the limitations of life and accept the reality that we do not get to live out every latent potential. In contrast, it is a mistake for youth to set their limits too tight. What a loss it is when a young person becomes so pragmatic that they give up their idealism, closing the door to the range of possible experiences that exist for their life. In the early years it is imperative to hold on to a sense of imagination and a vision of new possibilities (indeed, the future of the world depends upon it).

A quality particularly relevant to the Wood stage is what Zen Buddhists call the *beginner's mind*. This is an attitude of openness and a willingness to stay in the question that allows a person to remain vibrant. It stands in contrast to the expert's mind, which in its certainty at having the truth, becomes obstinate and stultified. As we know through observing nature, it is the flexible tree that survives the windstorm, while the rigid tree is the one that is uprooted. The beginner's mind is valuable at every turn, but is most essential at this stage. There is nothing more upsetting than someone with limited experience who claims to have all the answers or is so certain as to their reality that they restrict their expressions in the world. The Wood energy is intimately connected to coming forth into life, and the quality of openness allows a person in this phase to stay engaged in a healthy process.

I treated a young man in his late 20's for incapacitating migraine headaches who, eight years earlier, had joined an ashram. At the time I first met him, he had taken an Indian name, was meditating five hours a day, and was devoting himself to intense spiritual practice. As I looked at my chart of the Five Elements I wondered whether, in a certain sense, he was violating the laws of nature. It seemed that he had moved abruptly from the Wood stage of growth to the Metal phase of cultivation of the spirit - leaving out crucial steps in between. As we explored his situation together, it became increasingly clear that, in his commitment to what he considered to be his "right path," he had severely restricted his choices. He essentially had "unlived life." Gradually, as he listened to his dreams and intuitions, he became aware that there was a work which he needed to do, and that his letting go of involvement in the world was indeed premature. Basically, "he had to be somebody before he could become nobody." In time, he elected to leave the ashram, eventually enrolling in law school. The headaches, which were over the Gallbladder Meridian (the Official of Upright Judgment and Decision-making), disappeared once he had reached a decision that was more appropriate to his stage of life. It is important to note that this interpretation does not apply to everyone who joins a monastery, as there certainly are some individiuals who are karmically meant to drop worldly involvement in order to pursue spiritual matters, even at an early age. It was simply a matter of finding this young man's truth, and to help him become the person he was meant to be. Hopefully, his time in the ashram will serve him on his journey, and the qualities of spirit that he cultivated there will enrich his life work.

The beginning sets the direction for what will follow, and the seeds that are planted in the springtime will determine the harvest to come. For a young person, the challenge of the Wood phase of life is, like the oak tree, to grow according to one's inner law. Through an awareness of the Law of the Five Elements there is an opportunity to emulate the qualities of nature found in the springtime and plant seeds that will endure. *The I Ching* offers this advice for "movement under heaven":

> *If one does not count on the harvest while plowing,*
> *Nor on the use of the ground while clearing it,*
> *It furthers one to undertake something.*

Warrior Rites of Passage

BY GARY DOLOWICH, M.D., B.AC.

In the Jungian model of depth psychology, the Wood energy corresponds to the Warrior archetype. This is an image that symbolizes discipline, focus, skilled action, and dedication to accomplishing a task. It is the energy that allows us to defend our boundaries and to follow through on commitments, despite the temptation to take some easier course.

We will discover that the various archetypal expressions seem to be part of the inherited structure of the psyche. In essence, we are hard-wired for them. It is the function of a culture to provide the psychosocial mechanisms that allow these potentials to emerge at the appropriate stage. Young people have a built in need to express the Warrior inside. In traditional cultures, an initiation into this energy was typically provided through rituals and ceremonies conducted by the elders of the tribe. If a healthy expression is not provided by the culture, the archetype will still manifest, but may then find destructive forms, such as membership in a gang. In our Western world, sports typically can provide a positive initiation into what it means to be a Warrior. The martial arts also offer a healthy way to develop these qualities, especially when training is connected to a spiritual tradition. Although in the past, these avenues into the world of the Warrior have been more available for boys, shifts in cultural values now support girls, as well, in developing this archetypal potential.

It is apparent that the qualities represented by the Warrior archetype are essential to meeting the tasks presented by the springtime of one's life. During these early years, we universally face the daunting challenges of finding one's identity, planting seeds that can grow over time, and discovering a path that resonates with some deeper truth. Only through developing the qualities of the Warrior can these tasks be met. It is the inner Warrior that provides the ability to make a commitment, set the boundaries that provide focus, and cultivate the skills that allow a potential to come forth. It is comforting to discover that the resources for accomplishing the stages of the journey do not need to be created de novo but, rather, exist within as part of the energetic make-up of the individual, ready to be activated as life unfolds.

Be like a tree
in pursuit of your cause.
Stand firm, grip hard,
thrust upward,
bend to the winds of heaven,
and learn tranquility.

DEDICATION TO RICHARD ST. BARBE BAKER, FATHER OF THE TREES

Caring for Tiny Sprouts

Your child's home,
the human body,
is miraculously constructed from
water, food, oxygen and light!

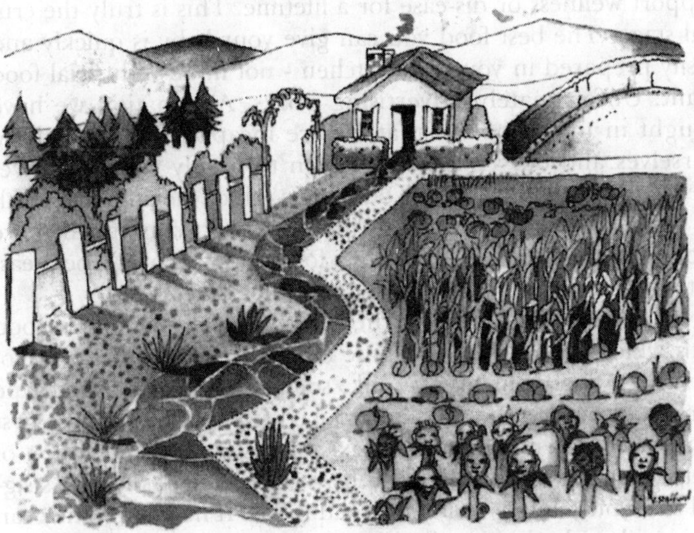

Enhancing Growth & Development During the Formative Years

What an incredible time in life, the birth of your baby! I can remember feeling completely overwhelmed and incompetent those first few days as I gazed down at my tiny daughter asleep in her crib. Would I be a good mom? Those nagging worries and fears were also accompanied by a sense of wonderment at nature's miracle of life. There is no joy greater than watching your little one grow. You are probably just like most other parents who want to give their children the very best - clothes, toys, a good education . . . but the greatest gift you can give them is YOU - your love, your time, your support, your respect for the unique individual they are and will become.

The next best gift you can give your child is that of great nutrition to build a strong healthy body. Your baby is in the springtime of their life - the Wood phase according to Traditional Chinese Medicine. Rapid growth and expansion is witnessed in all of nature during the months of spring and just like a young bamboo shoot or bean sprout, your baby is rapidly growing - reaching for the sun. These formative years are so important. Right now, the foods with which you nurture your baby go towards building a body and creating eating habits that support wellness or dis-ease for a lifetime. This is truly the crucial stage. The best food you can give your baby is quickly and easily prepared in your own kitchen - not in an industrial food plant. Unfortunately, advertising works. As a nation we have bought in to the notion that we are incapable of nourishing ourselves and our children; we turn to highly refined convenience foods that eventually take their toll on health. The truth is, besides being far more nutritious, it is actually much more economical to prepare your baby's food at home. You'll be pleasantly surprised; it really doesn't take that much time.

Your own breast milk is the most naturally healthful food with which to nourish your little one during their first year of life. To supplement breast milk, solid foods like mashed ripe banana, avocado, rice cereal or cooked sweet potato can be first introduced when your baby is six months old. The eruption of teeth, typically around six months, can be taken as nature's signal that your child is ready for solid foods. If necessary, they can be introduced a little earlier (but not earlier than four months) if your baby

- weighs at least 13 to 15 pounds;
- has doubled their birth weight;
- can sit with support so they are able to lean forward to accept another bite or move backward to refuse it;
- control their head and neck muscles so they can turn away, refusing food when they do not want it;
- no longer exhibits the extrusion reflex (if food pops out of their mouth when you spoon feed them, they are not ready);
- is drinking 32 to 40 ounces of formula in 24 hours and wants more; or
- is breast feeding 8 to 10 times in 24 hours, empties both breasts when fed and is still hungry.

Your baby's miniature immature digestive system just isn't ready for solid foods prior to four months of age. Their system does not begin to produce amylase, an enzyme required for the digestion of starches found in cereals until at least four months of age; and certain fats are a problem until they are about six months old. Starting solid foods too soon can create problems later in life such as food allergies, respiratory disorders like asthma and weight gain. However, it is also important not to wait more than eight months to start your baby on solid foods. After six months they begin to need additional nutrients such as vitamin C, protein, carbohydrates, water, zinc, iron, etc. They will need small amounts of water once they start eating solid foods.

An excellent book by Ruth Yaron, entitled *Super Baby Food* is literally jampacked with great tips for nourishing your child until age three. She includes over 300 easy, simple, inexpensive, nutritious recipes. For example, one wonderful time-saving tip involves freezing miniature entrees for your baby. Simply cook up a sizable portion of butternut squash, or sweet potato, or rice, or green beans, or chicken breast; then puree it in your blender; spread the food in ice cube trays (perfect size); once it has frozen, remove and place in freezer bags; date the bag and use within thirty days or so. It's important not to add sugar or salt to your child's food; these flavors are unnecessary and highly addictive; they cover the naturally delicious flavors of whole, nourishing foods.

Depending upon genetics, some children will do better on semi-vegetarian diets that include organic whole grain cereals, legumes, eggs, and predigested milk products like whole yogurt and cottage cheese. Others may require lean cuts of meat or fish. Never purchase frozen meat or fish to make frozen baby food cubes (foods must never be re-frozen). Fresh, preferably lean organic chicken, beef, turkey, lamb and fish like sole, cod and haddock can be introduced to your infant at 8 months of age; for fatty fish like tuna, halibut and salmon, wait until 9 months; and for shellfish like scallops, shrimp, lobster and crab wait until 12 to 14 months since these tend to be foods that frequently cause allergies. Be sure not to store your baby's meats in the refrigerator for more than 24 hours before cooking; remove all bones; cook the meat thoroughly; puree and freeze in ice cube trays immediately. Store the food cubes in freezer bags for up to one month; be sure the temperature in your freezer is at 0 degrees Fahrenheit or lower.

Regarding the best diet for your child - whether they will do better with semi-vegetarian food fare or if meat and fish will be necessary for a healthy metabolism - the best advice I can offer is to look at your genetics. If you or your spouse constantly battle with keeping off the bulge (averaging 20 to 40 pounds or more overweight) or members of your family suffer from Adult Onset Diabetes, the chances are that your child will do much better with plenty of fresh organic veggies, some whole fruits, lean meat or fish, legumes, nuts, seeds and whole grain cereals that are low on the glycemic index. (Note: the glycemic index is a measure of the speed at which sugars contained in carbohydrate foods enter the bloodstream - see page 365. For people who are sensitive to sugars, meaning that their pancreas reacts instantaneously to carbohydrate consumption by secreting excess quantities of insulin, it is important to limit the quantity of these foods eaten in a refined form. In simple terms, insulin is a fat-storing hormone and your body cannot burn fat as a fuel if the blood is loaded with it. For more information please see "Weight Problems" on page 356).

Your baby should be at least twelve months old before being introduced to citrus fruits like orange (frequently responsible for allergic reactions), tangerine, lemon, lime and grapefruit. Some foods that should be avoided until your baby is at least 18 months old include: Peanut butter, wheat, sugar, chocolate, corn, corn syrup, whole cow's milk, raw onions, garlic, cucumbers, cabbage, vanilla flavoring with alcohol added. These foods frequently cause digestive disturbances and/or allergies in babies. Sugary foods are incredibly addicting to tiny taste buds. My best advice is to avoid giving them to your youngster as long as possible. Once they start school it will be next to impossible to keep them away from sugar unless we, as a society, start making some serious changes. Hopefully, you will have been able to create a good nutritional foundation during the first years of your child's life so they will prefer to reach for life-promoting naturally sweet treats like fresh fruits, nuts and seeds. And, if you talk to other parents, maybe you can help change the tide by encouraging that healthful, nutrient-rich treats be provided for youngsters at school, for holiday celebrations and other social gatherings. Stevia is a natural herbal sweetener that comes to us from Paraguay; it can be used after your child reaches 18 months of age - a few drops will sweeten bitter herbal teas. It is best to never give them chemically altered foods that contain artificial sweeteners, margarine, colorings or preservatives, honey or corn syrup.

When introducing new foods to your baby it is important to wait five to seven days before introducing another new one. If your baby eats something to which he is allergic, the reaction may be immediate or it can occur up to several days later. If you give your child two or more new foods in a short period of time, he could have a reaction to one of them and you won't know which one was the source of the problem. Allergy symptoms include nausea, diarrhea, wheezing, a runny nose, hives or rashes. Please read the section regarding "Allergies" on page 324.

Food to Build a Body that Lasts a Lifetime

The doctor of the future will give no medicine,
but will interest his patients
in the care of the human frame,
in diet, and in the causes
and prevention of disease.

THOMAS EDISON

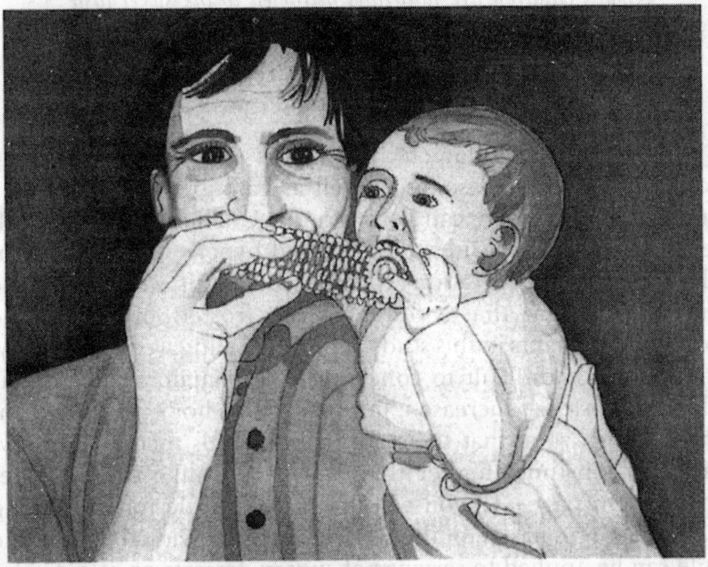

In nature, the very first lessons taught by animal mothers to their new offspring have to do with which foods to eat. In hunting and gathering societies, children followed the adults in search of natural foods, out of the ground or stream and off bush, stem, twig and tree; these natural foods maintained their health. In modern America we are teaching our children to hunt and gather at the corner convenience store or fast food restaurant. Unfortunately, in our society, it is easier to talk about religion or politics than it is to talk about diet. We all have our food preferences; we've been indoctrinated by advertising; we get stuck in our ways; and we get really grumpy about making changes. Many of our food preferences simply reflect a food addiction or allergy that keeps us hooked and coming back for more of the same - day, after day, after day. In this way our food becomes our poison.

Every day, in every way we are reconstructing our bodies by giving each cell the life-promoting fuel it needs to rebuild its walls and carry on its very specialized functions. Even our moods and cravings are incredibly affected by what we ingest.

Studies from the University of Michigan have demonstrated that your child's "sweet-tooth" in later life depends greatly upon how many sugary foods he receives as an infant. Small children are naturally attracted to the sweet taste but you can help form their preferences for whole foods by not serving them sweetened foods during their first few formative years of life.

One of our popular cultural myths tells us that drinking coffee or caffeinated sodas as well as eating sweets gives us a boost of energy so we can get more done. The truth is that caffeine and sweets provide scattered and hyper energy that actually impairs concentration. In one study, kids were given the amount of sugar that is found in two frosted cupcakes. The young participants in this study reported feeling weak and shaky; they found it difficult to concentrate or remain seated. Their blood sugar levels increased, just like adults, however the alarming findings were that their adrenaline levels increased an average of ten times higher than normal - unlike the adult response. On page 118 you will find Clark's Rule for calculating herbal dosages based on the weight of the individual. This same rule can be applied to servings of sugary desserts or cola drinks. If you weigh the average 150 pounds used in Clark's Rule and you take your 10 year old, who weighs 75 pounds, and your little 25 pound toddler out for a treat, say a double decker ice cream cone, this would be the result: You have two scoops, but for your

75 pound 10 year old that translates into four scoops and for your tiny tyke, it would be like you consuming 12 scoops of ice cream. For your 10 year old, the amount of caffeine found in one cola drink is equal to your drinking a whole cup of coffee.

Coping with Common Complaints of Babies and Youngsters to Age 12

During their first few years of life, little ones are coping with new experiences such as teething, new foods and infections. Since a tiny tot's metabolism races much faster than an adult's, with a quicker heartbeat and breathing rate, s/he will tend to become ill in a dramatic way. A fever can send a baby's temperature soaring. Most often, treatment at home with gentle herbs will solve the problem. However, it's important to seek medical assistance immediately if symptoms are acute or increase in severity.

You'll be amazed how quickly those early years pass - how soon your youngster will be all dressed up and ready for their first day of school. Before you know it they will be running in the door with wonderful pictures created just for you! Kids are naturally filled with the upward moving energies of Wood and Fire as described in Chinese medical wisdom - exploration, enthusiasm, and curiosity spurred by their desire to discover what this marvelous magical world is all about. At school your child will probably be picking up math and reading skills, as well as quite a few germs. Hopefully, they will have a great immune system to fight off the colds, flu and infections encountered. In Chinese thought, the immune system is often equated with Wood warrior energy since it is concerned with the ability to defend our boundaries from foreign invaders. Below you will find tips about tried and true, gentle, yet effective herbal allies to help soothe your child's formative years. Most frequently, I recommend very simple food grade herbs that will do the trick. In the tradition of Native American, Mayan, Aztec and Incan healers, let's keep it as simple as possible during your child's first two years of life - if one herb will do the trick for your youngster, then let's use just one herb. You can easily create a small herbal pharmacy composed of ten to twelve herbs that effectively treat a number of dis-eases. For example, you can purchase an ounce or two of the following herbs in dry form, or simply purchase them in tinctures at your natural food store. Here are some that I frequently recommend: Chamomile, Lemon Balm, Catnip,

Elder Flowers, Fennel Seeds, Ginger, Licorice, Slippery Elm powder. If you find it necessary to give your child stronger antibiotic herbs like echinacea, honeysuckle, forsythia, isatis, chaparral, or goldenseal, always be sure to include a few pieces of licorice root, jujube dates or ginger in the formula. These herbal harmonizers improve the flavor of bitter herbs as well as aid assimilation and utilization of the healing constituents of your formula.

Clark's Rule: Calculating Herbal Dosages for Kids

A standard formula used in calculating the correct dosage for little ones is called "Clark's Rule." It is assumed that the average adult weighs 150 pounds. If a child weighs 75 pounds, then the dosage would be 1/2 of the adult amount since 75 is 1/2 of 150. If the adult dosage is 1 cup of herbal tea, then the child would be given 1/2 cup of tea. If a child weighs only 25 pounds, this represents 1/6 of 150 pounds, and the child would receive only 1/6 cup of tea (4 tablespoons equals 1/4 cup, so 1/6 cup would be approximately 3 tablespoons). Be sure not to overdose. Infants and toddlers can benefit from a slightly higher dosage of extremely gentle herbs like chamomile, catnip, and lemon balm - up to 1/4 cup three to six times a day for a six month old. For herbal formulas that contain Oregon grape root, goldenseal, echinacea or other bitter antibiotic herbs, follow the dosage guidelines. You can make bitter herbal formulas more palatable for children by adding a few drops of stevia (see page 114). *NOTE: Never give honey or corn syrup to children under two years of age, they may contain bacterial spores which cause infant botulism. Even if the honey or corn syrup is cooked there is a possibility that the hard bacterial spores will survive the heat to wreak havoc in your child's body. Botulism is a rare but serious disease that can affect the nervous system of your infant.*

Bedwetting

Regular bedwetting can result for a number of reasons - urinary infections, emotional traumas, dietary deficiencies; or a minor physical problem affecting the urinary system. If it continues, it is important to get professional help to identify the source of the problem. In the meantime be very supportive of your youngster and give them plenty of hugs. A gentle herbal tea that could help would be made of one teaspoon of cornsilk (to soothe and heal the urinary tract); one teaspoon of lemon balm and/or 1/2 teaspoon of St. John's wort (to reduce anxiety and nervous tension) and 1/4 teaspoon licorice root; bring two cups of spring water to a boil; remove from heat and stir in herbs; cover and steep for 10 to 15 minutes; strain and serve. Refrigerate remaining tea in a glass container for up to 48 hours, warm before serving.

This is a common occurrence, often due to minor emotional upset, and is eventually outgrown. It is important not to traumatize your youngster around this problem. Since a full bladder would naturally aggravate the situation, avoid serving liquid close to bedtime. - *Dr. Gary*

Colds, Flu & Infections

The greatest discovery of any generation is that human beings can alter their lives by altering the attitudes of their minds.

ALBERT SCHWEITZER

These days, little ones are catching far too many colds, flu and chronic ear infections - we see them in our clinic regularly. Just notice how many children are afflicted with a runny nose most of the school year. Building immunity is truly the name of the game parents need to play during the elementary school years.

Immune building foods and herbs for children include ginger, onion and garlic (wait until they are over 18 months of age for the onion and garlic), as well as bitter flavored ones such as endive, dandelion and salad greens. Astragalus and codonopsis are two gentle Chinese food-like immune-building herbs that can be simmered with grains, soups or stews in the fall and winter months to help protect the whole family against colds, flu and infections. These are available at most health food stores.

If your child is frequently ill you might want to help boost his immunity by preparing the following tea: Bring two cups of water to a boil; stir in 1 teaspoon of chamomile flowers, 1/2 teaspoon of echinacea, 1/2 teaspoon schisandra berries and 1/2 teaspoon licorice root; cover, remove from heat and steep for 15 to 20 minutes; strain and refrigerate for up to 48 hours in a glass container. Give him a cup every other day (50 pound child) for three to four weeks.

Research has shown that it is best not to administer echinacea indefinitely, but rather use it in short "bursts" of several weeks. It will be more effective if given this way during the height of the flu season, if your child has been exposed to germs, or if there are actual symptoms of infection. - *Dr. Gary*

Here is a simple antibiotic formula you can prepare for your child if he does come down with a cold, flu or infection: Bring two cups of water to boil in a stainless steel saucepan; add 1/2 teaspoon Oregon grape root, 1/2 teaspoon echinacea root and 1/2 teaspoon licorice root; simmer for two to three minutes; cover, remove from heat and let the herbs steep for 15 to 20 minutes; strain. Give 1/4 cup per day to a 25 pound child (spreading it out over 3 to 4 servings) or 1/2 cup per day for a 50 pound child. You can mix this formula with an equal amount of organic, unsweetened apple, pear or grape juice to improve its flavor.

Most important is for your child to remain well-hydrated during an active infection. They can go without food for several days and be fine, but adequate quantities of clear liquids - water, tea, and juices - are essential. When a fever or diarrhea is present, fluid requirements are even higher. If nausea and vomiting occur, administer very small amounts (even one spoonful at a time) frequently. Obviously, rest is essential when fighting infection. A common problem (especially in the wintertime when the heat is on) is low humidity that dries out the respiratory system. This will create thickened, viscid secretions that are difficult to cough or blow out. Options to counter this tendency include: putting a pan of water on the heater (if possible); boiling water on the stove that contains chamomile leaves to soothe the mucosal lining and breathing these vapors directly; turning on the hot water in the shower (while your child sits in the bathroom); and using a steam vaporizer. - *Dr. Gary*

Colic

Rushed or tense feeding times can contribute to your baby's painful gut spasms which are characteristic of colic. An allergic reaction to foods can also be responsible for colic or stomach upsets - the more common allergy producers tend to be wheat, corn, orange juice, cow's milk, peanut butter, eggs, chocolate or hot spices. If you are breast feeding, you will probably want to remove spicy foods from your diet for awhile.

Chamomile is frequently given to infants to relieve colic (herbalists sometimes refer to it as the "band-aid for the stomach"). Highly regarded for its soothing, calming and digestive properties, chamomile is used to treat a wide range of discomforts ranging from nervousness and insomnia to diarrhea, colds and flu. Catnip is another gentle herb which is ideal for children; it eases colic and acts as a mild sedative. A soft cloth soaked in the remaining warm tea water makes an ideal compress to lay on your baby's abdomen to relieve colicky pains - remove once it has cooled. For a simple, effective one herb aide, add one tablespoon of chamomile flowers or catnip to 2 cups of boiling water; cover and remove from heat; steep for 10 to 15 minutes; strain and serve; refrigerate remaining liquid for up to 48 hours in a glass container; warm before serving. Offer 1/4 cup of the tea (in a baby bottle) to your infant every two or three hours until the symptoms subside. *(Note: Do not add sweeteners to the tea,* *see page 118)*.

Here are a few more tips from mothers around the world! Chinese moms traditionally gave their infants fennel tea to ease colic pains, while Lebanese and East Indian babies drank a gentle tea made of dill. In one study, Israeli researchers found that chamomile, fennel, lemon balm and licorice tea effectively relieved colic pain; the babies who were given plain water to drink continued to cry and fuss. Here's the recipe: Bring two cups of water to a boil, stir in 1/2 teaspoon each of licorice root and fennel (slightly bruise the whole fennel seeds before adding to the water); remove from heat and add one teaspoon each of chamomile and lemon balm; cover and steep for 10 to 15 minutes; strain and give this pleasant tasting herbal infusion to your little one in a bottle. Offer 1/4 cup to your baby every two or three hours until the symptoms subside. Refrigerate any leftover tea in a glass container for up to 48 hours; warm before serving.

Cuts and Scratches

Cuts and scratches are one of those inevitable parts of growing up, but hopefully they come about as the result of some fun filled game or childhood adventure. It is important to keep them clean, bandaged if necessary, and to discourage children from picking off the scabs. There are some excellent, antiseptic herbal ointments on the market. Products containing St. John's wort, tea tree or marigold are all perfect to help heal broken skin.

Do not use chemicals such as alcohol, methiolate, or Betadine on an open wound. They will kill healthy tissue in addition to bacteria. Clean with warm water, perhaps with an antibacterial soap (such as Physoderm or Dial). If there is a thick scab (under which bacteria can grow) remove by soaking in the same solution and gently rubbing with gauze. An antibiotic ointment will kill germs and also protect the area - an ointment (not a cream, which is drying) is especially recommended with an abrasion. Herbal remedies usually contain goldenseal or calendula. Synthetic antibiotics (such as Neosporin, Bacitracin, Bactroban) are also effective, providing there is no allergy to the chemicals in these ointments. Bandage only if there is going to be exposure to dirt. - *Dr. Gary*

Diaper Rash

Diaper rash can be the result of digestive problems or yeast infections; it can also be related to irregular or inefficient diaper changes. Gently cleanse the irritated skin with warm water; be certain the area is completely dry (gently pat dry or blow dry with a hair dryer on the cool setting) before applying a little comfrey waterproof ointment or oil. Comfrey speeds the healing of damaged tissue. Never use creams for diaper rash - they will soften the skin further. It is a good idea to let the area breathe by leaving the diaper off as long as possible.

The baby ointments and oils you find in most drugstores are made with mineral oil (petroleum). This stuff is, undoubtedly, great for machines but nature did not intend for it to touch your baby's delicate skin. Most commercial powders contain colorings, preservatives, artificial fragrances as well as other chemical compounds to make it pour evenly. One common ingredient, zinc stearate, will not harm your baby's skin but is harmful if inhaled; some of its side effects include vomiting, coughing, labored breathing and insufficient blood oxygen according to reports from Centers for Poison Control. Talcum powder has a sharp molecular structure that can injure delicate lung tissues. It occasionally contains traces of asbestos (a known carcinogen) and arsenic (an extremely poisonous compound). You can make your own safe, delicately scented baby powder by simply adding 1/4 teaspoon of lavender essential oil to 1/2 pound of potato starch, arrowroot powder or cornstarch. Put the ingredients in a self-sealing freezer bag and shake well to break up any clumps and evenly distribute the lavender oil.

Moisture is the biggest culprit in diaper dermatitis, so change diapers frequently and expose the skin to the air as much as possible. A plastic layer will hold water in and contribute to the problem. A powder can help absorb moisture; corn starch is a natural remedy that is often used. To help combat early infections, Caldescene powder will suppress yeast and bacteria. If a full blown Monilia (yeast) infection is present, suggested by diffuse redness with "satellite" papules, Nystatin or Clotrimazole Cream may be applied twice a day. - *Dr. Gary*

Diarrhea

Diarrhea occurs for any number of reasons including flu, over excitement, tension, microbial invaders, overeating, food allergies and antibiotics. A simple remedy to help stop noninfectious diarrhea is white rice. You can mash steamed white rice with a ripe banana to serve your child; it's delicious and usually does the trick. Other herbs that will help include chamomile, catnip, lemon balm or slippery elm powder. (You can mix a couple of teaspoons of slippery elm powder with plain yogurt; it will soothe the gut and help reestablish healthy intestinal microbes. Or, combine this mixture with the rice and banana for a tasty treat).

Standard advice for binding loose bowel movements is the A, B, C foods: apples, bananas, cheese. An old-time remedy for diarrhea is Kaopectate - 1 to 2 teaspoons with each loose stool. It's chief ingredient is pectin, a natural substance found in apples. Since Kaopectate is not absorbed from the gastrointestinal tract, it has no systemic side-effects. If diarrhea is due to antibiotics, replace healthy intestinal flora with a brand of yogurt that has a good bacterial culture or acidophilus. Again, the critical factor is to provide liquids to prevent dehydration. Apple juice, ginger ale (at room temperature without carbonation), rice water, or tea also offer some benefit in binding the stools. When nausea or vomiting is present, administer small amounts frequently. For diarrhea that is more severe, Pedialyte may be used to replace salts. If you are unable to keep up with the liquids needed, if there is bloody diarrhea, or if your child appears really ill, he or she may need to be seen by a medical doctor. In these cases, intravenous fluids and systemic antibiotics can be life-saving. - *Dr. Gary*

Earache

About 33 percent of all visits to pediatricians are the result of ear pain. Earaches sometimes occur after weaning and are frequently your baby's first encounter with a significant discomfort other than teething. Research conducted at Georgetown University showed that most of the children studied suffered from food allergies as well as chronic ear infections. Researchers concluded that food allergies can be at the root of many ear problems. Telltale symptoms that your child's ear is hurting might include a high fever and pulling on his ear. Children have very small eustachian tubes that connect the middle ears to the throat and allow the ear to drain. Germs can easily travel up these tubes from the throat causing infection. Infection or allergies create swelling which stops drainage, increasing the problem. For this reason, if the infections persist, pediatricians will insert small drainage tubes into your child's ears.

Unfortunately ear infections can turn into a chronic condition resulting in possible hearing impairment. Over the years, we have all become familiar with the problems associated with the frequent ingestion of antibiotics. They have no effect in combating virus infections and their effectiveness against bacterial infections diminishes with overuse, encouraging the growth of unfriendly microbes that have built up resistance to them. Physicians are recognizing that these important drugs need to be reserved for use when a true emergency arises.

What can be done herbally to help build resistance? Garlic, always easily available in fresh form, is one of nature's very best natural antibiotics. You can try adding it to your youngster's meals. There are many garlic supplements on the market if your child resists the fresh version. Ginger tea is another wonderful herbal remedy that many children find tasty. (Also please see the other herbs recommended for building immunity in the previous section on colds and flu). If the eardrum is not perforated you can put a few drops of mullein and garlic oil in the ear and cover it with a cotton ball. This oil will kill fungal and bacterial infections, stop pain and help reduce the inflammation. Fungal infections, while generally less serious than bacterial infections, can cause lots of itching. You can purchase herbal ear drops in most health food stores.

Chinese medicine offers a number of excellent herbal formulas for chronic ear infections; one that I have found particularly helpful in my practice is called Minor Bupleurum Formula. It is important to consult a health professional if your child suffers from chronic ear infections.

The key to prevention is supporting the drainage of liquid that may accumulate in the middle ear as a result of an allergy or URI. When the eustachian tube is blocked, a decongestant may keep it patent, preventing secondary bacterial infection. A common over-the-counter decongestant is Sudafed. Herbal decongestants generally contain ephedra (Ma Huang). Both these remedies act as a stimulant, so do not administer at bed time. A Chinese patent formula, Bi Yan Pian can also be effective and does not cause insomnia. Once fluid has stagnated in the middle-ear, and become infected, antibiotics are usually necessary. Antibiotics, though effective in eliminating bacteria, often leave fluid in the middle ear, which can impair hearing and lead to recurrent episodes of infection. If a chronic state of fluid persists in the middle ear (Serous Otitis Media), one therapy to explore before inserting tubes is Cranial Osteopathy - balancing the bones of the skull - to encourage drainage. In the hands of a skilled practitioner, it is successful about 50 percent of the time. - *Dr. Gary*

Fever

About 33 percent of all visits to pediatricians are the result of fevers. Actually, many pediatricians recommend forcing the fever down only if your child is exhausted, uncomfortable and the fever reaches: 101 degrees for babies; 102 degrees for toddlers; or 103 degrees for children over four years of age. A fever usually indicates that our body's natural defense system is busy battling some unwelcomed microbial visitors. Chief of Pediatrics, David Lang, M.D., at the University of Maryland Medical School advises, "The body is wiser than we; we shouldn't interfere with normal body responses to illness just because we can." However, it's important to be alert and call your pediatrician if your child's fever rises very quickly or goes over the guidelines listed above.

If you find it necessary to lower your child's temperature, lemon balm is a gentle, pleasant tasting herb that can help reduce it. Bring two cups of water to a boil; remove from heat and stir in one tablespoon of herb; cover and steep for ten to fifteen minutes; strain and serve. Lemon balm is also effective in treating nervousness, depression, upset tummies and gas.

A standard Western pharmaceutical for reducing fever is Acetaminophen (Tylenol), at a dose of 1 grain (60 mgm) for each year of age. It is generally safe and effective. If the temperature rises above 104 degrees, a cool bath can bring the fever down quickly, preventing more serious complications, such as seizures. A fever is generally a symptom of infection; in children, 90 percent will be viral in origin and clear by themselves, not requiring antibiotic therapy. However, if your child seems very sick, or is not keeping up with liquids, medical intervention is essential. - *Dr. Gary*

Hyperactivity

Typical symptoms of hyperactivity include poor attention span, sleeplessness, crying and aggressive behavior. It is possible your child is suffering from emotional problems. However, in my experience, poor diet, food intolerance or allergies are more frequently to blame. Sadly, every morning, before boarding the school bus, 3 to 5 percent of American children are given Ritalin (methylphenidate). This is a mind-altering drug - a stimulant that (paradoxically) functions to calm the child. Pharmaceutical products such as methylphenidate can cause serious long-term side effects such as insomnia, appetite and weight loss, irregular heartbeat and a docile, drugged state.

There are other ways to deal with hyperactivity or "Attention Deficit Hyperactivity Disorder" (ADHD)! People living in Europe regularly use herbs to treat this condition. A German study conducted with 100 hyperactive children demonstrated that after a few weeks of taking valerian root tincture, the children were less restless, less aggressive and less anxious. The great news is that in only a few weeks their learning skills and muscle coordination also improved. Valerian does not taste very good, so you will have more success giving it to your child in tincture form; half a dropperful two to three times daily for a 50 pound child. You might try putting the drops in a 1/4 cup of organic, unsweetened apple, pear, peach or grape juice.

Over 50 percent of the hyperactive children receiving treatment at the Pain and Stress Therapy Center in San Antonio, Texas, began to improve once foods and drinks containing sugar and caffeine were eliminated from their diets. Nutritional supplements such as vitamin C, magnesium and the B-complex vitamins were given to the children enrolled in this program.

Let me tell you about Josh, the son of a dear friend who came to California for a visit last summer. Lydia is a nutritionist who plans meals for patients in a small hospital back East; she has two wonderful children Trish, age 4, and Josh, age 7. Lydia and her children spent a week with us; we hadn't seen each other in years and it was great to get a chance to catch up. It was obvious from day one that Josh was having incredible problems; he was literally bouncing off the walls. Lydia would shake her head and apologetically say her pediatrician had recommended Josh be put on Ritalin before the new school year began. Josh, a really sweet toe headed Dennis-the-Menace type was begging for attention and, more than that, his tiny body was begging for some real food - which he would not eat because his addicted taste buds kept crying out for sugar. The first day I watched silently as he refused to eat the healthful breakfast I had prepared and demanded white toast, jam and orange juice. He had some candy around 11:00. For lunch his mom gave in to his demands and made him a cheese and mayonnaise sandwich on white bread with potato chips and a sugary soft drink; after that it was soda pop and candy all afternoon. Josh didn't want to eat dinner and demanded chocolate milk before bed; then there was some more chocolate candy. He couldn't sleep. It was obvious to me that Josh's hyperactivity and emotional outbursts were fueled by sugar induced highs and lows with which his little body was incapable of coping. During their stay I tried to prepare healthful meals and drop as many casual hints as possible about whole foods but, in the name of friendship and minding my own business, most of the time I was forced just to watch. During their seven day visit, the only real food that Josh ate was a few pieces of broccoli, a fast food hamburger and a few slices of pizza (these last two items don't score very high on my list of "real foods"). Before Lydia boarded the plane, I gave her a copy of Chapter 9, "Hugs, Not Drugs", from

John Robbins book titled Reclaiming Our Health. I don't know how Josh's story is going to end, but I do know that many patients have success in reversing their child's hyperactivity once diet is addressed. Please, before giving your child a drug to control hyperactivity, read John Robbins' insightful book. However, keep in mind that the vegan diet recommended by Robbins may not be the right one for your child - but a balanced selection of natural whole foods will be right.

There are any number of gentle herbal helpers to sooth your hyperactive child. But first, according to my naturalistic view, it is important to address dietary issues. Strictly control your child's intake of chocolate, soft drinks and sugar. Read labels and try to avoid food additives, preservatives and artificial colorings. This is not going to be easy, but we all know that many aspects of parenting can sometimes be downright difficult. Once your child regains his cheery optimistic disposition and joy for life you will realize that every moment of it was worth the effort. Be sure that your child's diet contains foods high in B vitamins (unsweetened whole grain cereals) and minerals such as zinc (pumpkin, sunflower seeds and oysters) and iron (apricots, dulse seaweed, mushrooms, green veggies like watercress, nettles and parsley).

A soothing herbal tea that most children enjoy can be made from catnip (which contains similar compounds to those found in valerian); other calming herbs that are extremely safe for children include chamomile, lemon balm, passionflower leaves, and spearmint. Linden (lime) flower is frequently used in France to help calm children - you can find it at most health food stores in the form of an herb tea.

Lice & Nits

It is fairly common to find youngsters infected with head lice in elementary schools - outbreaks tend to spread quickly. It would a good idea to check your child for the eggs, called nits, on the scalp or nape of the neck once or twice a month. If you find nits, the best herbal remedy is to comb the hair gently but thoroughly two to three times per week with a fine-toothed comb that has been sprayed with tea tree oil. You can follow-up by shampooing with a gentle tea-tree oil shampoo or simply add one teaspoon of tea tree oil to a full regular sized bottle of your favorite shampoo (shake well to mix thoroughly). Tea tree oil is one of the best antiseptic and antimicrobial herbs around and it doesn't irritate the skin.

If more gentle herbal approaches are unsuccessful, or only partially eradicate the lice, it may be necessary to use more aggressive therapy with insecticides. Although obviously more toxic, they are used topically and, if carefully washed off, the risks are small. Permethrin 1% cream rinse (Nix) can be bought over-the-counter. It is applied for ten minutes before being rinsed off with water; treatment should be repeated in one week. For more resistant cases, lindane lotion (Kwell) is commonly used. Be sure to wash and dry (at high temperatures) all clothes and bedding that comes in contact with infested areas. - *Dr. Gary*

Parasites

Pinworms are highly contagious and far more common in children than we imagine. Your child might complain of an itchy bottom, though many times these parasites produce no symptoms at all and, therefore, go untreated. When he is asleep at night, the worms lays eggs in the anus. Just before bedtime you can check his bottom if you suspect he's infected and gently remove worms where possible. Carrots are toxic for worms. In some cultures, youngsters are fed only raw, grated carrots for two days to clear the infestation. Here is a much simpler solution: Mix 10 drops of wormwood tincture (effective to clear worms but quite bitter) and 20 drops of fennel tincture (a pleasant tasting herb to help cover the bitterness of the wormwood) into 1/4 cup of carrot juice and have your child drink it before breakfast; repeat this procedure for four days. Exactly two weeks later you will need to repeat the treatment for four days since worms have a life cycle of two weeks.

Giardia is another intestinal parasite that is becoming more common. Some of its side effects include cramps, belching, diarrhea and weight loss. Probably one of nature's best herbal preventatives against giardia, pinworms and intestinal flu is garlic. For children over 5 or 6 years of age, you can cut a clove of garlic into 6 to 8 tiny pieces and wrap each piece in bread; be sure to make it small enough so your child can swallow it easily without chewing; also, it is probably a good idea to have a glass of water handy so he can wash it down. A clove of garlic ingested every other day or so will do wonders in helping to prevent a plethora of childhood illnesses. Another way to take advantage of the garlic cure is to cut a clove of garlic in half and rub it on the soles of your child's feet. No, this is not some strange healing ritual from a long forgotten culture - you will find plenty of those in the upcoming chapters! Believe it or not, garlic is absorbed through the skin. Give it a try on yourself; in about thirty minutes you can taste garlic on your breath.

There are a number of culinary herbs right on your spice rack that kill intestinal parasites. Researchers have shown that some of the compounds in ginger are more effective in killing these uninvited visitors than piperzine citrate, a drug frequently prescribed for parasite infestations. Other studies demonstrated that summer savory and thyme kill roundworms and hookworms; chamomile, elecampane, gentian and rosemary destroy parasites and soothe intestinal inflammation.

Prevention is the name of the game here. Worms thrive in the intestinal environment created by sugar and starchy refined flour products. Encourage your child to eat plenty of fibrous vegetables to help push the parasites out of the intestines.

Once again, we are faced with the choice of using more effective (and toxic) remedies, if natural therapies fail to eliminate the parasite. As with any potential treatment, we must ask whether the benefits outweigh the risks. Since allowing a chronic infestation to persist can have long range harmful repercussions to the health of the child and we are dealing with a short course medication, to my mind these agents certainly have a place in dealing with parasites. Be sure to confirm the diagnosis with a stool for ova and parasites or, in the case of pinworms, a scotch-tape slide test that pulls the eggs off the anus. The current recommendation is Vermox (Mebendazole) 100 mgm chewable tablet, one dose for pinworms and one twice a day for three days to treat most worms. Giardia requires Quinacrine for a week (Flagyl is contraindicated in children). Since pinworms are highly contagious, it is necessary to treat all family members and wash pajamas and bed linens. These medications require a doctor's prescription. - *Dr. Gary*

Sleeplessness

A sleepless baby or toddler can keep your whole household up at night making everybody cranky. Be sure your little one is comfortable - not hungry or thirsty or too cold or hot. It is also important to check in with slightly older youngsters to be sure that fears or nightmares are not creating the problem. Catnip tea is a simple yet effective remedy to help you and your little one catch some zzzzz's.

Teething

Teething is one of the really difficult stages that all infants must go through. Usually, their four front teeth appear without too many complications. However, the going can get rough in a couple of months when their flat molars start to appear. Teething biscuits will come in very handy at that time. Also, a soothing tea made of one teaspoon lemon balm and one teaspoon of chamomile will help. Bring 2 cups of water to a boil; remove from heat and stir in herbs; cover and let steep for 10 to 15 minutes; strain and give up to 1/4 cup of the mixture to your baby three to six times a day. You can also create an incredibly helpful oil to rub on your child's gums by thoroughly mixing no more than 4 drops of clove bud essential oil into a tablespoon of organic cold-pressed olive oil. Gently rub your baby's gums with a small amount of the mixture. (Note: Never apply undiluted clove bud essential oil to your baby's gums.)

Sucking on ice chips or a cold wash-cloth can also provide relief of symptoms. - *Dr. Gary*

Upset Tummies

A number of things can contribute to your tot's tummy troubles - tension, excitement, overeating, food sensitivities or antibiotics. Attacks of nausea and vomiting may be linked to food sensitivities that in later life will manifest as migraines. Ginger, chamomile, lemon balm, dill, fennel and slippery elm are all excellent herbal allies to ease your child's discomfort. Please see the previous "Colic" section for more tips that will help your youngster through bouts of stomach pain, nausea and indigestion.

Recognizing and Preventing Wood Imbalances Through Life's Phases

The supernatural forces of
spring create wind in Heaven
and wood upon the Earth.
Within the body they create
the liver and the tendons;
they create the green color . . .

and give the voice the ability to
make a shouting sound . . .
they create the eyes,
the sour flavor,
and the emotion anger.

THE YELLOW EMPEROR'S CLASSIC OF INTERNAL MEDICINE

On a physical level, if our Wood element is deficient or weak, we may experience some of the following symptoms: low self-esteem, inability to assert oneself, indecisiveness, poor immunity, blurred or weak vision, dry eyes, dizziness, restlessness, depression, pale or discolored nails and scanty menstruation.

If you are suffering from the deficient Wood symptoms listed above, try to increase your consumption of herbs and foods that are naturally high in mineral salts (like nettles, mushrooms, miso, seaweed, dragon bone, oyster shell, walnuts or pumpkin seeds), as well as full sweet earth protein foods such a fresh fish and poultry, legumes (mung and black beans are particularly good), whole grains as well as green and orange colored veggies. A very slight increase in sour fruits and herbs can help improve liver function - lemon, blackberry, strawberry or plum. Take it very easy with hot, spicy foods but a gentle formula containing some warm, sweet spicy herbs like dang gui can help build blood, warm cold hands and feet and move congestion. Be certain that you are getting your essential omega-3 fatty acids (see page 303); evening primrose oil can help balance hormonal fluctuations resulting in PMS.

An excess Wood condition is characterized by: Feelings of frustration, anger, irritability, moodiness, depression, allergies, PMS, menstrual cramps, high blood pressure, rigidity, stiffness, pain, red eyes, pounding headaches, tendinitis.

Increase your consumption of green vegetables and sour fruits dramatically, also add low-fat dairy, cold-water fish, legumes and whole grains. Eliminate processed meats, fried foods, highly-refined fatty foods like salami and ice cream, coffee and chocolate from your diet. Organic green tea is an healthful substitute to help you get over a coffee addiction. Dandelion, hawthorn and/or one of the extremely effective Chinese bupleurum formulations can help reduce excess Wood conditions. *(Note: If you suffer from migraine headaches, substitute cyperus for bupleurum).* To assist your body in detoxifying, you can choose from a number of herbs (like dandelion, bupleurum or cyperus) that range from neutral to cold energy. If you are plagued with boils or other infections (a hot condition), you will need to add cooling anti microbial herbs like coptis, forsythia, honeysuckle or scutellaria to the formula. Cooling, bitter or slightly spicy herbs like gardenia, peppermint, lemon balm and chamomile can help soothe your irritability. Persons suffering from a Wood Excess condition may be attracted to the idea of enhancing energy by taking warming tonic herbs like panax ginseng. They are not for you until your Wood element has come back into balance. Once in balance, you should never take panax ginseng alone, but always in an energetically balanced formula. However, a more neutral ginseng (like Siberian or American) will probably be more suited to your constitution.

Persons with symptoms of Wood imbalance might want to consider undergoing a one to three day "liver-cleansing" fast in the springtime and a lighter fast in the autumn (using organic, unfiltered grape juice diluted with spring water). Excess Wood types would probably do best to ease into a fast by first attempting half day semi-fasts of organic unfiltered apple-juice diluted 50/50 with spring water for the first four or five days - the evening meal should be light - vegetable soup or stir-fried veggies and tofu over whole grains. After three or four days, they can try a one day fast of lemon or lime juice diluted in spring water (add a touch of maple syrup, olive oil, cayenne pepper and garlic). Deficient types may benefit from a one-day fast; however, it is much more important for them to concentrate on consuming blood-building, nutrient rich produce as described previously. Plan on taking it easy during the fast - no driving, no shopping, no parties, no work, no marathons! It is best to stay home, read, relax and take short walks. You will be amazed at the new energy and mental clarity you feel after giving your body a break from its regular food fare! Be sure to drink plenty of spring water while fasting and always check with your health practitioner before undertaking a fast. Rigorous fasting is not recommended for debilitated persons or vegetarians.

Over the years, Dr. Gary and I have prescribed variations of the following Liver Flush, it should be taken FIRST thing in the morning on an empty stomach:

1) Blend 2 oz. (1/4 cup) of fresh squeezed lemon or lime juice with one clove of chopped garlic, 1 oz. (2 tablespoons) of

organic, cold-pressed olive oil, a dash of cayenne pepper and one teaspoon of organic raw honey or maple syrup (if desired).

2) Immediately drink the following tea: Bring 1-1/4 cups spring water to a boil and add one teaspoon of slightly crushed fenugreek seeds; cover and simmer on low heat for 10 minutes. Once it has been removed from the heat you can add two teaspoons of chamomile or mint (if desired); stir, cover and let steep for another five minutes; strain and drink.
3) Wait 45 minutes to an hour and eat one or two servings of naturally SOUR organic citrus fruit - orange, tangerine, grapefruit, or strawberries, etc.
4) Throughout the day consume only organic fruit, veggies or steamed grains like brown rice, quinoa or millet.

When our Wood element is in balance we experience stable moods, reacting with steadiness if we are under pressure or if difficulties arise. We have clear vision as to what needs to be accomplished and when it needs to be to accomplished so that our lives can move forward with fulfillment, purpose and direction in harmony with our unique vision and the divine plan.

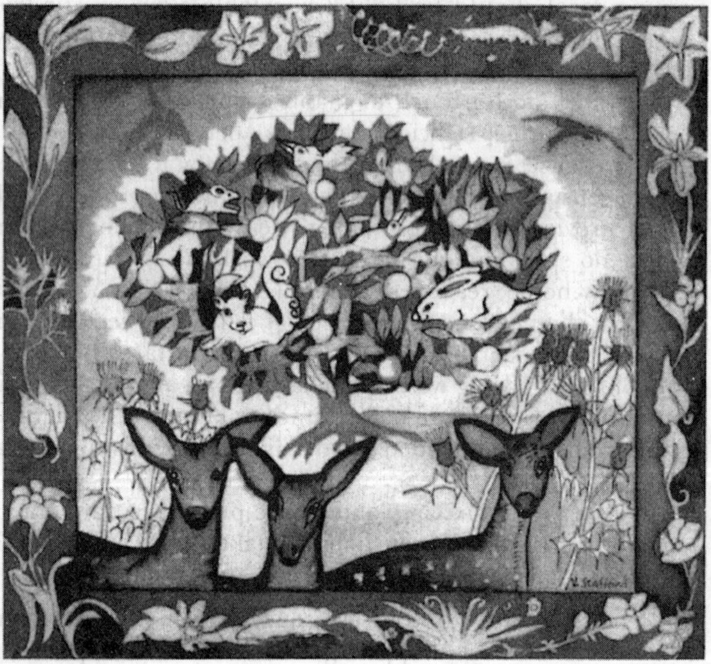

Tree of Life

Trees and plants are truly amazing life forms! Through the miracle of sunlight they transform earth's nutrients and water into roots, trunks, branches, twigs, stems, leaves, flowers, fruit and seeds. In a daily act of worship, God's green creatures stretch leafy fingers towards the firmament, linking Heaven and Earth, manifesting earthly form from heavenly energy. Just think of it - we breath in what plants breath out - maintaining a balance of oxygen and carbon dioxide in the world.

For many cultures around the world, the tree symbolizes life itself. In the Mayan world view, the green ceiba, or Yaxche tree grew at the center of their universe, supporting the four cardinal directions on its branches. The ancient Norse people also constructed their metaphorical reality with a tree as the central pillar of the cosmos. For ancient Celts, each tree was a spiritual being containing its own sacred knowledge; the Celtic word for "learning" was the same word as for "tree". While Japanese people plant a cherry tree to commemorate the birth of each child, Israelis plant trees when their loved ones pass from this world as an everlasting memorial to the time they spent on earth. Before attaining their powers, it is believed that the souls of Siberian Tungus shamen are reared in nests of the great Tuuru tree; during rites the shaman's soul ascends this tree to God - invisibly reaching the very summit of heaven. The African Dagara people believe trees shield and protect human beings from the Other World. From antiquity, Christmas trees have commemorated the winter solstice (the birth of light during the winter season) and the birth of Jesus Christ. The Bo tree (ficus religiosa) represents spiritual attainment for Buddhists since Buddha became enlightened while sitting beneath this tree.

In Chinese Five Element thought, plants and trees (or the Wood element) represent birth, growth and development. Trees sink roots deeply into earth's dark rich crust; their growth depends upon the environment around them. Always tending towards the light, trees reshape themselves, twining, turning, and twisting around any obstacles that inhibit their growth. Trees are flexible - gently swaying in the wind or graciously bending in the torrent. A tree follows the unique vision contained in its original seed - a pine seed becomes a pine; an acorn becomes an oak - it couldn't be otherwise. Human beings are the same. Depending upon the family and culture into which we are born, our belief systems and growth may be shaped by those around us - but the original plan contained in our unique seed seeks to unfold itself. We each have a special purpose and vision that can, should, and must be unfolded during our precious time on this earth.

Just as a picture is drawn by an artist,
surroundings are created by the activities of the mind.

BUDDHA (BCE 568-488)

Not only our surroundings, but every single detail of our daily lives has been created by the activities of our mind. What is your vision? What did you love to do as a child? What brings joy to your heart? Perhaps your parents wanted to mold you after themselves or for you to live out their unfulfilled fantasies; maybe you did not receive the encouragement you needed as a youngster to pursue your dreams. But, those dreams, your vision, still live within you.

The health of our Wood element depends largely upon how closely we are following our personal truth. Do you feel stuck, irritable, cranky with stiff neck and shoulder muscles? Is your body flexible? Can you bend with the winds of change or do you feel threatened when your viewpoint is challenged by new ideas with which you are not familiar? Can you make decisions, create plans for your future and follow through? Can you let go of unwise plans or do you stubbornly cling to them to prove your point? Can you stand firm when you see injustice and protect those who are not yet able to defend themselves?

It is this ideal tension between flexibility and firmness that defines the health of our Wood element. We must be able to defend our own boundaries but not violate the boundaries of other living beings - for they too have their unique plan to unfold on this earth. Our personal vision must be one that is in harmony with life-promoting, health-enhancing, joy-producing values not only for ourselves, our family, our culture, but also for the earth and all of earth's inhabitants - leafed, frond, finned, feathered, furred, four-legged . . . . . . or two-legged.

4

The Fire Stage of Life Adolescence & Early Adulthood

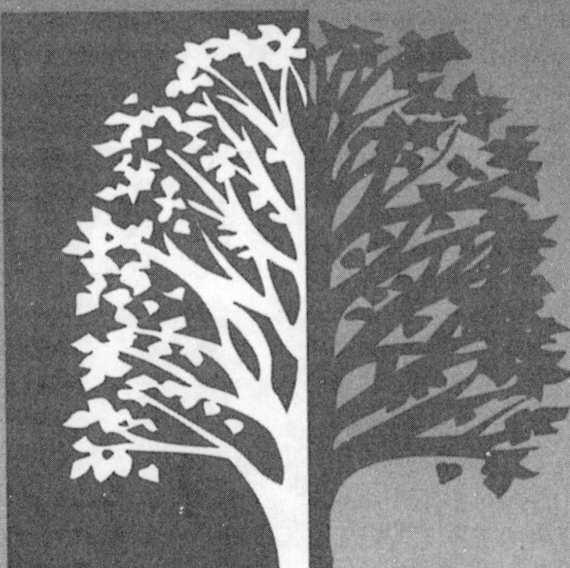

Summertime/Fire Element

BY GARY DOLOWICH, M.D., B.AC.

Not only all the dawns of summer,
not only the days, so tender around flowers and above,
around the patterned treetops, so strong, so intense.
Not only the reverence of all these unfolded powers,
not only the meadows at sunset . . .
but also the lofty summer nights, and the stars as well,
the stars of the earth.
. . . Look, I was calling for my lover.
But not just she would come . . .
for how could I limit the call once I called it?

RILKE

In nature, summer represents the time when the plant world comes to its fullest expression. It is known in the Chinese classics as "the period of luxurious growth," when the potential that was prefigured in the seed now becomes manifest. The sun is high overhead providing, in addition to heat, the light that allows everything to be seen with great clarity. The Fire element is an image of these attributes, and we find that this energy, which exists in the natural world, is also a vital aspect of what it means to be human.

In our lives, to be in the Fire phase of young adulthood means expressing all that is within us. Whether we consider the cellular level, where metabolism is essentially a slow burning fire, or the level of the organism, Fire is a life principle. It involves connection, joy, warmth, relationships, and the full manifestation of our being. The task is to come out fully into life and become all that we are capable of. If there is something that needs to find expression, this is the time to do it - and not hold anything back. Rumi, the Sufi poet from the 13th century, implores us to "burn it all up."

> *"You have the energy of the sun in you,*
> *but you keep knotting it up at the base of your spine....*
> *You've gotten drunk on so many kinds of wine.*
> *Taste this. It won't make you wild.*
> *It's fire. Give up,*
> *if you don't understand by this time*
> *that your living is firewood."*

Fire, like Wood, is an active, rising energy. We can see the Shen cycle (the Mother-Child relationship of the elements) operating here, as it is the growth of spring that leads to the full manifestation in summer. And it is only through meeting the challenges of the Wood stage, which includes finding one's direction and path, that the expression in the time of Fire becomes possible. In turn, living out the Fire stage will allow a person to move into the Earth phase, the time of harvest, which follows.

These are the years when we come to maturity. During the Fire stage we develop a career, discover meaningful relationships, and find our expression in the world. It is a time of clarity, as we allow ourselves to be seen. In this active time it would certainly be a great loss if a lack of Fire prevents a person from coming forth, leaving them cut off from life. It is also common for someone with an imbalance in this element (specifically in the Heart Protector official) to feel vulnerable and easily hurt; this too can isolate them and stifle expression. On the other hand, the Fire phase is inherently an intense, busy time, which presents its own challenges for us as we navigate its territory. People are often swept along in the frenzy of activity that can be associated with this element, forgetting the value of rest. When we neglect to allow our energies to replenish an imbalance is often created in the body. Symptoms such as migraine headaches, insomnia, or high blood pressure may then appear, reflecting an excess in the Fire element. As always in Chinese medicine, the ideal is balance.

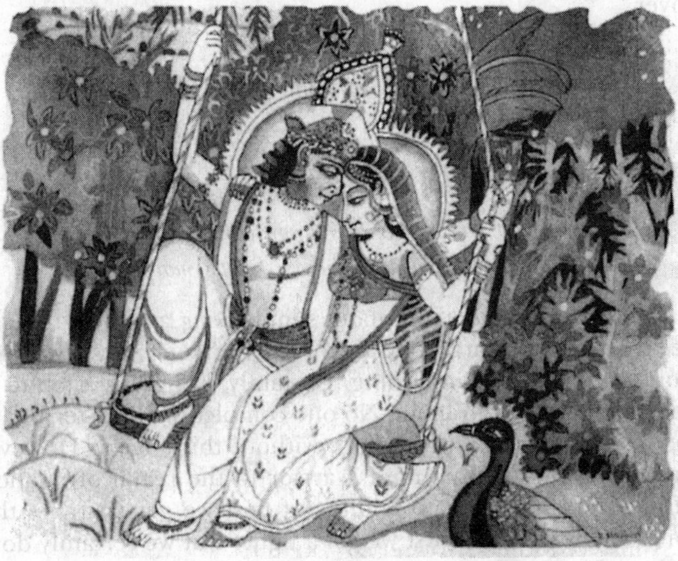

In the Garden of the Lover

BY GARY DOLOWICH, M.D., B.AC.

On the archetypal level, the Fire element can be compared to the image of the Lover. This is an energy within that allows us to simply appreciate life; to delight in the senses, and to enjoy the world around us. It is an aspect that draws us into life, keeping us involved and connected. It is the world of relationships that is the province of the Lover - and this includes relationship to nature, to other people, and to our own inner self. The deepening of our connection to the world within, which comes as we mature, is the beginning of self-knowledge and a prerequisite for healthy external relationships. Only when we are in touch with our moods and feelings can we express ourselves more honestly to others.

A very special expression of the Lover archetype is found in an intimate, committed relationship to another human being.

Here, behind the walled garden, in the realm of Aphrodite, there is the possibility of experiencing a level of communication, sexuality, and deep connection that truly brings the Spirit present. In learning the lessons of love, and discovering what it means to be there for another soul over time, we fulfill a very important task of this stage of life. Rumi is very much the poet of the Lover.

Look at her face.
Open your eyes into her eyes.
When she laughs, everyone falls in love.
Lift your head up off the table. See,
there are no edges to this garden.
Sweet fruits, every kind you can think of,
branches green and always slightly moving.

The Lover is essentially about simply *being* and delighting in life. It stands in sharp contrast to the Warrior energy, which is about *doing* and accomplishing. Certainly, if there is a job to be done, we need our Warrior. No one completes a long-term task, such as training in a profession, without this energy. However, if we bring the task-oriented Warrior to the realm of relationships, we are doomed to failure. At best we get partners that work side by side, at worst we get a fight - but we certainly don't get love. In some ways our modern world has become so focused on the accomplishments of the Warrior that many people have lost the ability to be in touch with the joy that comes from the Lover. Even our leisure time has taken on the quality of endless doing and we fail to realize the simple pleasure that can only be found in stopping to take in the wonder of being alive.

Mature relationships demand a different consciousness - one that can appreciate another person and allow things *to be* without needing *to fix it*. The maturation process involves developing access to the energy that is appropriate for a given time, and one of the challenges of the Fire stage is to develop the qualities of the Lover. It seems to be part of the human condition for this energy to emerge as we move into full adulthood. If it has been dammed up for too long, however, there is the risk that its appearance can be truly overwhelming. We observe this pattern in the mid-life crisis, when Fire energy can erupt like a volcano - destroying structures in its path. In Jungian psychology this is known as a *possession*, a situation where one archetype literally takes over a person's life. The goal is rather to integrate the new energies in a balanced way that builds upon what has come before. As we learn about the Lover archetype in the Fire time, it is important that we not lose the Warrior qualities that were so integrally related to the purpose of the Wood phase.

If we approach the tasks of each stage with awareness, we find ourselves on a journey of continual development. Life experience asks us to expand the range of expression - and this inevitably leads to a connection with a number of archetypes. The increasing ability to be in touch with these internal resources is an essential element in *individuation,* the term Jung used for the process of becoming the unique, whole person that is the culmination of a life well lived.

Fueling Potential and Building Immunity for Teens & Young Adults

To be nobody-but-yourself . . .
in a world which is doing its best,
night and day,
to make you everybody else . . .
means to fight the hardest battle
which any human being can fight;
and never stop fighting.

E.E. CUMMINGS

The energy of the Fire element is one of transformation. Cultures around the world associate fire with divinity, destruction and purification. In the Old Testament, God's voice came from a burning bush; the flames of Hawaiian volcano goddess Pele consume those who displease her; heretics and witches were burned at the stake; and the furnaces of hell await sinners. During the teen years, when the Fire energy is on the rise, we human beings are rapidly transforming physically, emotionally, intellectually and socially. Adolescents are relentlessly driven by their burning desires - for love, for knowledge, for freedom, for sex, for justice. For real growth to occur, it couldn't be otherwise. The restless fire of youth can be all-consuming, causing endless pain as young adults search for meaning and their unique place under the sun. Once children reach their teen years, the inevitable desire to stretch their wings and fly from the home nest starts to surface. Many times they form friendships or romantic relationships that are far more powerful than family ties - as they reach out to the world to pursue activities and relationships that interest them. This is such a vulnerable time for both parents and children. As concerned parents, our continued desire to protect, direct and guide can sometimes work in the opposite direction, creating rebellion. Hopefully, by the time our kids have reached their late teens, we have helped them build a good strong foundation for making wise decisions and feeling confident about themselves and their abilities. They're going to make some mistakes - it's inevitable. But, all in all, if we can just manage to keep the lines of communication open, these can be positive years. The act of parenting is a difficult and challenging dance that requires us to be a step or two ahead of our fleet-footed, bright and rebellious teenagers. Personally, I am looking forward to the role of being a gray-haired grandmother watching the parent/teenager dance as a spectator!

It is said that the task of the adolescent is to *kill* the parent (at least psychologically) and the task of the parent is not to retaliate. For the adolescent to make the transition from child to adulthood, they need to find the means to extricate themselves from the parent's control. Being one down in the power relationship, their acting out may be the way that they declare their autonomy and free themselves from the parent's "field of energy." This is where the adult needs to hold the bigger picture in mind and, rather than being personally offended, support their teenager's emancipation. To give your blessing at this crucial stage and allow your son or daughter to discover their own path, which likely includes making mistakes, is truly a gift of love. One can only pray that life will be forgiving and the mistakes not damaging. When a parent can take this position it frees the youngster to become their own unique person. They can then move into the Fire stage of life and express themselves in the world. - *Dr. Gary*

The sons of a father who rules with force
soon scatter to the wind.

ANCIENT CHINESE PROVERB

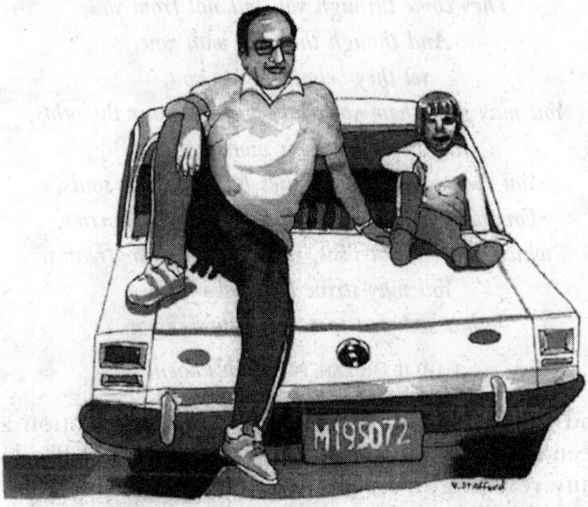

One of the most important gifts a parent can give their kids is to encourage their interests. And, just because of life's little ironies, don't be surprised if their special interest involves something that you never cared one iota about. It might be sports or bugs or stars or photography or music or medicine - whatever it is that makes your child's eyes twinkle with enthusiasm - do all you can to help them immerse themselves into it completely. What we love most helps give our lives meaning, purpose, focus and direction. These are the years in which your teenager is deciding what s/he will do for the rest of their life; be sure to let them make a decision that they can live happily with for a lifetime.

Last year Shelly, a bright and lively 17 year old, came with her mom to see me due to chronic asthma. We talked for a long while. When asked what she enjoyed studying, Shelly immediately lit up and replied enthusiastically, "I love learning about other cultures and wish I could be an archaeologist!" Her mom immediately interjected, "But she is going to study accounting next year in college because she knows she can't make a living as as archaeologist. Isn't that right?" Shelly literally sank into her chair. As a practitioner of wholistic Chinese medicine the first question that came to my mind was, "are Shelly's asthmatic symptoms simply a reaction to a suffocating mother?"

Your children are not your children.

They are the sons and daughters of Life's longing for itself.

They come through you but not from you,
And though they are with you
yet they belong not to you.
You may give them your love but not your thoughts,
for they have their own thoughts.
You may house their bodies but not their souls,
For their souls dwell in the house of tomorrow,
which you cannot visit, not even in your dreams.
You may strive to be like them,
but seek not to make them like you.

KAHLIL GIBRAN, FROM *THE PROPHET*

Good nutrition, once again, is the best prevention against most teenage and young adult physical complaints like lowered immunity resulting in frequent colds and flu. However, this is the time kids will be attracted to junk foods more than any other stage of their life. So here is the big question! How do you encourage your teenager to focus on good nutrition? It's difficult but not impossible. If they are accustomed to taking herbs throughout infancy and childhood to treat minor complaints, the herbs will continue to be a part of their lives - no big deal. Diet is a little more difficult to contend with at this age, but with a little luck they will still enjoy your simple, nutritious home cooked meals. It is only natural for them to eat their share of fast foods, but if truly nutritious meals are available once or twice a day it will certainly help to even the score. Following are a few tips:

- *Kelp* tablets and *nettle* capsules or tincture can help supply vital minerals missing from a junk-food diet.
- *Zinc* is an incredibly important mineral for hormone development - encourage your adolescent to snack on nuts and, more specifically, pumpkin seeds which are very high in this nutrient.
- *Siberian ginseng* (also known as eleuthero ginseng) is an excellent tonic to increase stamina and help the system cope with stress (see page 166).
- There are some excellent tonic Chinese herbs you can throw into soups and whole grain dishes to help build your family's immunity before school starts and through the chilly winter months. At our home, around the first of September we

slowly simmer soups and grains with two or three slices of *astragalus root* - a mild, slightly sweet tasting food grade root that comes to us from Asia. *Codonopsis root* is another gentle herb that can be added to soups and stews. Western studies have confirmed the immune-building properties of both astragalus and codonopsis.

- An easy trick to help build immunity is to cook with more *garlic* and *onions* as the cold and flu season approaches - they are filled with nature's natural antibiotics.
- A gentle effective Chinese classic formula called *Jade Windscreen* is frequently prescribed to help build immunity. *(For more information on cooking with Chinese herbs, please see my book entitled* Herbal Healing Secrets of the Orient*).*

Common Health Complaints of Teenagers & Young Adults

Food Fads & Dietary Issues

Eating disorders such as anorexia and bulimia often surface during life's Fire stage. Teenagers are particularly prone to dietary irregularities and disorders. Fear about being overweight starts early in our culture. Investigators from Iowa State University found more than 60% of the 4th graders they were studying weighed themselves almost every day; wished they were thinner; and worried about being fat. Consider this: 81 percent of 10 year old girls were already dieting and unhappy about their weight according to a University of California study.

Diana, a 22 year old university student came to me complaining of bleeding stomach ulcers, dizziness, heart palpitations, anxiety attacks (to mention only a few of her symptoms). When asked about her diet she handed me a list and said, "This is what I will eat." On the list was: broccoli, raisins and soy milk - that was it. Diana, when questioned, confided that she was plagued with bouts of anorexia and bulimia. She joined a support group for persons with eating disorders while receiving acupuncture treatments. Four years later, while Diana doesn't inhabit a body composed of 10% fat, none of her fears of becoming truly overweight have manifested. She eats three healthy meals a day, exercises, and enjoys a blossoming career as a music teacher.

So many of my patients, women who are of normal weight but of poor health, come with one idea in mind - and that is to shed 5 to 15 pounds, never giving a thought to the importance of enhancing their general wellbeing. Sadly, they think by dropping 10 pounds - it doesn't matter what the means (the current fad diet) - that they are improving their health. The thin body has become equated with the healthy body - this is not necessarily true. Even more alarming, like Diana, I see many women and some men with eating disorders. Sadly, our society has not given its young men and women the necessary tools to make the mental connection between food and its positive life and health-giving qualities. Food (in the form of fat, or carbohydrate or protein, depending upon the current dietary trend) has become the number one enemy in America's ever-escalating battle against fat. Here are a few fat factoids that seldom make the press:

- To date, no research has been able to convincingly demonstrate that overweight is an independent cause of ill health.
- Medically "obese" premenopausal women have a 40 percent lower risk of breast cancer.
- Marilyn Monroe wore a size 12; the "average" American woman wears a size 14.
- Worldwide, 28 percent body fat is the average for healthy 20 to 50 year old women.
- The thinnest elderly women have a death rate that is 50 percent higher than their average-weight counterparts.
- The *New England Journal of Medicine* published a study on seventeen thousand Harvard alumni: Men who gained the most weight (25 pounds or more), but stayed physically active, had a better chance of living longer than their thinner, less active counterparts.

Children learn from our examples. Are you happy in your body or are you constantly fretting about losing weight? One of the best gifts we can give our children is parents who are happy and secure about themselves, regardless of their weight or physical defects as defined by a culture that makes judgments based solely on appearances. The truth is that all of nature's creations - dogs, flowers, leaves and birds - come in a great variety of sizes, colors and shapes. So do human beings. If you point out these differences to your child in a positive way from the beginning you will be giving them the gift of self esteem and a respect for human differences - so necessary for living a happy life. It is also essential for children to feel that they are loved unconditionally so they can love themselves and others. Being critical of them about being too thin, too fat, too dark, too light, too tall, too short, having a long nose, big feet or funny ears only undermines their feelings of self-worth.

Weight problems are terribly over-simplified in our society. Unfortunately, it does not reduce down to a simple caloric equation that 3,500 calories equals one pound of body fat. Genetics and hormonal balances play a major role in determining how much we weigh. Please see Chapter 13 for much more detail on this important topic. It is essential to get professional help if you feel that your child has an eating disorder. If you suspect your child is suffering from anorexia or bulimia, I recommend an excellent book on the subject by Peggy Claude-Pierre entitled *The Secret Language of Eating Disorders.*

Moodiness, PMS & Menstrual Problems

As the teen years approach, hormone levels begin to soar for both boys and girls. It's an incredibly confusing time for adolescents to say the least. Their bodies are changing, their interests are changing, the opposite sex and sexuality is being discovered. Do you remember what coping with puberty was like? The trials and tribulations of growing up can create mood swings that range from depression and tears to giddiness and euphoria.

Girls have to contend with their monthly cycle accompanied by its fluctuating hormonal levels. The name for the female hormone estrogen comes from the Latin word *oestrus*, which means "frenzy." Estrogen certainly has a beneficial side - it makes you feel energetic and keeps your skin soft. However, excessively high estrogen levels can cause insomnia, anxiety, poor concentration and sensitive skin. A number of things tend to increase estrogen levels in the body including a lack of healthful fats (particularly omega-3 essential fatty acids), sugar, alcohol, stress, cortisone and some antidepressants. High estrogen levels can further complicate matters by causing water retention and slowing your body's ability to burn fat. Studies conducted in the 1980s and 90s demonstrated that there is a connection between high estrogen levels and more serious health concerns such as breast cysts, breast cancer, uterine cancer, uterine fibroids, cervical dysplasia and endometriosis.

Progesterone is the important female hormone that balances estrogen. It calms uterine spasms (relieving cramps), reduces water retention, decreases stress, and helps control sugar, food and alcohol cravings. PMS and menstrual irregularities frequently result from too little progesterone compared to estrogen. Researchers at Johns Hopkins University gave women participating in one study 800 IU's of vitamin E for ten weeks. Results of the study showed that menstrual cycles normalized and estrogen-progesterone levels balanced with vitamin E supplementation.

In addition to associating hormones and sexuality with the Fire stage, the Wood element, and specifically the Liver official, is intimately connected to these cycles. Herbalists will frequently look to improving liver function in cases of excess moodiness, PMS and menstrual problems. The liver deactivates estrogen produced in the body as well as the estrogen compounds that come to us through many other avenues, particularly commercially grown foods. *(Note: Exposure to excess estrogen is a problem that needs to be addressed in our nation as a whole. Commercially produced fertilizers and pesticides are estrogen-based chemicals which end up in our food supply. Is there a correlation between exposure to chemical estrogens and the increased frequency with which we see young girls prematurely starting their menstrual cycles at eight to ten years of age?).*

There are many herbs and foods that improve liver function, these include mung beans (help remove pesticides from the system), milk thistle seed, burdock and dandelion roots. Vitex berries, also known as chaste berries, are one of the few single herbs known that directly balance hormonal levels relieving irritability, water retention and breast tenderness (see page 173). Vitex can be taken when coming off contraceptive pills or other hormone replacement therapies - however, it should not be ingested in conjunction with progesterone. *(Dosage: Take 20 to 30 drops of Vitex tincture once daily before breakfast.)* Both Ayurvedic and Chinese herbal medicines gently and effectively regulate gynecological disharmonies through various herbal formulas that are chosen based on your unique constitution. Please see Chapter 5, *Gynecological Disorders*, for more information.

Mononucleosis

Symptoms of mononucleosis include achy muscles, fatigue, sore throat and tender, swollen glands that can remain enlarged for three or four months. Previously mentioned herbs that help boost immunity and build energy to prevent the occurrence of mono include astragalus, codonopsis and Siberian ginseng.

To treat an acute case of mononucleosis, make the following antimicrobial formula that will also help to reduce swollen lymph nodes: Bring two cups of water to a boil; add 1/2 teaspoon of each of the following dried herbs - echinacea root, mullein leaves, red clover flowers, cleavers leaves, prickly ash bark and ginger root; cover and simmer for two minutes; remove from heat and steep for 20 minutes; strain and drink the remaining liquid throughout the day at regular intervals. You could also purchase tinctures of these same herbs; mixing equal quantities (1/2 or 1 teaspoon of each herb) - take 1/2 dropperful 5 to 8 times daily during an active infection. Be sure to consult a health professional if symptoms persist.

Mononucleosis is an acute infectious disease caused by the Epstein-Barr virus, the same virus that has been implicated in Chronic Fatigue Syndrome. Characteristic symptoms include malaise, fever, sore throat, lymph enlargement, and extreme fatigue. Since there is no specific Western medical treatment available, herbal approaches are very appropriate. - *Dr. Gary*

Finding Ourselves

Just imagine the intensity of noontime sunshine on a hot summer's day, or the leaping flames of a bonfire on the beach at night - such is the unbridled excitement that fuels us throughout the Fire phase of our lives. Life is extremely busy for people in the summertime of their lives as they seek their unique destiny, a lasting relationship and meaningful career. During our teens, 20s and 30s, the Fire stage of human existence, we frequently take good health for granted - literally burning the candle at both ends. Who has time for regular meals, exercise or sleep when there is so much to see, do, and accomplish? However, too much alcohol, caffeine, nicotine and junk food accompanied by too much stress, too little relaxation and lack of exercise can set the stage for long-term health problems. As a good investment for our later years, this is the time to adopt a healthy lifestyle.

While lifestyles have changed dramatically over the past hundred years, based on our gender, there are some basic underlying biological patterns that distinguish the direction our live's can take during the Fire phase. In fact, throughout this time of expansion, when we are reaching out - struggling to find ourselves, our career and our partner - it frequently seems that men and women are psychologically, or emotionally, going in completely different directions.

In men, unbridled Wood warrior energy can lead to an expression in the Fire stage dominated by the drive to accomplish, succeed and make a mark on the world. In contrast, during the Fire time of life many women feel the natural instinct to create a home and have children, tasks which interfere with furthering their education and beginning a career. Often women have to defer their Warrior side in order to honor these Fire (relationship) and Earth (nurturance) expressions and fulfill their responsibilities as a wife and mother. It is common for these same women to experience an activation of their Wood warrior energy once the kids are raised, at which time they may go back to school or begin an entirely new profession. It is just at this same mid-life period that men are typically awakening to their Fire/Lover energy and find themselves moving in the opposite direction. No wonder relationships can be so challenging! - *Dr. Gary*

You have probably noticed that there is no distinct cut off in the phases of our lives when viewed through the cycle of Five Elements - the stages overlap. The beauty of this system of thought lies is its fluidity - you may be involved in any number of cycles simultaneously. For example, while in the Metal phase of your life (roughly between the ages of 55 to 75) you could be creating the vision for a new project (Wood element); and, having lost your spouse you may be starting up a new relationship (Fire element). The Five Element cycles are interwoven and perpetually in motion. They can be used to describe musical compositions, works of art, personalities, social movements, inanimate objects or office politics. They can be used to describe dynamics in relationships bringing much insight in to life's daily experiences. Life's inevitable stresses can be reduced by being aware of the patterns described in the cycle of Five Elements.

Recognizing and Preventing Fire Imbalances Through Life's Phases

The supernatural forces of summer
create heat in the Heavens
and fire on Earth;
they create the heart
and the pulse within the body . . .
the red color, the tongue,
and the ability to express laughter . . .
they create the bitter flavor,
and the emotions of
happiness and joy.

THE YELLOW EMPEROR'S CLASSIC OF INTERNAL MEDICINE

On a physical level, if our Fire element is deficient or weak, we may experience some of the following symptoms: anxiety, insomnia, palpitations, weak or erratic pulses, cold hands and feet, pale complexion, lack of joy and vitality, fatigue, poor concentration, stuttering or impaired speech, and difficulty maintaining close relationships.

If you are suffering from deficient Fire symptoms listed above, try to increase your consumption of herbs and foods that naturally add heat to the body: small portions of protein foods like lean cuts of lamb, beef, chicken, salmon, anchovies, trout. Flavor your foods with warming herbs, spices and roots such as anise, basil, cardamom, carrots, chives, cinnamon, cloves, cumin, fennel, garlic, leeks, onions, parsnips, rosemary. Full sweet Earth foods will help calm and center: basmati rice, buckwheat, corn, oats, spelt, quinoa, black beans, acorn, butternut and kabocha squash, pumpkin, yams. Bitter leafy green veggies tonify your Fire element (but they should all be cooked): arugala, bok choy, broccoli, chard, dandelion greens, purslane, kale and spinach. Sprinkle the following fresh seeds and nuts on casseroles and stir fries: flax, sunflower, pumpkin and sesame seeds, pine nuts, almonds and walnuts. Pitted fruits like apricots, cherries, nectarines, plums and peaches help tonify the Fire element; however, they are cooling in nature and should be consumed in moderation. Have your beverages without ice and avoid cold, raw foods and salads right out of the refrigerator.

An excess Fire condition is characterized by: anxiety, hyperactivity, insomnia, ruddy or purplish lips and complexion, pounding pulses, high blood pressure, heart disease, inappropriate laughter, compulsive talking, pressured speech, and manic episodes.

Excess Fire can be controlled by ingesting foods associated with its flavor - bitter. Dramatically increase your consumption of cooling bitter green veggies and cooling fruits - dandelion greens, arugala, kale, purslane, bok choy, zucchini, endive, sprouts and other salad greens, mushrooms, watermelon, cantaloupes, lemons, limes, nectarines, plums, apples, bananas, pears as well as sea veggies such as kelp, arame and nori. Until that Fire is under control you will do much better if you eliminate all processed meats, fried foods, alcohol, highly-refined fatty foods like salami and ice cream, coffee and chocolate from your diet. Concentrate on consuming cooling protein foods such as tofu, aduki and mung beans, non-fat dairy, cold-water fish, and whole grains. Use small amounts of grape seed oil or clarified butter when cooking; olive oil and lemon make a tasty dressing for vegetables and salads. Drink at least 8 to 10 glasses of fresh spring water daily. Avoid icy cold foods and drinks - they create contraction that only seals in the heat.

Hawthorn is a remarkable, extremely safe herbal food and medicine that has been used in the treatment of disorders associated with an excess Fire condition (such as arteriosclerosis and heart disease) for centuries. Traditionally, in the countryside, tasty young leaves of the hawthorn were added to sandwiches like lettuce - which gave it the common name "bread and cheese." Modern medicinal extracts use its leaves and flowers while traditional preparations use the ripe fruit. Hawthorn is currently utilized to treat angina pectoris, atherosclerosis, congestive heart failure and high blood pressure. Hawthorn should be considered a long-term therapy; it may take 4 to 8 weeks for its maximum effect to take hold - this herb/food is extremely safe for long term use. The best news is that there are no known interactions of hawthorn with prescription cardiac medications or other drugs. It is even safe to use during pregnancy or lactation. *(For more information, see page 207)*.

If you are plagued with boils or other infections (a Hot condition), you will need to add cooling anti-microbial herbs like coptis, forsythia, honeysuckle, isatis or scutellaria to your herbal pharmacy. Cooling, bitter or slightly spicy herbs like gardenia, peppermint, lemon balm, catnip and chamomile will aid digestion and bring peace of mind. Persons suffering from a Fire excess condition should not ingest warming tonic herbs like panax ginseng. However, small amounts of mildly warming spices like ginger, onion and garlic will encourage perspiration - helping to drain excess Fire.

Heartfelt laughter is the sound of the Fire element. When it is in balance, we can take delight in the moment at hand; we express our thoughts and feelings clearly and experience love in all its forms. Healthy Fire gives us warmth, zest, the ability to trust and reach out to others while protecting ourselves from those who may be hurtful. It gives us the enthusiasm to fulfill the vision provided by our Wood element. Fire symbolizes awareness and the development of compassion. The human heart not only propels red blood through the vessels, it houses the Shen (which is translated as both Mind and Spirit). The presence of Shen is that sparkle you see in the eyes of a wise, compassionate soul!

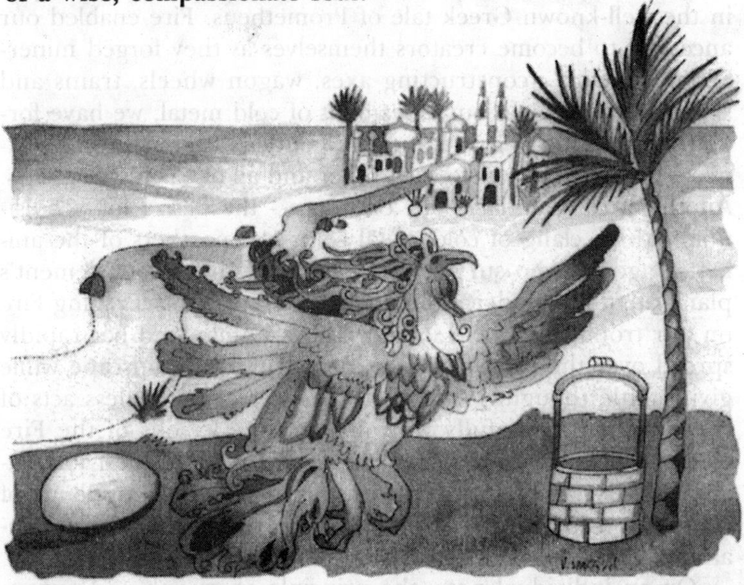

. In Greek and Egyptian cultures, the mythological phoenix *(its name means "red" - the color associated with fire)* represents the transformative nature of fire symbolizing immortality, resurrection and life after death. As the story goes, this solitary bird, servant of the fiery sun god, resides in Arabia near a cool well. It greets each dawn with a song so beautiful that the sun god must stop his chariot just to listen. When the phoenix feels its death approaching (every 500 or 1461 years, depending upon the myth) it constructs a nest of aromatic wood, sets it ablaze and is consumed by the leaping flames. Once the embers die back and only ashes remain, a new phoenix springs forth from the pyre. Ashes of its ancestor are embalmed by the new phoenix in an egg of myrrh which is flown to Heliopolis (city of the sun) to be left on the altar of the sun god.

We find similar associations between fire, the sun, a bird and transformation in other mythologies. The Chinese phoenix known as "Feng", depicted with the head of a pheasant and the tail of a peacock, represents the fiery yang primordial energy of the heavens. In East Indian mythology, Garuda is the king of birds who is associated with the all-consuming rays of the sun. Fire represents the very essence of the sun on this earthly plane. In many myths around the world it was an element stolen from the gods, the creators, to be used by humankind as, for example, in the well-known Greek tale of Prometheus. Fire enabled our ancestors to become creators themselves as they forged minerals into metals - constructing axes, wagon wheels, trains and skyscrapers. Now, in our cities built of cold metal, we have forgotten the Source of life and the gentle warming fire of connectedness that ties us to each other and all of earth's creatures. Another fire dominates our existence - the desire for acquisition with its clang of cold metal coins. As members of the animal kingdom who survive by consuming the Wood element's plant kingdom, modern human culture represents a raging Fire on our troubled globe. Like a wildfire, humankind has rapidly spread over the earth's surface, devouring the landscape while giving little thought to the consequences of its endless acts of consumption. Hopefully we will learn the lessons of the Fire element, before it is too late, so that our restless quest for material goods can be replaced with the steadily burning flame of compassion for all of creation - Fire's true gift from the Creator.

On an individual note, the principle of growth and expansion which begins with the Wood element in our youth reaches full potential when sparked by the Fire element during young adulthood. While the Wood element gives us the vision and the plan to carry out our unique purpose on earth, it is the Fire element that gives us the power to fulfill that destiny. There our many phrases that express this peaking of power or activity, such as "full steam ahead," or "full throttle," or "fired up." The Fire element corresponds to the summer season, a time of intense heat and activity - all of nature is deliriously engaged in life. Insects and hummingbirds dart amid the bright profusion of blossoms that have exploded in our gardens. Similarly, whenever we are thoroughly immersed in any creative project, we call upon the energy of Fire to bring the work to maturity.

Fire is nature's agent of transformation and rebirth. In much the same way that lightening can ignite a forest fire whose leaping flames burn and destroy all life in its path - clearing out the old so that new seedlings might sprout - life's transformative lessons forge us into fully realized adults. Fire is the element of connection - we experience real connection only when we have achieved a reasonable degree of self-awareness, connecting to our inner self. True self-awareness opens the door to genuine feelings of love and compassion for our partner, family, friends, humanity and all of earth's creatures.

Individuation, life's transforming journey to wholeness, described by Jung in the West and comparable to the Eastern concept of "enlightenment," becomes reality when we are finally fully present - each waking moment. Instead of thinking about reality, which separates us from experience, thought is experienced as a tool for navigating our way. When the mind slows we begin to joyously live simply and directly, moment to moment, in the peaceful heart center. Certainly, there are many gradations in consciousness as our individual paths lead us to this ultimate unity.

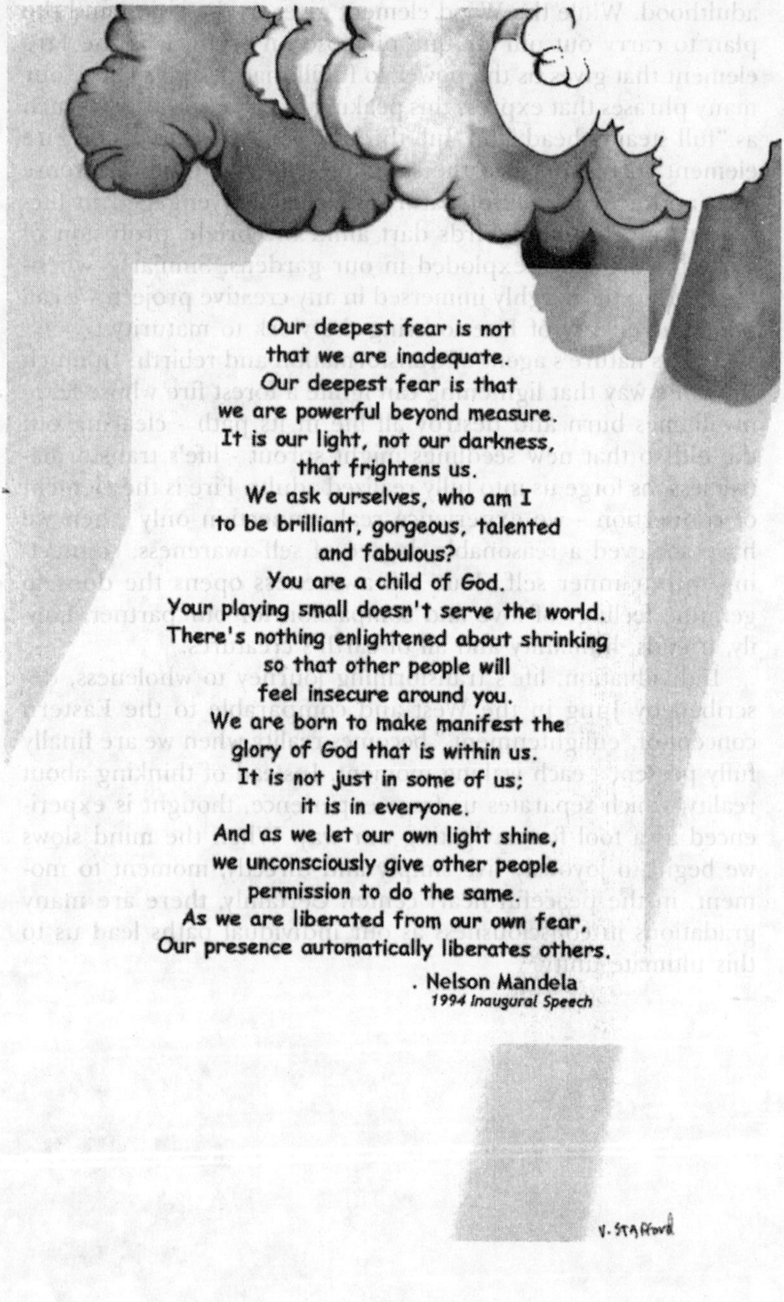

Our deepest fear is not
that we are inadequate.
Our deepest fear is that
we are powerful beyond measure.
It is our light, not our darkness,
that frightens us.
We ask ourselves, who am I
to be brilliant, gorgeous, talented
and fabulous?
You are a child of God.
Your playing small doesn't serve the world.
There's nothing enlightened about shrinking
so that other people will
feel insecure around you.
We are born to make manifest the
glory of God that is within us.
It is not just in some of us;
it is in everyone.
And as we let our own light shine,
we unconsciously give other people
permission to do the same.
As we are liberated from our own fear,
Our presence automatically liberates others.

. **Nelson Mandela**
1994 Inaugural Speech

5

The Earth Stage of Life The Householder & Reproductive Years

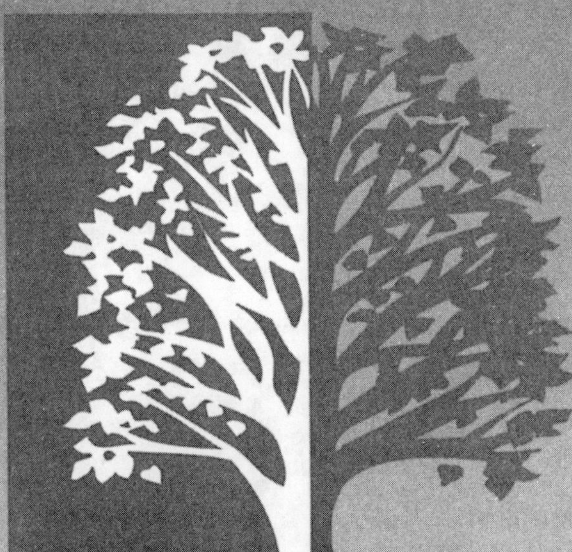

Harvest time (Late Summer)/ Earth Element

BY GARY DOLOWICH, M.D., B.AC.

Teach your children what we have taught our children,
that the Earth is our Mother.
Whatever befalls the earth
befalls the sons and daughters of the earth....
We did not weave the web of life,
We are merely a strand in it.
Whatever we do to the web, we do to ourselves.

CHIEF SEATTLE

No phase in the cycle of the elements can last forever - and so the Fire phase gives way to the late summer, the time of the Earth element. There is a decrease in the light energy; the sun is not quite as high in the sky and this offers a welcome relief from the intensity of summer. The fruits and vegetables are now full on the vine and ready for the harvest. It is a time of fulfillment as we feel ourselves supported by the abundance of nature. The nourishment provided at the harvest time brings with it a sense of security and grounding. Here is how the German poet Rilke describes it:

Lord, it is time. The huge summer has gone by.
Now overlap the sundials with your shadows,
and on the meadows let the wind go free.
Command the fruits to swell on tree and vine;
grant them a few more warm transparent days,
urge them on to fulfillment then, and press
the final sweetness into the heavy wine.

For humans, the stage associated with the Earth energy represents the harvest of our lives. We can see the work of the springtime, the planting of the seeds and the growth, coming to full maturity and expression in the summer, and then leading to its natural culmination in the late summer. Now is the time to reap the harvest and experience the fulfillment of the cycle of the elements. It can certainly be a great loss when people at this stage don't stay grounded in their lives, perhaps switching careers or relationships too easily, and fail to bring things to completion. And so, we find that a different set of rules apply to this time than were true for the Wood stage when it was crucial to explore a number of possibilities. The qualities of stability and containment, basic to the Earth element, are needed in order to meet the tasks of this stage. If we live according to the natural cycle, there is a feeling of support and security as we are held by the Earth Mother.

One of the most important ways the Earth phase is expressed in our lives is in raising a family. Again, we can see the *Shen* cycle of the elements operating, as the relationship work of the Fire phase leads to its fulfillment in the Earth stage of nurturing new life. In this time we face the many tasks of parenthood in order to help our children unfold and become who they need to be. There is a strong sense of being an instrument of nature, as we learn to sacrifice personal needs to a force bigger than ourselves. For women in particular, there are specific issues that are inherent in the childbearing years. In many ways the process of pregnancy, birthing, and breast-feeding the newborn requires that the woman herself embody the qualities of the Earth. For the man, the challenge of fatherhood asks him to go beyond the controlling male ego and develop another more gentle side, bringing with it the possibility of considerable personal growth.

It is in the time of the Earth element that the harvest of a career can be experienced. We have now reached a stage where we have something of value to share and can contribute to the betterment of the world. If there is a work that needs to become manifest, this is the time to bring it forth. Life also presents us with an opportunity to assist others, as we find ourselves in a position to mentor and support those who are younger than ourselves. Individuals just beginning on a path desperately need to be acknowledged; the encouragement of those further along can be critical for their success. It is amazing how stingy older people can be with words of praise, especially since it doesn't cost them anything. This is usually due to the fact that they did not receive such positive support in their own lives and, specifically, blessings were not forthcoming in their immediate family. It is an important aspect of the Earth stage to bring things to harvest on many levels and contribute to the development of those around us. Through holding these tasks with an expanded consciousness, we have a choice to express the positive side of this energy, rather than repeating dysfunctional patterns. This brings with it an opportunity to heal wounds that may have been around for generations.

The Archetype of the Great Mother

BY GARY DOLOWICH, M.D., B.AC.

Just as the earth is boundlessly wide,
sustaining and caring for all creatures on it,
so the sage sustains and cares for all people
and excludes no part of humanity.

I CHING

In the archetypal realm the energies of the Earth would correspond to the image of the Queen, the embodiment of infinite compassion and understanding. Whether we are speaking of Mary, the symbol of mercy in the Christian tradition, Shechyna in Judaism, the Sabbath Queen who brings rest and peace, or Kuan Yin in the Chinese pantheon, it is the same. This is the Goddess that allows people to feel secure and nurtured, regardless of their position in life or monetary status. As with all the archetypes, we first come in contact with this energy from the outside, perhaps through an image or story. Later, we can develop the ability to hold it as an inner quality. Whether within or without, it is the archetype of the Great Mother that brings faith and trust in life, enabling us to be receptive and, in the words of the Beatles, "let it be."

As we travel along the journey of life, we inevitably reach a time when our personal parents are no longer with us. One way to overcome this loss and find the courage to go on is through a connection to the universal Earth Mother and Heavenly Father. Through making a shift from the personal to the archetypal, we receive support from an eternal source of strength outside our own egos. Establishing this sort of "religious perspective" in the householder years is a vital step. The humility that comes from honoring our archetypal parents keeps us from becoming self-absorbed adults who take ourselves too seriously. In this way, it is possible to grow older and still retain the openness and freshness that is such a wonderful hallmark of children.

In dealing with the people we meet along the road, the essential question for the Earth stage is whether we can find ways to nurture and to give our blessing to their process. Through developing a connection to the Great Mother archetype, there comes the quality of compassion and a genuine concern for the plight of others. This may be expressed in work, charitable efforts, or in a kind gesture - but the essential thing is that we now extend our concerns beyond personal issues and give back to the community. The archetypes are powerful resources, but they depend on our lives to be expressed in the world. Without us, they are two-dimensional. Indeed, the Goddess becomes manifest when we can give our support to those with whom we have contact and help them flourish. In the Earth phase we have the opportunity to experience the culmination of all that has come before, as we bring forth the fruits of a lifetime and encourage a harvest in the world around us.

Common Complaints that Accompany the Responsibilities of Householding & Parenting

If there is light in the soul,
There will be beauty in the person.
If there is beauty in the person,
There will be harmony in the house.
If there is harmony in the house,

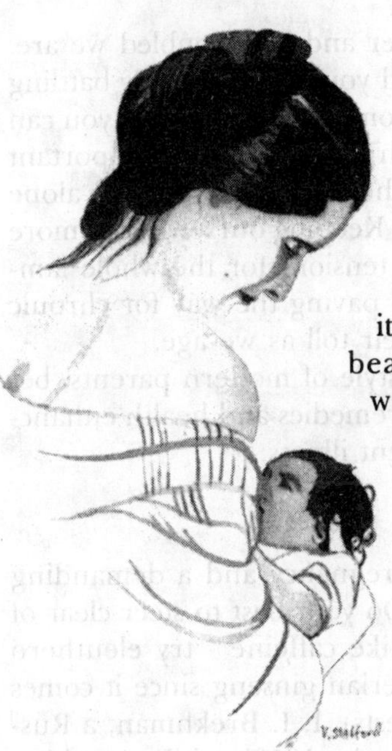

There will be order in the nation.
If there is order in the nation,
There will be peace in the world.
ANCIENT CHINESE PROVERB

While the ancient Chinese proverb above paints an ideal picture, it's fairly difficult to think about light, beauty, harmony, order and peace when you are not sure if you can make the mortgage payment; your toddler has taken all of the pots and pans out of the cupboard and is banging on the lids with a spatula; your husband can't find a clean pair of socks; the phone's ringing; and, after putting in a hard day at the office you've got a splitting headache; then there's dinner - still to be made. But somehow you always manage to pull it all together. Believe me, I've been there!

While the true full Earth phase of our lives, the harvest, usually comes a bit later on in life - when the kids are grown - pregnancy and providing for our family is certainly an Earth element function. In a way, early parenting and householding duties could be viewed as an Earth expression within the Fire stage of our lives. Most frequently in our society, young parents combine full-time jobs with caring for little children without much outside help. In traditional societies grandparents or relatives were usually on hand to help nurture the little ones. Modern lifestyles create time limitations and financial pressures which result in personal needs being neglected . . . leading to fatigue, frustration and worry.

In anthropology we talk a lot about "perceived reality" versus "lived-in reality". Perceived reality is how we imagine our lives and ourselves to be - you know the perfect mother, wife, father, husband, lover, housekeeper, provider, son, daughter and employee versus the down to earth, "plain-truth-of-the-matter" reality that we find ourselves living every day. The greater the distance between these two realities, the greater is the tension and stress we feel in our lives. The closer our perceived reality is to our lived-in reality, the happier and less troubled we are. Are you a perfectionist? Do you find yourself constantly battling with what you think you should accomplish versus what you can humanly and humanely accomplish? It is especially important during this stage in our lives to schedule "private time" alone with ourselves and with our partner. Keeping ourselves in a more relaxed, centered state will reduce tensions for the whole family. Too frequently stress builds up, paving the way for chronic physical problems that will take their toll as we age.

Keeping in mind the hectic lifestyle of modern parents, below are some suggestions for quick remedies and health enhancers to help reduce stress and prevent illness.

Exhaustion

Commutes, long working hours, pregnancy and a demanding family life would exhaust anyone! Do your best to steer clear of energy-robbing, fast pick-me-ups like caffeine - try eleuthero ginseng instead (also known as Siberian ginseng since it comes to us from the Eastern Russian forests). I. I. Brekhman, a Russian medical doctor, discovered it in the 1950's while searching for a source of Panax ginseng. Brekhman extensively studied this herb for over 20 years, concluding that eleuthero helps the human body adapt to stress and normalize all its functions. If blood sugar is too low, eleuthero will bring it up; if it's too high, eleuthero lowers it. Studies indicate that this herb helps to protect us from environmental pollutants while enhancing immunity and supporting the kidney-adrenal complex. A true adaptogenic herb in every sense of the word, eleuthero is frequently used by athletes to enhance endurance and performance, enabling them to recover more rapidly after strenuous exercise. Eleuthero even assists us in adapting to time zone changes (jet lag) or higher elevations.

When the healing qualities of Eleuthero ginseng are compared to those of Panax ginseng, eleuthero is preferable if you are under stress. However, if you are recovering from a chronic illness, surgery, or childbirth and your energy is extremely low then Panax ginseng would be best suited for you for a short while. Eleuthero is a more neutral/less stimulating herb than Panax ginseng and it can be taken for a much longer period of time. For an energy boost, take two Siberian ginseng capsules (200 mg) or 20 to 30 drops of tincture up to three times daily; it is a good idea to ingest tonic herbs only 5 to 6 days a week and then rest from them for two weeks after taking a three month round. *(Note: Avoid ingesting Siberian and Panax ginseng if you suffer from high blood pressure or a heart disorder).*

Indigestion

Missed or rushed mealtimes, tension and stress can quickly lead to chronic digestive problems such as pain, gas, heartburn and ulcers. During pregnancy changing hormonal levels and the growing fetus frequently wreak havoc with digestion. In Asian medical thought, the Earth element is related to our digestive organs located in the center of our body (the Stomach and Spleen/Pancreas). The Earth element was placed in the center of the first Chinese Five Element chart, with the Fire element above, the Water element below, and the Wood and Metal elements on either side. To be "centered" we must nourish our center.

In the same way that the soil of our earth collects nutrients and moisture so that they are available to sustain roots and seeds, our personal Earth element gathers resources through the food we take into our bodies to be stored and disbursed at precisely the right time - when our cells call out for sustenance. Just think of the earth and its rhythmic cycles - seasonal changes, the 28-day cycle of the moon and the 24 hours of daylight and darkness that compose one day. Our personal Earth element also follows a natural cadence, requiring that it be nourished in a rhythmic way to avoid drops in blood sugar signaled by hunger, mood swings, feelings of fatigue, anxiety, irritability and lack of mental clarity. Mealtimes mark transitions throughout the day - from a time of sleep to one of activity (breakfast); from morning to afternoon (lunch) and from afternoon to evening (dinner). Try to schedule meals and light snacks throughout the day at regular intervals devoting adequate time to truly relax for a few moments to thoroughly enjoy them.

Some helpful herbal digestive aides include:

- Chamomile is an excellent tea to drink after meals; peppermint tea aides digestion, eliminates gas and will help settle frazzled nerves. A cup of lemon balm tea soothes digestion and relieves depression.
- Twenty drops of gentian root tincture in 1/3 cup water taken 10 minutes before a meal helps increase the flow of digestive enzymes to break down food more thoroughly.

- You can make your own herbal remedy to relieve heartburn and acidity by filling gelatin capsules (available at most health food stores) with a mixture composed of 1/2 marshmallow root powder and 1/2 slippery elm bark powder - take one to two capsules as needed.
- In East Indian Ayurveda, fennel seed is commonly used to fend of digestive disturbances. Simply chew on a teaspoon of fennel after each meal.

Irritability

It is only natural to feel irritable when you are being pulled in ten different directions all at the same time. Try to take some time off for personal pampering. Instead of coffee, you might brew up a cup of wood betony tea (avoid during pregnancy). It is a natural nervine that is used to reduce anxiety, irritability, insomnia and for chronic headaches. Bring 1-1/4 cups spring water to boil; stir in 1 tablespoon of wood betony; remove from heat, cover and steep for ten minutes; strain and add a little milk to the brew plus some honey if you like; then sit down, put your feet up and enjoy. If you prefer, take 20 to 30 drops of wood betony tincture. You might like to experiment with some Bach Flower Remedies - impatiens can help with general irritability while beech eases intolerance.

Loss of Libido

Unfortunately, life's hectic pace results in exhaustion that ultimately can take its toll on a couple's intimate life. Once or twice a month try to schedule quiet time away together *(with music, a little chocolate, a few rose petals and lots of romance - but no kids, no friends, no pets, no in-laws!)* to rekindle the fire and renew the bonds of love that brought you together in the first place. Be sure to read the section on "Aphrodisiacs and Love Potions" in Chapter 13.

Stress and Worry

Occasionally it's incredibly important to come to a complete stop and re-evaluate our lives. If you find yourself in an over-extended situation, try to answer the all important question, "Is it really worth all this trouble?" Sometimes we manage to get in over our heads - so it is essential to take time out to make a plan; if not, we feel like hamsters hectically running in an exercise wheel. Do you need to purchase that new car or will the old one get you around for a few more years? Does your child really require that new expensive toy or would he be much happier playing one-on-one basketball with his dad? What would happen if you just cut up those credit cards and made every effort to systematically wipe out the debt? Worry dissipates if you can see light at the end of the tunnel.

In the overall scheme of things what is truly important to you? By making a plan we are calling on our Wood element to help control troublesome Earth worry syndrome. Just as trees keep a hillside from eroding, the law of the Five Elements teaches us that the structure of Wood can bring control to an Earth element that is mothering everyone. Life was meant to be a pleasant journey; try to take the pressure off yourself so you can enjoy its meaningful moments.

When we are over-extended our Earth element tends to go out of balance and we are inclined to worry more. Repetitive or obsessive thought patterns are a signal that our Earth needs tending. Following are a few stress reducing tips:

- Are you consuming regular, nutritious meals? Before we can nurture others, we must nurture ourselves.
- Regular exercise, even if it's only a daily brisk walk around the block, will reduce stress and help maintain physical and mental health.
- Treat yourself to a regular massage. You might be able to talk your partner into swapping neck and shoulder rubs with relaxing lavender scented oil.
- Complex carbohydrates found in whole grains such as brown rice, oats, millet, kamut and barley as well as potatoes promote production of serotonin, the neurotransmitter which creates feelings of well-being and relaxation. Serotonin is actually produced from the amino-acid tryptophan found in protein foods, but your body requires complex carbohydrates to help move this important chemical to your brain. For best results, have foods for lunch that are high in tryptophan (like low-fat turkey or chicken); then try snacking on a piece of whole grain toast, rice cake or plain popcorn around 4:00 p.m. You can top the toast or rice cake with a little honey or jam if you like; avoid butter or any oils since fat will slow its assimilation. If you suffer from sugar sensitivity, alcoholism or depression, you will discover helpful pointers in an ex-

cellent book by Kathleen DesMaisons, Ph.D. entitled *Potatoes Not Prozac*. (Note: If you are extremely sugar or carbohydrate sensitive you will have to proceed with caution when consuming this type of snack; see page 363).

- Increase your celery consumption. The Chinese traditionally drank fresh celery juice mixed with a touch of raw honey as a remedy for stress.
- Lettuce contains lactucarium, a calming substance, so why not enjoy a nice big salad before dinner?
- Rosemary has a high calcium content and has been used for centuries by European, Arabian and Chinese people to calm stress. It is as effective as aspirin in relieving stress-related headaches and it won't upset your stomach. Simply add 2 teaspoons of rosemary to 1 cup of boiling water; remove from heat, cover and steep for 10 minutes; strain and drink.
- Indian snakeroot *(Rauwolfia serpentina)*, also known as serpentwood or *sarpagandha* in *Sanskrit*, has been used for over 4,000 years in India to soothe the mind. Mahatma Gandhi, Hindu spiritual leader and nationalist, is said to have drank snakeroot tea regularly for its calming effects.

Female Health: Special Support During the Childbearing Years

G-d could not be everywhere, therefore,
He created Mothers.

JEWISH PROVERB

During pregnancy and breast feeding mothers literally become the earth for their offspring. Our infant draws nourishment from us in the same way a sprout extracts sustenance from the soil. For a healthy seedling to grow to maturity, it must be planted in a rich, fertile location with just the right amount of sunlight, moisture and drainage. It is no different for a tiny human sprout! Pay special attention to diet during your reproductive years; mother nature will pull all available resources from your body to nurture your little one - those resources must be replenished or your health will suffer in the long run.

The act of parenting the upcoming generation is probably

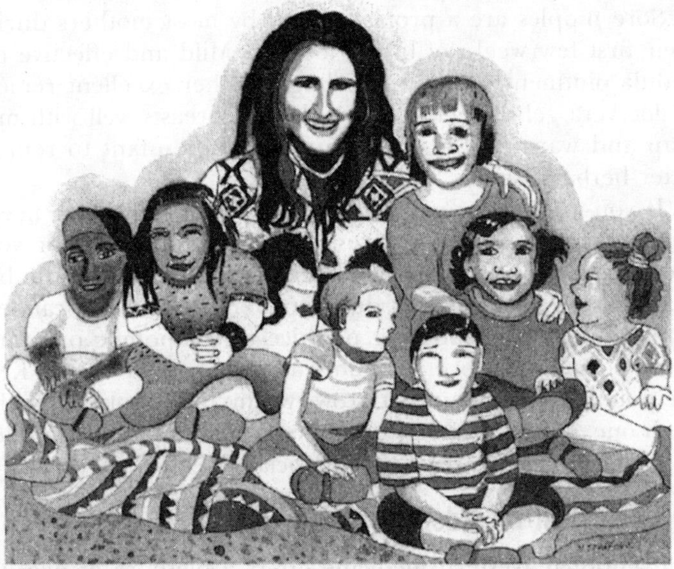

one of the most important and meaningful roles anyone can play in their lifetime. Take time to relax and enjoy your very own miracle of creation.

Breastfeeding

While blessed thistle should not be ingested during pregnancy (it could cause uterine bleeding), after your baby's birth it can be one of your best herbal allies to increase milk production if you can't keep up with your hungry infant's demands for nourishment. Frequently, stress is one of the prime culprits in reduced milk flow. A calming, nutritive tea of the following herbs will come to the rescue: Combine equal parts of blessed thistle, chamomile, nettles and oat straw (all are packed with naturally occurring minerals like calcium, silicon, and iron) with a pinch of fennel seed; bring 1-1/4 cups water to a boil; stir in 2 teaspoons of the blend; remove the pan from heat and cover, steep for ten minutes; strain and enjoy (up to three or four cups daily). You can use only one of the above ingredients for your tea or combine two or three. It is always best to rotate herbs if you are taking them over a long period of time, so change the formula regularly and ingest it six days per week, resting from it the 7th - after three months take off two weeks and then repeat the round if desired.

Sore nipples are a problem faced by most mothers during their first few weeks of breast feeding. Mild and effective calendula ointment promotes healing; another excellent remedy is aloe vera gel. Be certain to wash your breasts well with mild soap and warm water before nursing your infant to remove bitter herbal residues.

If you are producing more milk than your little one needs, it is very important to express the milk completely or your breasts can become engorged. Prevention is definitely the best practice since blocked milk ducts are very painful and can lead to mastitis. A cool soothing poultice of chamomile or grated white potatoes can bring comfort to an engorged breast. Keep the poultice in place until it grows warm, then replace it with a fresh one. If your breasts become red, hot, tender and swollen, be certain to check with your physician.

Gynecological Disorders

Conventional Western medicine offers a plethora of over-the counter and prescription drugs to relieve our monthly menstrual woes - from pain and cramping to bloating or headaches - however, these remedies rarely address the underlying issues that are creating the problems in the first place. Following is a listing of time-honored women's herbal helpers with their special healing characteristics noted, as well as any contraindications. You can pick and choose, creating your own herbal brew, tailored to your unique constitutional problems by simply mixing 2 to 6 of the herbs listed. Normally, combine herbal tinctures or raw herbs in equal parts and add 1/8 to 1/6 part of an herbal harmonizer - either licorice or ginger. Be patient, while many women notice immediate improvement, sometimes it takes six to eight weeks before you begin to feel the full effect of herbal treatment. *Take 20 to 30 drops of your tincture 2 to 3 times daily; or brew up three or four cups of tea (1 to 1-1/2 teaspoons dried herbs per cup); take them six days per week, rest the seventh. After taking any herbal formula for three months, rest from it for two weeks. You might want to make up two separate formulas to help with problems affecting the different phases of your cycle. For example, if anxiety is a problem during the first half, you might add herbal relaxers like skullcap, valerian or passionflower during that time; during the second half of your cycle, you might prefer to add herbs that promote circulation and relieve cramping.*

- **Chaste berry**, also known as vitex, is a crunchy, grayish-brown seed that comes to us from the Mediterranean. Over 2,500 years ago Greek women prepared a special wine with chaste berries to relieve menstrual problems. Today in Europe, it is widely prescribed by gynecologists to treat PMS and irregular periods. It is one of the few single herbs known that directly balances hormonal levels relieving irritability, water retention and breast tenderness. Vitex can be taken when coming off contraceptive pills or other hormone replacement therapies - however, it should not be ingested in conjunction with progesterone since it seems to work by increasing progesterone levels. One word of caution, some herbal experts feel vitex may interfere with the effectiveness of birth control pills; others believe it has no effect. *(Dosage: Add 2 parts of chaste berry to your herbal brew or take 20 to 30 drops of vitex tincture once daily before breakfast.)*
- **Dang Gui** *(Angelica sinensis)*, also known as tangkuei, tonifies and invigorates the entire female system. Frequently referred to as the "queen of women's herbs," the use of this tonic root dates back to about 200 CE in China. During the 15th century, one of its close relatives, A. archangelica, was so widely used in Europe that it was considered the "most important" of all herbs. Reputed to cure every imaginable ailment, including the plague, angelica also used to ward off evil spirits. Dang gui helps build blood, eliminating anemia and constipation due to anemia; it regulates menses, and is used for almost all gynecological problems, including irregular menstruation, painful or absent periods. Dang gui treats other symptoms such as dry skin and blemishes, palpitations, ringing in the ears (tinnitus), blurred vision and abdominal pain. Dang gui increases circulation reducing rheumatic pains and pain from traumatic injury in both men and women. When shopping for dang gui, look for large, plump main roots with pále yellowish flesh. Most herbalists use slices of large roots for herbal preparations while small whole knobs make a delicious addition to your chicken soup. Be certain to purchase roots with a strong penetrating fragrance reminiscent of celery - angelica's close cousin. There are a number of varieties of angelica used medicinally, specify that you want Angelica sinensis. *Note: Persons suffering from diarrhea, chronic water-retention, poor digestion, chronic infection, night sweats or skin rashes should use dang gui with caution.*

- **Dandelion root** is one of the best herbal aides in treating hepatitis and eczema and is a possible preventative for breast cancer. Research has shown that bitter dandelion leaves stimulate bile secretion by as much as 40 percent - greatly aiding digestion. By assisting liver and digestive functions, dandelion helps breakdown circulating hormones that worsen PMS symptoms. Dandelion leaves are rich in vitamins and minerals - including potassium. Troubled with water retention during your cycle? It's probable that dandelion is the only naturally occurring potassium-sparing diuretic - although its diuretic action is likely different from that of pharmaceutical drugs. The leaves relieve constipation, indigestion, heartburn and are delicious when steamed and seasoned with garlic, olive oil and a squeeze of lemon. *Note: Dandelion leaf and root should be used cautiously by persons with gallstones, obstruction of the bile ducts, gastritis or stomach ulcer.*
- **Skullcap** *(Scutellaria lateriflora)*, a native North American herb, soothes jangled nerves and eases the anxiety that frequently accompanies PMS. Used by Cherokee women to promote menstruation, skullcap was first listed in the U.S. Pharmacopoeia in 1863 as a sedative and antispasmodic. Research has confirmed that one of its constituents, scutellarin, has antispasmodic and sedative properties treating insomnia, irritability, neuralgia and muscle spasms. You might try adding skullcap to your formula 7 to 10 days before the onset of menses to prevent PMS.
- **Black Cohosh** *(Cimicifuga racemosa)* was frequently used by Native American women to treat feminine problems. Traditionally, pregnant women ingested a tea of black cohosh, raspberry leaves and other parturient herbs two weeks before their delivery date to facilitate childbirth. It was added to 19th century patent medicines to lift spirits and relieve menstrual distress. Studies have demonstrated that one of its constituents, formononetin, mimics estrogen, helping to balance hormones by binding to estrogen receptor sites on cells. Black cohosh improves circulation, reduces cramping and helps relieve depression. *Note: This herb should not be ingested during pregnancy since it stimulates the uterus; it should not be taken while breast feeding.*
- **Pau d'Arco** *(Tabebuia impetiginosa)*, sacred trumpet flower of the Incas, also known as lapacho or taheebo in South America, is considered a "cure-all" by descendants of the ancient Mayas

and Incas. Herbalists frequently view this herb as one that enhances liver-function and thus add it to women's formulas. It contains lapachol, a natural antibiotic and is used in the treatment of chronic degenerative diseases, as well as fungal infections such as candidiasis, ulcers, cysts, venereal, rheumatic and skin diseases (such as herpes, scabies and eczema). *Note: If taken in excess, pau d'arco can cause dizziness, nausea, vomiting and/or diarrhea.*

- **Wild Mexican Yam** *(Dioscorea villosa)* contains substances very similar to progesterone. A number of different species have been used in East Indian Ayurvedic and Asian medicine for hundreds of years. Yam is used specifically to relieve menstrual cramping as well as to treat cramps associated with the pain of kidney and gallstones.
- **Ginger root** is an important ingredient in approximately 50 percent of all Ayurvedic and Oriental herbal prescriptions. Its name in Ayurveda, *vishwabhesaj*, means "universal medicine." If you suffer from deficiency symptoms like cold hands and feet, warming ginger can help by boosting circulation. Simply add 1/8 to 1/6 part ginger root to your formula; it is known as an herbal harmonizer - meaning that it reduces the toxicity or irritant effects of other herbs in the formula.
- **Licorice root** is another important herbal harmonizer that has been used to antidote poisons throughout history. This sweet tasting herb relaxes muscle spasms (particularly of the abdomen and legs); reduces pain and inflammation, balances blood-sugar levels, stimulates adrenocorticol hormones, regulates and normalizes hormone production. Instead of warming ginger root, you can add 1/8 to 1/6 part neutral raw licorice root to your formula to harmonize and direct the effects of the other herbs. *Note: Taken in excess, licorice can raise blood pressure and cause water retention. It should not be ingested during pregnancy, or in cases of hypertension, kidney disease, or for persons taking digoxin-based medications.*

Menopause: Those Hormones Again!

Traditionally, Chinese thought divided a woman's life into seven year cycles while men's life cycles were based on eight year increments. For a woman, age 49 marked the end of her reproductive years and the start of menopause. Technically speaking, you are in menopause when you have not had a menstrual cycle for 6 to 12 months. However, well before cessation of menses your body has begun to change in many subtle ways - this phase, which can last for a few years, is referred to as perimenopause.

Perimenopause, like puberty, is a transition in life's stages. It can be accompanied by mood swings, night sweats, hot flashes, changes in the intensity and duration of your menses, insomnia, fatigue, dizziness, palpitations, reduced libido. The great news is that as you pass into true menopause the wonderful mental clarity and zest for life of those early childhood years begins to surface once again! This is frequently referred to as "post menopausal zeal."

But let's back up to perimenopause with its changing hormonal levels. This is what is happening in your body: Estrogen production begins to decline, while output of other hormones (follicle-stimulating hormone and luteinizing hormone - known as FSH and LS) increases by 30 to 60 percent. By the time we reach 50 years of age, a woman's body has produced approximately 400 mature eggs. However, at age 50 there are very few remaining eggs, and without active egg follicles, our bodies produce lower levels of estrogen and progesterone. Nature, in a last hurrah, tries to jump-start egg production by releasing copious quantities of LH and FSH. Finding no egg follicles to stimulate, these hormones act on our ovaries and adrenal glands creating increased production of androgen. These changes are a normal part of aging, however, decreased estrogen levels can increase our risk of heart disease and osteoporosis. All that estrogen circulating in our systems kept our bones strong and helped protect our hearts by controlling cholesterol levels.

Menopause is not an illness, it is a natural process; however, conventional medicine tends to treat it like a disease by prescribing hormone replacement therapy (HRT) for protection against osteoporosis and heart disease. While HRT may be appropriate for women suffering from severe menopausal symptoms or for those with osteoporosis, they come with some unpleasant side effects that impact an estimated 50 percent of all women who ingest them. Problems associated with HRT include bloating, weight gain, headaches, abnormal uterine bleeding, cramps, irritability and breast tenderness. Estrogen replacement therapy doubles our chances of developing gallbladder disease. (For many years HRT was thought to decrease the risk of coronary artery disease. A recent study tips the scale away from using hormones in menopause. Taking estrogens at this stage of life has now been shown to actually slightly increase the risk of coronary events, while greatly increasing the risk of breast cancer. - *Dr. Gary*)

In making your decision about HRT, it is important to consider the differences between natural and synthetic forms of estrogen. Synthetic estrogens tend to accumulate in the body, causing metabolic changes in the liver which has the difficult job of breaking them down - side effects include fluid retention, blood clots and high blood pressure. Natural estrogens are chemically identical to those produced by our ovaries. Equine estrogen (sold as Estratab and Premarin) is made from the urine of pregnant mares; it is effective but extremely potent and may also cause metabolic changes in the liver. This form of estrogen is best avoided by women who smoke, are overweight, suffer from varicose veins, high blood pressure or high cholesterol. Estropipate (Ogen) and estradiol (Estraderm, Emcyt and Estrace) are the most natural estrogens available and are easily metabolized. Some physicians recommend taking the smallest dosage of estrogen that provides relief from menopausal symptoms every other day, rather than daily.

You can see why some women, those with light menopausal symptoms, may fair better without hormonal replacement. Recent studies suggest that progesterone replacement may be more appropriate for many women. Natural progesterone creams are available at most health food stores.

It's time to check out the herbal helpers that mother nature has to offer!

- Consume foods containing **phytoestrogens** which act like estrogens created by the body - these include: soybeans, tofu, miso, dates, pomegranate and flaxseeds. One article featured in *The Lancet*, a British medical journal, reported that Japanese women experience fewer menopausal symptoms than their Western sisters. It is speculated that one of the reasons for this is because Japanese ladies regularly ingest more plant-based estrogens, such as those found in soybean products.
- Create your own healing brew with **herbs that contain natural estrogen** promoters: anise, black cohosh, dang gui, fennel, licorice, raspberry, sage, sarsaparilla and wild yam root. *(Note: Sage reduces night sweats but should not be ingested if you are afflicted by any type of seizure disorder; in large amounts, it can*

cause irritability. Avoid licorice if you suffer from high blood pressure or edema; it should not be ingested for more than seven days in a row and is usually best taken in conjunction with other herbs in a balanced formula).

- An **Ayurvedic formula** which helps balance hormonal levels consists of equal parts of *shatavari* (Asparagus racemosus) and *vidari* (similar to wild yam which can be used in its place): Ingest 1 teaspoon of the powdered herbs two times daily after lunch and dinner. *Take the formula six days per week and rest from it on the seventh.*
- An excellent **Chinese patent formula, Zhi Bai Di Huang Wan** (Temper Fire) relieves hot flashes while supporting the Kidney/adrenal organ system, helping to balance hormonal levels.
- **Herbs and foods which are naturally rich in calcium** can help prevent osteoporosis: Amaranth, bok choy, chickweed, dandelion greens, nettle, seaweed, sesame seeds, water cress, as well as low or non-fat organic milk products such as yogurt or cottage cheese. Most studies suggest an intake of 1500 mgm calcium per day to prevent osteoporosis. Since diet normally supplies about 500 mgm, taking a 500 mgm calcium carbonate/250 mgm magnesium supplement plus vitamin D (to help absorption into the bones) twice daily with meals is a good idea. Remember that weight bearing exercise helps keep the bones strong.
- **Avoid acid producing foods** which stimulate the bones to release calcium as a buffering agent, these include: coffee, black tea, caffeinated cola drinks, sugar, refined foods, excess animal protein.
- **Avoid tobacco** - studies have shown a close association between early menopause and smoking.
- **Hawthorn** is an excellent herbal ally to aide in the prevention of heart disease (see page 154).
- **Damiana** is an herbal aphrodisiac that enhances desire and pleasure. If intimate relations are unpleasant due to dryness, try lubricating with aloe vera gel, vitamin E oil, or comfrey ointment. Good news for you and your partner - regular intimacy increases blood circulation to vaginal tissues - improving their tone and lubrication. For vaginal itching, Abkit offers a very effective product - Natureworks Marigold Ointment.

- **Don't forget exercise!** Swedish research has demonstrated that regular exercise helps lower the frequency, as well as the severity of hot flashes. A simple 30 minute walk daily can aid immensely.

Morning Sickness

The first three or four months of pregnancy can be challenging if you have to deal with morning sickness. Ginger can come to the rescue! It is one of the safest and most effective anti-nausea herbs around. Brew up a pot of tea in the morning by simmering a 4 inch long chunk of fresh ginger (that has been cut into several smaller pieces) in 4 cups of spring water; add the root to boiling water, cover while simmering on low heat for ten minutes; remove from heat and let steep for another 10 minutes, strain and sip throughout the day. You can also purchase ginger in tea bag or tincture form at most herb or health food stores.

You may find it useful to rotate herbs - try gentle meadowsweet tea by stirring one tablespoon of herb into 1-1/4 cups of boiling water; cover, remove from heat and steep for 15 minutes; strain and enjoy.

Aniseed is another herbal ally that can help settle the stomach; it has also been used by traditional cultures to encourage milk production. Simply chew on three or four aniseeds at the first sign of discomfort.

Inhaling the fragrance of fresh peppermint leaves or peppermint oil can also help relieve queasiness.

Vitamin B6 (Pyridoxine) at 50 mg a day also reduces morning sickness.

Male Health: Tips for Maintaining a Healthy Reproductive System

The prostate, a walnut-sized gland located at the base of the bladder, surrounds the urethra - the tube that carries urine out of the body. It produces the fluid that nourishes and carries sperm. While 80 percent of all cases of prostate cancer occur in men over the age of 65; studies project that 13 percent of male babies born in the U.S. today will develop this disease at some point in their lives. Prostate enlargement (benign prostatic hypertrophy) affects approximately 50 percent of men over age

50 and 75 percent of males over 70 years of age. Symptoms of prostate enlargement include frequent urination, urgency to urinate, increased night time urination, reduced size and force of urine flow, and, when extreme, inability to urinate. Prostate cancer may produce similar symptoms, however, in most cases, there are no symptoms at all until the disease has reached an advanced stage. The most simple and cost-effective means for diagnosing prostate cancer is a careful rectal examination along with a blood test for Prostate Specific Antigen, which becomes elevated if there is cancer. The American Cancer Society recommends that starting at age 40, men undergo an annual exam.

A 1994 report in The New England Journal of Medicine revealed the results of a study on a large group of men who refused traditional therapy. Interestingly, they fared as well, if not better than men who underwent treatment. Some physicians believe that prostate cancer is over treated here in America; European MD's have taken a more conservative approach in treating this disease, with similar results.

It is never too early to start prevention!

- Zinc nourishes the prostate gland and is a component of over 300 enzymes essential for boosting immunity, repairing wounds, synthesizing protein, preserving vision and protecting our cells against free radicals. Increase your consumption of foods naturally high in this important mineral: pumpkin seeds, sunflower seeds, mushrooms, seaweed, seafood, spinach and whole grains. *Supplement your diet with one 30 mg tablet daily, taken with a meal to avoid stomach distress, 6 days a week.*
- Consume whole foods - raw nuts and seeds, flax seed (2 to 3 tablespoons daily), whole grains, fresh fruits and vegetables, legumes (such as lentils, mung beans, black beans), low or non-fat organic dairy products (such as cottage cheese and yogurt), cold-water fish and lean cuts of poultry.
- Reduce your consumption of convenience and fast foods. A high-fat, low-fiber diet is linked to both prostate cancer and heart disease. Read about the differences in the types of fats you consume in Chapter 13.

Do It Yourself Herbal Checklist

Choose from the following herbs and make your own healing blend - **use one to two parts of saw palmetto, one part pygeum and nettles; add 1/2 part of two to four herbs of your choice,**

then combine with 1/8 to 1/4 part ginger or licorice root to harmonize the formula. *To make it simple, you can purchase tinctures and mix them together; taking 20 to 30 drops, three times daily, 6 days a week. Alternate the herbs in your formula regularly.*

- *Saw Palmetto*, usually the chief herb in most men's prostate formulas, is specific for helping to maintain a healthy prostate function; use up to two parts. *If taking capsules, the usual dosage is 160 mgm two times a day.*
- *Pygeum* is normally prescribed in conjunction with saw palmetto. Studies conducted in Europe suggest it may help prevent prostate cancer. If desired, add one part to your formula.
- *Nettles* is considered a plague by farmers because it absorbs valuable minerals from the soil; herbalists love it for the very same reason! This remarkable herb is rich in Vitamins A and C and is a treasure trove of minerals that help to build strong bones and support kidney/adrenal function. *Nettle tea can be taken daily as a general tonic to relieve low energy and fatigue. You can add 2 tablespoons of this delicious herb/food into soups (let it simmer for 20 minutes with other veggies). If desired, use one part in your formula.*
- *Dodder seeds*, also known as cuscuta, is an excellent food grade herb that is used to treat prostatitis, impotence, low back ache, rheumatoid arthritis, cold knees. In Chinese medicine, it is considered both a yin and yang tonic. Its energy is considered sweet and neutral, neither hot nor cold.
- *Dandelion root* and *red clover* cleanse the liver and blood of toxins.
- *Gravel root, parsley root, yarrow, oat straw* are diuretics that can help dissolve stones.
- *Carnivora*, a substance derived from a South American plant, is utilized by German cancer specialist Dr. Hans Nieper to treat prostate cancer. *(Note: I have not worked with or prescribed this substance but it is certainly worth investigating.)*
- *Pau d'arco, buchu, goldenseal* and *echinacea* have antimicrobial and anticancer properties; if desired, add 1/2 part to your formula but alternate frequently.
- *False unicorn root* is a general tonic for genitourinary disorders, treating dull aching pain in the lumbosacral region and impotence. Known for its aphrodisiac properties, damiana

is frequently used to treat frigidity in women and impotence in men; it also improves digestion and relieves constipation. If indicated, add 1/4 to 1/2 part of your formula.

In Asian medical thought walnuts are considered an excellent tonic food for the Water element (which includes the kidney/adrenal, urinary bladder and reproductive organ systems). Consume 3 or 4 walnut halves with your breakfast or for a snack in the afternoon. Small servings of shrimp, oysters and lean white pork are also considered excellent foods to support the Water element. *See Chapter 7 for more information.*

Recognizing and Preventing Earth Imbalances Through Life's Phases

The mysterious forces of the Earth
create moisture in the Heaven and
fertile soil upon the Earth;
they create the flesh within the body
and the stomach (and spleen/pancreas).
They create the yellow color . . .
and give the voice the ability to sing . . .
they create the mouth,
the sweet flavor,
and the emotions of anxiety and worry.

THE YELLOW EMPEROR'S CLASSIC OF INTERNAL MEDICINE

On a physical level, if our Earth element is deficient or weak, we may experience some of the following symptoms: fatigue, loose stools, abdominal noises, gas, difficult weight loss, poor appetite, pale lips and tongue, mental spaciness, frequent bruising, poor muscle tone, varicose veins, water retention, diabetes, hypoglycemia, cravings for sweets, poor concentration, feelings of being overwhelmed.

Deficient Earth disharmonies often benefit from an increase in full sweet earth foods (small portions of lean cuts of beef, poultry and fish). Cookies, cakes, chocolate, coffee and other refined sugars weaken the digestion, creating more deficiency and fatigue - try to eliminate them. Consume small portions of healthful complex carbohydrates found in whole organic rolled oats, barley, quinoa and amaranth, aduki, mung and black beans, yams, sweet potatoes and yellow squash. Flavor your foods with warming herbs, spices and roots such as cardamom, chives, cinnamon, fennel, garlic, leeks, onions, and parsnips. Aid digestion by increasing the Bitter flavor in the form of herbal bitters and/or steamed greens. Cold, uncooked foods create dampness and phlegm in the body and tax digestion that is already weak. Consume moderately-sized, warm meals on a regular basis in a peaceful setting. Pay special attention to chew well - digestion begins in the mouth. Avoid all cold foods - especially iced drinks, fruit juices, sodas and ice cream. Small amounts of cooked fruit can be spiced with cinnamon or ginger to aid digestion - pear or apple are probably best. Warm ginger tea stimulates digestion and warms our center.

An excess Earth condition is characterized by: feeling of heaviness in the head or limbs, dull headache, overweight, nausea, vomiting, belching, constipation, nodules or lumps under the skin, swollen glands, sinus congestion, yeast infections, tender or bleeding gums, respiratory phlegm, mental fuzziness (one patient described it as "fog on the brain"), obsessive or repetitive thoughts, tendency to worry, tendency to take care of others at the expense of oneself.

Excess Earth conditions can be aided by cutting back on Earth engendering full sweet foods and increasing the consumption of the Sour *(Astringent in Ayurvedic thought, see page 256)*, Bitter and Spicy Flavors to eliminate dampness. Consume plenty of cooked greens to drain dampness. Small lean portions of meat, poultry and fish will be helpful unless there are Fire signs (infection, irritability, fevers, throbbing headaches and a yellow tongue coat) - in which case, try to eliminate animal products as well as warming herbs like garlic and onion for one to two weeks until the Heat signs are eliminated. Aduki or mung bean vegetable soup with a very small portion of whole grains (1/2 cup) like brown rice or millet would be good during this phase. Eliminate refined carbohydrates and alcoholic beverages which increase dampness. Once heat symptoms are eliminated, see the recommendations above for Earth Deficiency symptoms - but keep grains at no more than 1/2 cup serving per meal.

If you have an extremely difficult time maintaining your weight, read the section entitled "Weight Problems" which can be found in Chapter 13.

Humming or singing is the sound of the Earth element.

When our personal Earth element is in balance we resonate with the unique song in our heart - feeling content, peaceful and grounded. Healthy Earth gives us the ability to first nourish ourselves and from that solid core, reach out to share with others. It fills us with a quality of openness, fairness and concern for those in need. Once we are centered and stable in our sense of HOME (our Earthly body), with a clear mind we can turn to the all important work at hand - that of compassionate service.

Our Earth phase of life corresponds to a time when we have put down roots and become established. This is a time of fulfillment, a time of home, family, and community. In choosing a profession we offer our unique talents in exchange for Earth element's money. In creating a home filled with family, a partner, children, friends or pets, we learn to refine the gentle rhythmic Earth dance of giving and receiving, nurturing and being nourished. As the years pass and we become more established - secure in our center - it is only natural to expand our interests to reach out to those in our community who are less fortunate.

Hopefully, by the time we reach the Earth stage of life, we see ourselves not only as an Asian, Hispanic, African or Caucasian; Protestant, Catholic, Jew, Buddhist, Hindu or Muslim, but FIRST and foremost as a member of the human family. The Earth element is about relationships - about cooperation, concern, caring and sharing. One story which illustrates the spirit of the Earth element goes something like this:

Aunt Hattie had passed on to the other world - upon awakening to her new reality - she was very pleased to find herself in a gorgeous garden filled with fountains, flowers, butterflies and singing birds. A radiant being dressed in white approached and asked if she would like to be escorted to the banquet. Known for her rather cranky disposition, Aunt Hattie sighed in relief to find herself in heaven. She joyously followed the being to an elegant banquet hall built of gold, silver, pearls and shiny jewels. She could smell the sumptuous banquet . . . the golden doors slowly swung open . . . Hattie was amazed at the sight. The long table was filled with every imaginable delicacy but the scene was terribly chaotic with food flying through the air in every direction. Three foot long spoons were strapped to the hands of the guests. In attempting to get the spoons to their own mouths, the poor souls kept banging them against their neighbors. In the feeding frenzy, food was spilled everywhere . . . yet no one was fed . . . mean-

while, the hungry guests were shouting profanities at each other. Hattie gasped and asked, "If this is heaven what is hell like?" The being smiled and graciously asked Hattie to follow him. Next door was another beautiful banquet hall. The golden doors swung open to reveal exactly the same scene. However, everyone was smiling and conversing as they offered food to one another with the long spoon strapped to their wrist. The being gently explained, "This is heaven . . . now it's time to get back to the other banquet."

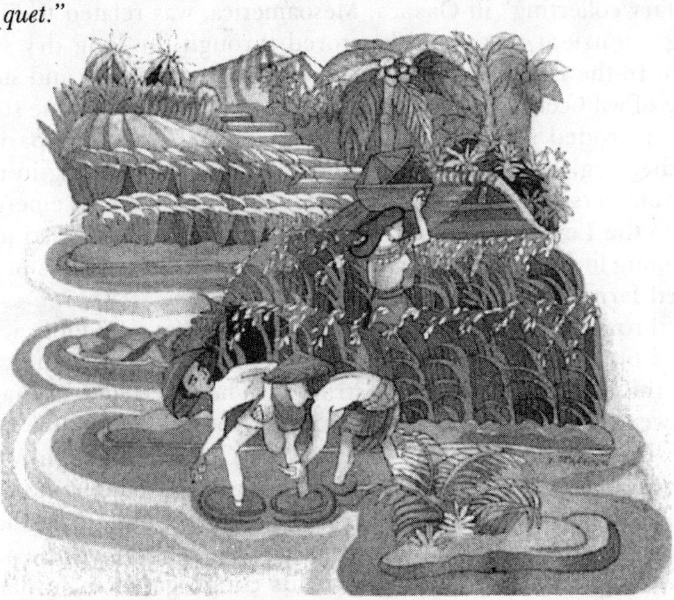

From Foraging to Farming

Will you come on another anthropological journey with me? It is a very important one to help us understand where we human beings have been, where we are and where we are going. I briefly want to take you through the transition from foraging to farming that took place on our planet in Mesoamerica and the Near Eastern Zagros Mountain and Levant area in what is now modern day Turkey and Iran. Always fascinated by the question, "Why do I think the way I think?", I find it particularly intriguing to follow societal changes that accompanied the transitions in lifestyle and human consciousness throughout history. **The following journey corresponds to the Earth element because it tracks the ways in which we human beings have nour-**

ished ourselves and others from the beginnings of time.

By approximately 10,000 BCE, most human groups had territorial rivals on all sides, creating a barrier against long-range migration. Not as free to pick up and move in the face of adversity, mobile foragers turned to utilization of food storage facilities in case of climatic changes or natural disasters. This risk reduction tactic dramatically impacted their subsistence patterns. According to Dr. Kent Flannery, archaeologist, the "key to sedentary collecting" in Oaxaca, Mesoamerica, was related to finding a nutrient that could be stored through the long dry season. In the Levant, sedentism, based on the collection and storage of wild cereals, preceded agriculture - grain or legume storage provided security against the unknown. When comparing archaeological data regarding the beginnings of farming in the Levant versus Mesoamerica, two very distinct sequences emerge: 1) in the Levant, sedentary foragers gradually transitioned to a farming lifestyle, while 2) in Mesoamerica, mobile foragers practiced farming and later became sedentary.

From before 9000 BCE to 3500 BCE, native people who lived in the semiarid basin and valleys of Mesoamerica survived on the basis of a collecting strategy. They moved seasonally between the floodplains, dry alluvial slopes and montane forest. During the long dry season, from October through May, bands of 4 to 8 people subsisted on deer, wild boar, cottontail rabbits, cactus leaves, acorns, pine nuts, maguey and avocado - native food sources of the higher elevations. During the wet season, June and July, larger bands congregated in lowland settlements, subsisting on mesquite pods (legume family), small game and wild plants from the nearby alluvial slopes. Natives began limited cultivation of primitive maize (teoscinte), beans and chile peppers in their natural habitats (highland canyons) by 5000 BCE. From 3500 to 2000 BCE, there was a rapid change in Mesoamerican subsistence patterns from mobile foraging to fully sedentary village-based farming. Small, one-room houses formed village settlements found on alluvial plain areas of the major rivers. At this time, domestication of maize, beans, squash and avocados was fully in place. Villagers scheduled highland hunting visits to procure wild game and plants at times of the year when it would not conflict with their intensive lowland cultivation practices. Archaeological sites from this period, characterized by rapid population growth, give artifactual evidence of long-distance trade systems.

Now, let's journey half-way around the world to the Levant area in the Near East. From 10,000 to 8,000 BCE, the climate was becoming more warm and moist. Human populations increased and the first stone huts with associated outside storage pits provide evidence of semi sedentism. The dead were buried in pits under the floor of huts and analysis of their skeletal remains give evidence of dietary changes to a more plant and shellfish based diet. Few plant remains have been preserved from this period and there is no clear evidence of domestic forms. Bones of wild game have been found at sites - including pigs, cattle, gazelles, sheep and goats, as well as migratory waterfowl.

A big population boom characterized the period from 7600 to 6000 BCE. Some of the largest settlements cover over 20 acres, and for the first time we witness **storage pits moving inside the patios** of the square houses which were built of stones or mud brick and composed of several rooms. While wild plant and animal remains are common, domestic sheep and goats dominate faunal assemblages with domestic barley, einkorn and emmer wheat, lentils and peas present at the earliest sites. From 6000 to 5000 BCE the climate became hotter and more arid and the human population moved into woodland zones. A decrease in hunting implements implies a depletion of wild game and an increased dependence on domesticated sheep, goats, cattle and pigs.

Did you notice the very significant change that occurred sometime between 8,000 and 7, 000 BCE? **Storage pits moved from outside the house to inside the patio.**

> **At this point in history, according to University of California - Santa Cruz, Professor Diane Gifford-Gonzalez, humankind, in the Levant area, permanently abandoned their sharing forager mentality, to embark on a path of personal accumulation and the subsequent hoarding mentality that accompanies it - the hallmark of sedentary food producing societies.**

Let's take that last statement and dig a little deeper. Lifestyles and value systems among mobile foragers are quite different, if not diametrically opposed, to those of food producers. Most foragers live in small communities composed of seven to ten households. The rule of "generalized generosity" is the norm and all individuals expect to share food and other belongings quite freely with members of other households. In fact, sharing is the key word in all forager interactions. Hoarding and arrogance are considered the two most dangerous human characteristics in these societies. It is understood that no one will starve unless everyone starves. Meat from cooperative hunts is divided among all persons; just as a successful individual hunter must equally divide the spoils of a good hunt (or even a bad hunt, for that matter) between all households in the community.

Births in forager households usually occur less frequently than those of sedentary food producers. A birth space of approximately five years between children is quite common due to the great physical demands an infant places on the very active nursing forager mother who must carry it wherever she goes. In forager society we see women exercising control over their own destiny in many ways including decisions regarding marriage, divorce and reproduction. In food producing societies, the egalitarian social structure of forager society is replaced by human hierarchies (usually patriarchal). Land owners always need more hands to work the soil or tend the herds - children become a valuable commodity. Females frequently lose their freedom and power to make decisions in food producing communities as their human value becomes measured in terms of infant production and domestic service. Wives are jealously guarded just as possessions are hoarded. *(Note: Today, in some countries, women are still bought and sold, others must hide their faces behind veils. In America, we witness remnants of this same mentality where women, frequently single mothers, receive less wages for doing the same job as their male counterparts.)*

Individuals living in food producing communities have a vested interest in the crops and animals they tend. While hunted animals do not have owners, tended plants and animals require considerable human energy output. This energy expended in caring for crops and herds becomes justification for individual ownership of land and animals. Just as seeds must be saved for next year's sowing, resources must be guarded to protect one's immediate family against an unsure future. Embarking on a path of accumulation (originally intended to prevent starvation in case of a drought or other unforeseen disaster) food producers develop a hoarding mentality. Privacy is sacred. Under no circumstances should other members of the community be privy to family secrets regarding wealth. Indeed, wealth represents status and power in food producing communities, and this status and power is passed down from generation to generation.

In transitioning from foraging to food producing societies, humankind experienced many demographic and social consequences. Contrary to popular beliefs that cultural changes from foraging to farming and animal husbandry offered human beings an improved standard of living that resulted in improved health, researchers Cohen and Armelagos site twelve studies that indicate quite the opposite is true. Data gathered from the examination of skeletal remains demonstrates that infection was a much more serious problem for farmers than their hunting/gathering ancestors. The sedentary lifestyle, which accompanies a food producing way of life, brings with it a much higher rate of infection for fairly simple reasons. Bacterial counts escalate in areas where human and animal feces and refuse accumulate. Small forager groups just pick up and leave an area before epidemics can occur.

Also, both New and Old World studies show an overall decline in quality of nutrition accompanied the adoption of farming with marked changes in bone morphology, including the thinning of longbone cortices and increased porosity of the skull and orbit (indicative of anemia). Poor nutrition undoubtedly contributed to the increase of disease witnessed in the archaeological record.

Depending upon their ecological niche on our planet, most of humankind once enjoyed an incredibly varied diet - several thousand plant species and several hundred animal species were used for food. But with the agricultural revolution, all of that was to change. According to Dr. Jack Harlan, Biology Professor at Tulane University, today, the earth's population is completely dependent upon four crops - wheat, rice, maize and potatoes - with the next 26 highest produced crops put together contributing less tonnage to the world than these four crops. We human beings, the domesticators, are hopelessly dependent on the very plants and animals we have domesticated - the tables have been turned. Due to human selection, favored species proliferate while the genes of many potentially valuable foods die out. As witnessed in the famous potato famine, reliance on one or two major food items can spell disaster.

Have you ever thought about the number of distinct nutrients you consume? If you start making a list, you will discover that you normally eat between 20 to 30 different foods (excluding the chemical additives!) that are combined and recombined in many ways to form different meals that are virtually the same.

Why not support your local organic farmer who is trying to bring healthful foods to your community? How about experimenting with other types of whole grains, beans and vegetables - like kamut, spelt, millet, barley, rice, quinoa, rye . . . or aduki, black, mung beans or lentils . . . or arugala, bok choy or dandelion greens? While in today's world it would be next to impossible to return to a foraging lifestyle, we can seek out a variety of healthful whole foods.

When addressing the Earth element, we cannot talk about nourishing ourselves without talking about feeding all of Earth's children. Isn't it fascinating that by the year 1500, the Incan people had already devised a system in which no one had to go hungry? - yet in the 21st century such a safety net still alludes us. Grain shipments to the impoverished are only a bandaid - the problem goes much deeper - the problem involves democracy. According to Webster's Dictionary, democracy is the "principle of equality of rights, opportunity and treatment, or the practice of this principle." True democracy cannot exist in any country, where the homeless walk the streets, or in our world until all persons are fed, clothed and have a means to make a respectable living (not to be confused with income). But how is that possible on our over-populated planet?

To answer that, we need to look at the real relationship between population density/population growth and hunger. Population density and hunger are not correlated in many countries. For example, compared to India, China has only 50 percent of the crop land per person; however, hunger is widespread in India but not in China. According to Oxford University scholar Keith Griffin, "less than three percent of China's population suffers from undernutrition." At the same time, significant food resources coexist with extreme hunger in countries like Brazil or Senegal. An interesting statistic to ponder comes from a World Bank study of 64 countries - when income of the poorest people went up by one percent, the general fertility rates dropped by nearly 3 percent. High birth rates are frequently linked to economic insecurity.

The Green Revolution was supposed to be a cure for world hunger. In this system of agriculture, the Earth is treated like a mining project, as maximum crop output is "extracted" in the shortest length of time. Such modes of food production result in soil erosion, pesticide contamination and ultimate desertification of once fertile farm land. Traditional farming intercropping wisdom is lost in the roar of industrialized farm machinery. But, is lack of food the ultimate reason for world hunger?

Over the past 25 years food production increased 16 percent while mountains of unsold grains glutted the market, pushing prices constantly lower during the same time span. There is not a scarcity of food on our planet, but a faulty distribution system to blame. Millions of small land-owners have been pushed off their land and do not have ways to feed themselves, or the means to purchase foods. Their land, gobbled up by large conglomerates, is used to raise luxury foods demanded by the wealthy elite. In Mexico, for example, 2/3's of the population is chronically undernourished. Sorghum, a grain used for poultry and livestock feed, was unknown in Mexico in 1958. However, by 1980, twice as much sorghum was being grown as wheat. Lappe & Collins tell us that livestock consumed 6 percent of Mexico's grain in 1958 but now 33 to 50 percent goes to animals - 25 million Mexican people are too poor to ever purchase meat, poultry or eggs.

As long as food is bought and sold like other commodities and societies continue to condone vast inequalities in landholdings and income, mountains of food can never eliminate hunger. The roots of famine will be eliminated only once conscientious capitalism, informed consumerism and true democracy exist in our world - and that will occur when economic democracy becomes a reality.

Let's talk briefly about "conscientious capitalism". After the birth of my daughter, I had a birth control device inserted; my doctor told me it was the safest and most effective apparatus on the market - the Dalkon Shield. To make a long story short . . . after feeling violently ill for a week, I visited the emergency room at our community hospital. The young intern sent me home saying it was probably just a gall bladder attack and I should "weather it out." Only a strange quirk of fate took me to work the following day - my two co-workers were absent and someone had to cover the office. Otherwise, I would have been home alone when the ectopic pregnancy ruptured. Luckily, someone found me slumped over the computer - in time to call the Fire Department that was only a couple of blocks away. They rushed me to the hospital for emergency surgery. The anesthesiologist said it was a miracle - five more minutes and I would not have survived. Though the Dalkon Shield and surgery left me incapable of having more children, I was lucky . . . other women lost their lives.

Now for the incomprehensible part of this story . . .

When this defective device was banned for sale in the United States, its manufacturer swiftly and mercilessly sold 700,000 Shields to USAID's Office of Population for overseas distribution. A 48 percent discount off standard prices was given to USAID and the deadly Dalkon Shields were bulk packaged, 1,000 unsterilized devices per box with one applicator for every ten Shields (greatly increasing the possibility of infection). Only one set of instructions was included in each box; it was translated into three languages English, Spanish and French - though the devices were being sent to many Asiatic and mid-Eastern countries where these languages are not spoken. The Dalkon Shields, paid for with dollars from the U.S. Treasury, left America's shores, destined for clinics and innocent, unsuspecting women in Indonesia, Chile, Israel, Kenya, Paraguay, Thailand and 36 other developing nations. It is estimated that the Dalkon Shield has taken the lives of hundreds, if not thousands of women living outside the United States due to serious infections, ruptured ectopic pregnancies, perforated wombs and septic abortions.

Our shareholder system of capitalism dictates that corporate enterprises are "morally" obligated to protect the interests and profits of its investors. This mentality has resulted in faulty U.S. products, pesticides and other chemicals, banned by the FDA, being swiftly and criminally dumped into developing nations to cut losses. Don't you think we, as consumers, investors, and human beings are morally obligated to be informed of such acts and to prevent them at all costs?

In comparing forager communities to food producing societies we find two diametrically opposed systems of existence - simply stated - one is based on sharing while the other is based on hoarding. At the beginning of the 21st century we Westerners still seek to export our goods, lifestyles and belief systems to other peoples and cultures, with the notion that they will be much better off because of them. This is not necessarily true. In our society, things are more important than people; dollars are more important than people. We separate ourselves from other human beings by objectifying them, or even worse, patronizing or matronizing them. Sadly, in today's profit-oriented market, human life is objectified like all other material goods -

it is bought, bartered and sold to the highest bidder.

What to do? Change starts with individuals. We can all help in simple ways - they really add up. Here are some ideas: 1) volunteer once or twice a month to serve food to the homeless in your community; 2) purchase foods that are organically grown by small enterprises; 3) recycle paper, plastic, glass and aluminum, 4) clean out your closet and garage - donate the goods to charity - they are probably just cluttering up your life anyway! 5) become an informed consumer - are you purchasing foods produced by conglomerates with interests in questionable enterprises like the tobacco industry? 6) before purchasing stocks in a company, find out about its interest and holdings in developing nations. The spirit of the Earth element is about fairness, equality, compassion and service.

Rain Forest Facts

Almost 90% of West Africa's
rain forest has been destroyed;
since the late 1700's, 75% of Australia's
tropical rain forest has been cleared;
over 90 different Amazonian tribes are thought
to have disappeared this century.

Now, it's time to move on . . . Once we have established a secure, grounded relationship with our mother, the Earth, then our aspirations naturally turn to the heavens, as we seek the archetypal father, God, G-d, Allah, the Creator or Prime Source represented by the Metal element in Chinese Five Element thought.

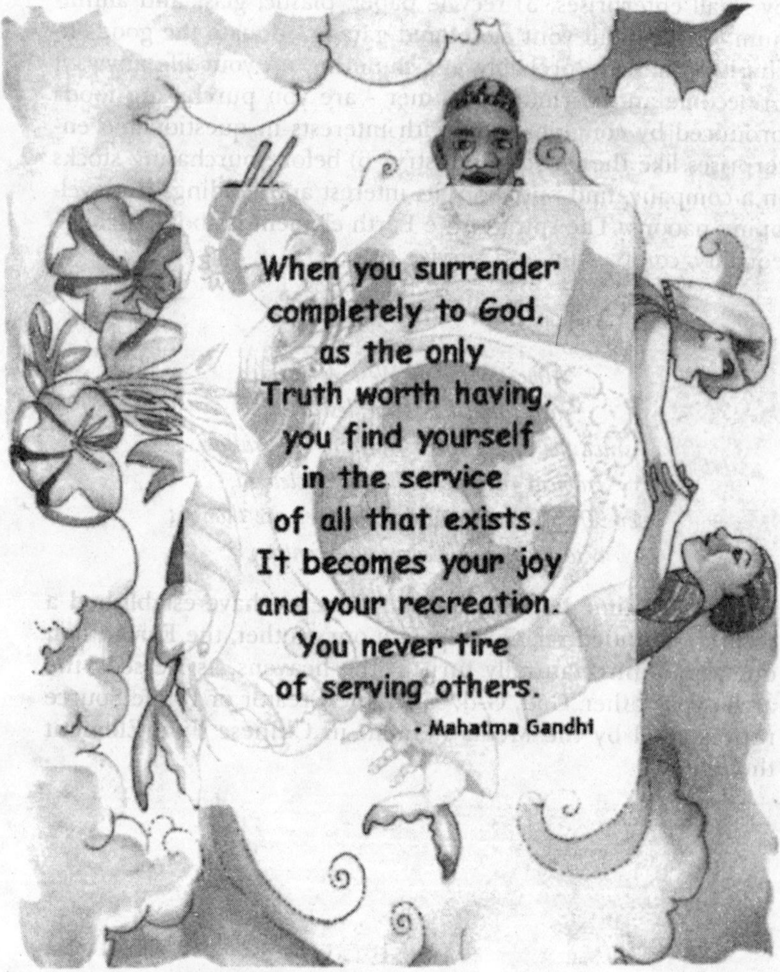
When you surrender
completely to God,
as the only
Truth worth having,
you find yourself
in the service
of all that exists.
It becomes your joy
and your recreation.
You never tire
of serving others.
- Mahatma Gandhi

6

The Metal Stage of Life The Wisdom Years

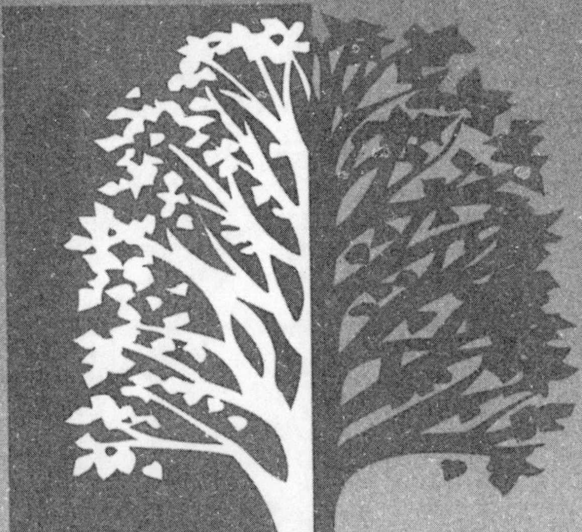

Autumn/Metal Element

By Gary Dolowich, M.D., B.Ac.

Bend and you will be whole.
Curl and you will be straight.
Keep empty and you will be filled.
Grow old and you will be renewed.

Lao Tzu

In nature, the autumn season is the time of letting go, as witnessed in the leaves falling from the trees. Clearly, the life cycle is no longer expanding; there is instead a contraction of the energy. As a Chinese poet once observed, at this season "no leaf is spared for its beauty." Rather than a concern with quantity, the autumn brings with it a sense of quality. From Earth, our thoughts turn towards Heaven; this is the season for connecting to the Spirit. Having completed the active stages of the elements, it is time to turn inward and be in touch with the essence of things.

For the human condition, the autumn of our lives is the season for finding tranquility and peace. Our work in the world concluded, we can now withdraw attention from outside involvement and turn towards cultivation of the Spirit. Again, we see the Mother-Child progression of the elements operating, as we move from the tasks of growth, expansion and harvest, to uncovering the hidden meaning. Like the autumn leaves, we must embrace the process of letting go, as we face the limits of life. It is now clear that, even with the best of intentions, there are paths that will not be traveled, dreams that will not be fulfilled. Often, the task at this stage is to make peace with how our lives have gone, and find acceptance. One way to facilitate this process is through a "life review" that allows re-examination of what may previously have been considered regrets or mistakes. From the perspective of this stage of life, we may discover that certain actions were not mistakes at all, but indeed necessary for the lessons that were needed. When we can reframe events and see them as essential aspects of our development, it brings meaning to the journey.

An appreciation for the officials of the Metal element is helpful here. The Colon is responsible for releasing, in addition to food that cannot be utilized by the body, all aspects that no longer nourish us. This is a function that is essential if we are to let go of old judgments and embrace how events have unfolded. We can see why the ancient Chinese associated grief with an imbalance in Metal, and how a healthy Colon allows us to flow with life's changes so that we don't succumb to depression at this stage. There is also a letting go that is required for us to detach from things of the world. It now may be useful to lighten our burden and give away material possessions. Once empty, it is possible to bring things in on another level. It is the Lung official that then allows us to take a deep inspiration, which is to say "bring in the Spirit." It is no accident that self-esteem, as well, depends upon the Metal element. For example, a person who is too attached to their physical body at this stage is doomed to disappointment, no matter how many cosmetic surgeries are performed. Only by meeting the task of the Metal stage, and transitioning to a non-material perspective, can a person accept growing older with all its inherent challenges.

Carl Jung, through his own inner explorations and work with clients, was deeply aware of these natural cycles. He stated that, in his experience, no patient in the second half of life was truly healed unless they re-established a connection to a religious outlook. In his essay, *The Stages of Life*, he describes the process of growing older in a way that reflects Five Element wisdom:

> **Aging people should know that their lives are not mounting and expanding, but that an inexorable inner process enforces the contraction of life. For a young person it is almost a sin, or at least a danger, to be too preoccupied**

with themself; but for the aging person it is a duty and a necessity to devote serious attention to himself. After having lavished its light upon the world,the sun withdraws its rays in order to illuminate itself."

What a beautiful metaphor for the patterns we are describing. It is only through fully expressing the Wood, Fire and Earth stages that one can rest in the peacefulness of the Metal time.

Awareness of these cycles allows us to embrace the rhythms of life and brings a perspective that is in harmony with the way things are in nature.

I treated a woman in her early 70's who was well known in our community as a singer in chorales and church groups, and had some professional experience in opera. She had brought inspiration to many through an ability to transmit the Spirit through music and yet, before she came in for treatment, had decided to give up singing completely. As her physician, I wondered whether this indicated a problem and if her retirement was a sign of depression. When I explored this with her, she was able to state with clarity, "I have done that work, it was fulfilling and now it is over." Knowledge of the Five Element model allowed me to see that she had indeed completed the harvest and this transition was healthy. Her "letting go" was very much in harmony with her stage of life. Had she not lived her path, and still had "unlived life," it would have been different; in this case her work in the world was over and she was accepting the autumn time. Chinese medicine provided a lens that confirmed what this woman intuitively knew to be the natural pattern.

It is important to emphasize that the Metal phase does not preclude a person from undertaking a new project, developing their creativity, or even returning to old expressions. What is essential is that the endeavors be approached with an attitude more appropriate to this stage of life. In fact, about a year later, this patient developed diarrhea and bronchitis, indicators from a Five Element perspective of a possible imbalance in the Colon and Lung officials. As we together evaluated what the symptoms were saying about the functions of letting go and taking in, it led to reconsidering her decision. Eventually, she came to the conclusion that it was now right for her to resume singing, and even told me, "I am having a springtime within the autumn." This statement implied that her creativity (Wood) was being expressed with the quality of Metal - and it was remarkable to observe the sense of ease she brought to her musical expression. She was far less concerned with issues of achievement or success, and was able to sing for the enjoyment of herself and a few close friends. Instead of bursting forth into new activities, as would be suitable in the springtime of life, she simply allowed the Spirit to move through her and gave it voice. The wisdom of life experience was reflected in the "calmness within the activity" apparent in her work.

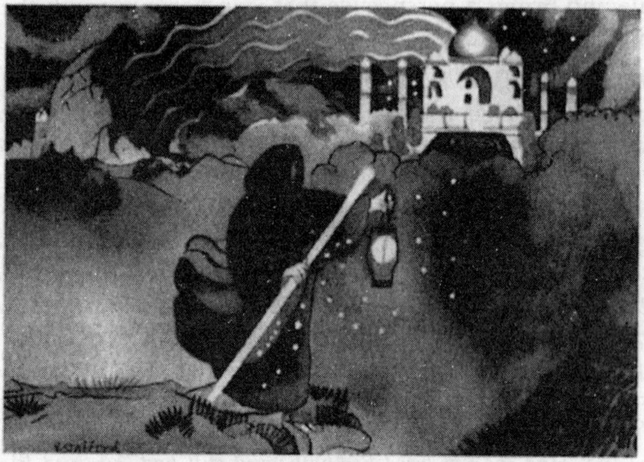

The Sage, The Archetype of Awareness

BY GARY DOLOWICH, M.D., B.AC.

In the Jungian model, the Metal element, so preeminent in the autumn of life, corresponds to the Sage archetype. This is the embodiment of wisdom and awareness, the image of the magician or wise elder. It is Merlin in the Arthurian legends and, in a modern day archetypal epic, Yoda in the Star Wars movies - the master of esoteric knowledge who deals with the world of the Spirit.

As with each of the archetypes, the Sage is an energetic potential within. However, we often first become aware of its existence on the outside through the psychological mechanism of projection. For example, we may first see this inner quality in the guru (or any teacher), who makes us aware of its existence and holds this energy for us. The goal ultimately is to reclaim this archetype for ourselves, and the person in a mentor role, if truly serving a greater purpose, will empower their students in this direction. Likewise, in the healing arts, we also operate under the image of the Sage, as we draw upon highly specialized information not generally available to the common person. When the health care provider claims to be "the healer" (an over identification with the archetype), it relegates the client to the role of the sick, dependent patient. For healing to take place, the practitioner needs to be able to own their own humanness, which includes their wounded side. The recipient of the care can then constellate their healer within (the inner Sage). This is the true goal of the therapy, as it brings growth and freedom from the constraints of the illness.

Certainly, the Sage is needed at every stage, providing the wisdom that allows the other archetypes to function optimally. For example, the history of warfare is full of magnificent warriors who fought and died for the wrong cause because they lacked awareness. When it comes to relationships, wisdom is needed in order to avoid naïveté and assess the other person realistically, keeping one's balance in the challenging world of Lover energy. It is worth noting that, in most cases, the ability to integrate these qualities develops only through making the "mistakes" that are an unavoidable part of life experience. And so we find there to be an interdependence between the archetypes, each is needed for the others to function well. Rather than a progression of separate functions, they all must work together at every age, though, as we have seen, there is an emphasis on a single archetype for each stage of the journey.

In traditional cultures, we find the Sage represented in the ritual elder who brings in the ceremonies that create a "sacred space." This is a valuable contribution to the life of the tribe, allowing regeneration through connection to the Spirit. It is understandable that this role will usually be reserved for someone later in life, as the Sage archetype can only become fully manifest after a person has experienced the spring, summer, and harvest time. It is indeed tragic the way our culture devalues the qualities that come with the elder years when, in societies more in touch with natural cycles, those in the autumn stage of their lives were honored for bringing the community meaning and wisdom.

Herbal Support to Increase Stamina & Longevity

The Metal years can be some of the most fulfilling ones we pass on this earth. By the time we reach our sixties, we know the score and a great amount of peace comes with the "knowing". Have you ever felt the calm of a quiet autumn afternoon touched by golden light? Autumn light has a special quality - it is truly magical. Our Metal years can be graced with this same quality as we sit back to tranquilly witness the elements dancing through the ever-changing seasons.

Life is never without its challenges, and retirement can usher in a period of major readjustment - especially for the workaholic. Regular, gentle exercise - walking, gardening, dancing, golf, bowling, cycling, swimming, tai chi or yoga will help maintain a positive outlook and keep us moving and flexible. This is the time to look into some of those activities that always called out to us but for which we never had time! How about taking a writing, language, astronomy or art class at the local community college? Have you always dreamed of taking a trip to the Grand Canyon, Alaska or Australia - but never made it?

In the East, age and the wisdom that accompanies it is so venerated that old Chinese people tend to stretch the truth by adding a few years to their age. Here in the West we might be tempted to knock a few years off our age when asked! In our youth-oriented society, the autumn years are devalued and frequently associated with physical difficulties like failing eyesight, aching limbs, memory loss, wrinkles and fatigue. East or West, now is the time to adopt a healthful lifestyle and look to tonifying herbs to boost immunity and build stamina. *(Note: If possible, consult with a practitioner of Traditional Oriental Medicine who can make recommendations specifically for your unique constitution).*

One of the following herbal aides might be right for you:

- **Astragalus:** Used for over 5,000 year in the East, astragalus is considered a superior herb in Traditional Chinese Medicine. Modern studies have confirmed its immune-enhancing properties. When combined with codonopsis (see below), the compound increases the activity of killer T-cells and reduces the generation of T-suppressor cells. Astragalus lowers blood pressure and is used in treating diabetes (it helps control blood-sugar levels), kidney problems and prolapsed organs.

It relieves edema, promotes urination and boosts energy.

- **Codonopsis:** This sweet, soothing herb strengthens the immune system, fights fatigue, lowers blood pressure, helps alleviate anemia and improves appetite and digestion. Also known as Dang Shen, codonopsis is less stimulating and less expensive than ginseng. It strengthens the lungs, treats bronchitis and is frequently combined with astragalus to create a powerful immune-enhancing formula.
- **Glehnia:** Sometimes referred to as the "white ginseng", this herb is not related to ginseng. However, it is an excellent tonic that is cooling (instead of warming and stimulating like ginseng). Frequently prescribed for persons who feel parched and dehydrated, glehnia strengthens and moistens the lungs. Considered a superior herb by the Chinese, it relieves dry, hacking coughs as well as constipation that accompanies this condition; it is also used to treat arthritis, rashes, acne and headaches. Glehnia is contraindicated for persons who feel chilled or who suffer from weak digestion.
- **Polygonum:** Also known as "he shou wu" or Fo-ti, this longevity herb is valued in the Orient as a kidney, liver and blood tonic that preserves youthful energy, reduces wrinkles and increases sexual potency. Fo-ti reduces cholesterol, lowers blood-sugar levels, relieves constipation in the elderly, reduces swollen lymph glands and has antibacterial properties. If taken in excess, polygonum can cause skin rash and numbness of the extremities. It should not be ingested by persons with diarrhea or weak digestion. Traditional sources caution against taking Fo-ti with chives, garlic or onions.
- **Panax ginseng:** In America, the use of ginseng has rapidly increased over the past 30 or 40 years; however, it might not be right for your particular body type. For overstimulated persons with strong constitutions, this herb can cause heart palpitations and/or insomnia, as well as feelings of anxiety. It should never be taken by those who have high blood pressure. Panax ginseng is often the herb of choice for persons who are weak or those recovering from chronic illness. It is ideal for elderly persons to increase appetite, improve digestion and aid in assimilation of nutrients. Ginseng should not be ingested with caffeine, tea, alcohol, bitter or spicy foods. It should not be taken for more than a few weeks at a time.
- **American ginseng:** This herb is considered to be the most

balanced of the Panax ginsengs and serves as both a yin and yang tonic. It is used in the recovery from infectious diseases like tuberculosis and chronic bronchitis. While Panax ginseng is warming, American ginseng is cooling and should not be ingested by persons suffering from weak digestion or diarrhea. This herb counteracts weakness, fatigue, irritability and thirst associated with chronic, low-grade fevers.

- **Eleuthero (Siberian) Ginseng:** Eleuthero is considered a more neutral herb than Panax ginseng and can be taken for a longer period of time (from two to eight months; ingest it six days per week - then rest from it for two weeks after three months). This adaptogenic herb stabilizes blood sugar levels; enhances immunity, protects us from environmental pollutants, supports the adrenals and is particularly indicated for individuals under stress. Athletes use it to enhance performance and endurance. *(For additional information, see page 166.)*

Common Complaints Associated with the Autumn Years

Circulatory Problems

Many disorders are associated with poor circulation. Stress, cold, smoking, poor diet, a sedentary lifestyle and other factors can contribute to the problem. Fatty deposits on the walls of arteries cause them to harden and constrict, resulting in arteriosclerosis. If this condition occurs in the coronary vessels, it can lead to angina pectoris (chest pain) or heart attacks; in the brain it can cause strokes. Another circulatory problem, *Buerger's disease* is seen in smokers and results in a chronic constriction of the blood vessels in the extremities. *Varicose veins* develop from faulty valves in the walls of the veins. *Raynaud's phenomenon* is a circulatory condition that most commonly affects women; blood vessels in the extremities constrict and spasm in cold weather, resulting in blanching of the extremities. Below are some recommendations to help in the care and prevention of circulatory problems:

Since poor circulation can result from a variety of different causes it is important to consult with your healthcare professional.

- **Shark cartilage: DO NOT** take any preparations containing shark cartilage if you have circulatory problems unless directed to do so by your physician. This substance inhibits the growth of new blood vessels.

- **Ginkgo & Gotu Kola:** Tribenoside is the standard drug prescribed to improve circulation in the legs - studies have shown that the combination of ginkgo & gotu kola is even more effective. Ginkgo encourages circulation of blood to the brain; gotu kola is renowned in Ayurvedic medicine as a superior herb that enhances mental clarity and calm. Both gotu kola and ginkgo are considered to be extremely safe herbal medicines that can be taken indefinitely. Research has shown that the combination of these two herbs is far more effective than either taken alone. However, over-dosage or sensitivity to ginkgo can cause dizziness, headaches or abdominal aches. If you experience any of these symptoms, reduce the amount of ginkgo you are taking.

Ginkgo also inhibits blood clotting, much like aspirin, and can decrease the risk of thrombosis leading to a stroke or heart attack. Since the effects are additive, it should not be taken together with aspirin if a person is on daily low dose aspirin therapy. - *Dr. Gary.*

No side-effects have been reported from ingestion of gotu kola. *(Additional information on ginkgo and gotu kola can be found in Chapter 7).*

- **Salvia:** Known as Dan Shen, Chinese sage or "red ginseng" (though not a member of the ginseng family), this herb is used to stimulate circulation while controlling bleeding and to strengthen the immune system. It is ingested to treat poor circulation, palpitations, bruises, menstrual pain, insomnia, coronary heart disease, breast abscesses and mastitis. It should be used cautiously in cases where blood stasis is not the issue.

High Blood Pressure

Hypertension affects more than half of all Americans over sixty-five years of age according to the U. S. Public Health Service. African-Americans have a 1/3 higher incidence rate for high blood pressure when compared to their Caucasian counterparts. This can be partly attributed to a genetic factor related to salt intake. Many African-American people have inherited a "salt-thrifty gene" from ancestors who lived in inland Africa. Salt was a scarce commodity in this area and the human body adapted to protect its reserves. High sodium intake triggers hypertension in these individuals.

A number of risk factors that contribute to high blood pressure have been identified, including: stress, cigarette smoking, excessive use of coffee, tea or other caffeinated beverages, high sodium intake, being overweight, the use of oral contraceptives, and a family history of high blood pressure.

Since high blood pressure usually causes no symptoms unless extremely elevated or complications set in, it is important to have it checked on a regular basis - three or four times a year would be a good preventive measure. Below are other suggestions to help prevent and control this all too common disorder. Many deaths associated with high blood pressure, stroke and heart attack can be prevented - be certain to consult with your healthcare professional:

- **Fiber:** Consume a healthful diet that is high in fiber from fresh fruits and vegetables such as apples, asparagus, bananas, beans (aduki, mung, black, lima, pinto, etc.), broccoli, cabbage, cantaloupe, celery, eggplant, grapefruit, winter squash, green leafy vegetables and whole grains (brown rice, millet, buckwheat, barley, oats). Avoid processed foods. See Chapter 5 for further dietary recommendations. Oat bran helps lower cholesterol levels.

- **Garlic:** Used by Egyptians over 3,000 years ago to cure tumors, heart problems, worm infestations and headache, this herb was even found in Tutankhamun's tomb. It helps thin the blood, lower blood pressure and strengthen the heart muscle. Several studies also show garlic to be a valuable anti-cancer agent. It stimulates the immune system and increases the activity of natural killer T-cells that halt the spread of cancer and other diseases. It is used by herbalists worldwide in the treatment of allergies, arthritis, arteriosclerosis, cancer, diabetes, fungal diseases, colitis, asthma, bronchitis and pneumonia. Since nature offers us an abundance of garlic and onions in the autumn season, it is always good to increase our intake of these foods during the colder months. Kyolic garlic undergoes a 20 month aging process which enhances its therapeutic properties beyond those of raw garlic. Take two capsules of Kyolic garlic three times daily with meals - six days per week.

- **Maitake, reishi and/or shiitake mushrooms** can help to reduce hypertension and prevent heart disease.

- **Hawthorn** (see page 154) is an extremely safe herbal food and medicine that has been used for centuries in Asia to treat disorders associated with an excess Fire condition. Modern medicinal extracts use its leaves and flowers while traditional preparations use the ripe fruit. Hawthorn is currently utilized to treat angina pectoris, atherosclerosis, congestive heart failure and high blood pressure. Hawthorn should be considered a long-term therapy; it may take 4 to 8 weeks for its maximum effect to take hold - this herb/food is extremely safe for long term use. The best news is that there are no known interactions of hawthorn with prescription cardiac medications or other drugs. It is even safe to use during pregnancy or lactation.
- **Coenzyme Q10:** Helps lower blood pressure and improves heart function. Ingest 100 mg daily.
- **Selenium:** Take 200 mcg daily. Our soils and foods are depleted of this important nutrient. A selenium deficiency has been linked to heart disease.
- **Calcium/magnesium:** Deficiencies in these important minerals have been linked to hypertension. Take 1,500 to 3,000 mg calcium carbonate (combined with 50% magnesium) daily.
- **Herbs to Avoid:** Licorice, Panax ginseng and ephedra (ma huang) can elevate blood pressure.

Prostate Health

Prostate enlargement (benign prostatic hypertrophy) affects approximately 50 percent of men over age 50 and 75 percent of males over 70 years of age. For more information see Chapter 5, the section entitled "Male Health: Tips for Maintaining a Healthy Reproductive System."

Recognizing and Preventing Metal Imbalances Through Life's Phases

The forces of Autumn create
dryness in Heaven and metal on Earth;
they create the lung organ
& the skin upon the body . . .

and the nose,
and the white color,
and the pungent flavor
the emotion grief,
and the ability to make
a weeping sound.

THE YELLOW EMPEROR'S CLASSIC OF INTERNAL MEDICINE

On a physical level, if our Metal element is deficient or weak, we may experience some of the following symptoms: frequent colds or flu, dry skin and hair, constipation, exhaustion, asthma or weak cough, overly bright or shiny complexion, shortness of breath on exertion, inability to let go of grief, excess or lack of perspiration.

Deficient Metal conditions require an increase of full sweet nurturing foods such as yam, winter squash, millet, barley, tofu, tempeh, black beans, salmon, halibut, and leans cuts of chicken, turkey or beef. Gentle warming spices such as ginger, cinnamon and garlic can help warm and dry clear mucus. Hearty stews filled with autumn vegetables such as daikon radish, turnips and parsnips nourish the Metal element. Apples and pears stewed with a dash of cinnamon or clove, a few raisins and pieces of walnut can provide a tasty treat. Since dryness is also an attribute of the autumn season, if symptoms such as constipation, dry hair or skin are present, it is important to increase moisture by consuming more sea veggies as well as healthful oils such as grape seed oil, olive oil, ghee (clarified butter) and sunflower, pumpkin and flax seeds.

An excess Metal condition is characterized by: dry skin and/or mucus membranes, swollen tonsils, deep mucus-producing cough, profuse nasal or respiratory mucus (may be yellow, green or gray in color), constipation or diarrhea, skin rashes, acne, hives or psoriasis, stuffiness in the head or chest, sinus headaches, judgmental behavior, inconsolable grief.

In treating excess Metal conditions, it is always important to first drain any heat (indicated by high fever, infection, yellow or green mucus, red rashes, sinus headaches) with antibiotic herbal formulas. Small amounts of spicy foods such as ginger, onions and garlic can help push out heat by promoting perspiration - however, take extreme care because this flavor can worsen heat conditions. Small amounts of the spicy roots like ginger, onions and garlic, in addition to burdock root, cabbage and cilantro in a light tofu or mung bean/barley/miso soup would be beneficial. A cooling peppermint/chrysanthemum/dandelion tea is appropriate at this time. Small portions of Metal fruits (those with thick skins) like grapefruit, lemon, lime, and orange will help cool and drain phlegm. Eat lightly until the heat has cleared and then add more Water element tonifying foods (to further drain Metal) like walnuts, pine nuts, sesame seeds, sea veggies, mushrooms, shellfish.

When our Metal element is in balance we have the ability to discern what contributes to our growth on all levels (body, mind and spirit) and release anything that no longer serves a purpose - acknowledging that which came before with gratitude, respect and integrity. Clear and precise judgment helps us determine the best actions to take in any given circumstance. We recognize the higher truths - social or spiritual - transcending individual pettiness. We honor grief and mourn each loss recognizing it is only by fully experiencing all of life's emotions that we can truly move ahead as a fuller, deeper and richer human being.

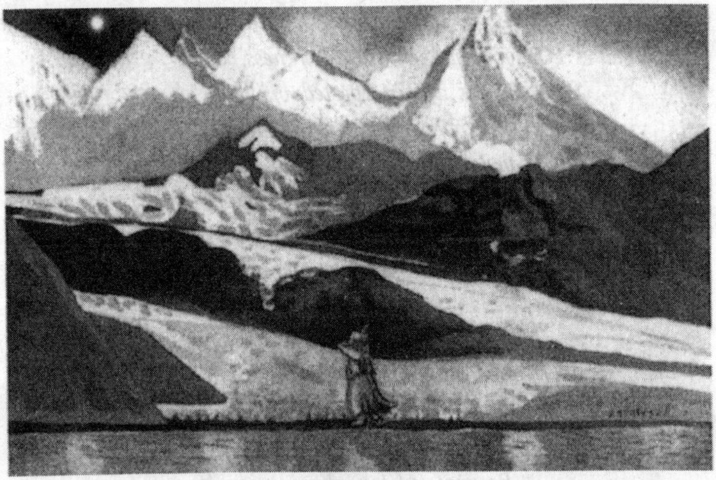

The Seeker

In mythology from cultures around the world, valiant seekers of truth venture forth on perilous journeys to unearth precious metals and jewels. Whether the quest be for the Holy grail, pearls from the dragon's lair, or the alchemist's gold - the treasure sought, interpreted symbolically, represents our internal gem of wisdom. Each of us, as we venture along life's winding path into the mountainous heights of self-knowledge, will encounter treachery, diabolical creatures and evil magicians; as well as integrity, angelic beings and fairy godmothers - each being offers a valuable lesson about our inner selves. We might be tempted to embrace only the light and run from the dark side of our psyche, but . . . we will probably just keep meeting the same archetypal forces in our external world (in the form of a friend, foe, boss, teacher, lover, partner or spouse) until we are fully open to embracing their existence within ourselves. *(For example, if we have not realized the Warrior archetype within us we might seek people out who exhibit this quality).* Have you ever finally managed to escape from one unhappy or extremely challenging relationship to find yourself in the exact same predicament - different time, different place, different person - same scenario? Life is full of surprises and potentials . . .

The Guest House

This being human is a guest house.
Every morning a new arrival.
A joy, a depression, a meanness,
some momentary awareness comes
as an unexpected visitor.
Welcome and entertain them all!
Even if they're a crowd of sorrows,
who violently sweep your house
empty of its furniture,
still, treat each guest honorably.
It may be clearing you out
for some new delight.
The dark thought, the shame, the malice,
meet them at the door laughing,
and invite them in.
Be grateful for whoever comes,
because each has been sent
as a guide from beyond.

RUMI

Through eons, deep within Earth's molten layers, precious Metals were formed and refined by Fire's capacity to melt, purify and merge. Later, our human ancestors forged their first crude implements from those hard, shiny metals. Axes, knives and swords were used to separate what was deemed pure from the unpure - mold from bread or life's breath from a foe.

If our Metal element is not balanced, individuals or nations can become self-righteous and judgmental. When our minds become cold and rigid with fundamentalisms, Metal becomes a hard taskmaster - it is used as a tool for punishment. Throughout our world's history, legions marched out to conquer the infidels and acquire their treasures - the gods of the conquered become the devils of the conquerors. At the beginning of the 21st century nations still forge weapons from Metal - tanks, guns and missiles. Hopefully humankind will soon learn Metal's higher truths, that is, a spiritual quality to be found on the inside, before our Earth is destroyed in the name of God and greed.

If we do not change our direction,
we are likely to end up
where we are headed.

ANCIENT CHINESE PROVERB

The true gems that come from the Metal element are not gold, silver, diamonds or rubies . . . but pearls of wisdom. With the sharp sword of wisdom we can cut through nonsense, superstition, prejudice and discrimination to make informed decisions. When we have been burnt, hammered and chiseled through life's struggles, our heart and spirit become transformed by the pure gold of understanding. We realize all the material and mental "stuff" we have managed to accumulate and hoard over the years may only serve to weigh us down. Metal's purified essence is one of grace, refinement and innocence. We recognize that the Creation is, after all, perfect - that each one of Earth's inhabitants has the right to exist with their unique destiny to fulfill. And, no matter how weary or weak we may become . . . as long as there is breath, there is hope.

The Way is perfect like vast space
where nothing is lacking and nothing is in excess.
Indeed, it is due to our choosing to accept or reject
that we do not see the true nature of things.
Live neither in the entanglements of outer things,
nor in inner feelings of emptiness.

Be serene in the oneness of things
and such erroneous views will disappear by themselves.
When you try to stop activity to achieve passivity
your very effort fills you with activity.
As long as you remain in one extreme or the other
you will never know Oneness.

FROM HSIN HSIN MING, BY SENGSTAN

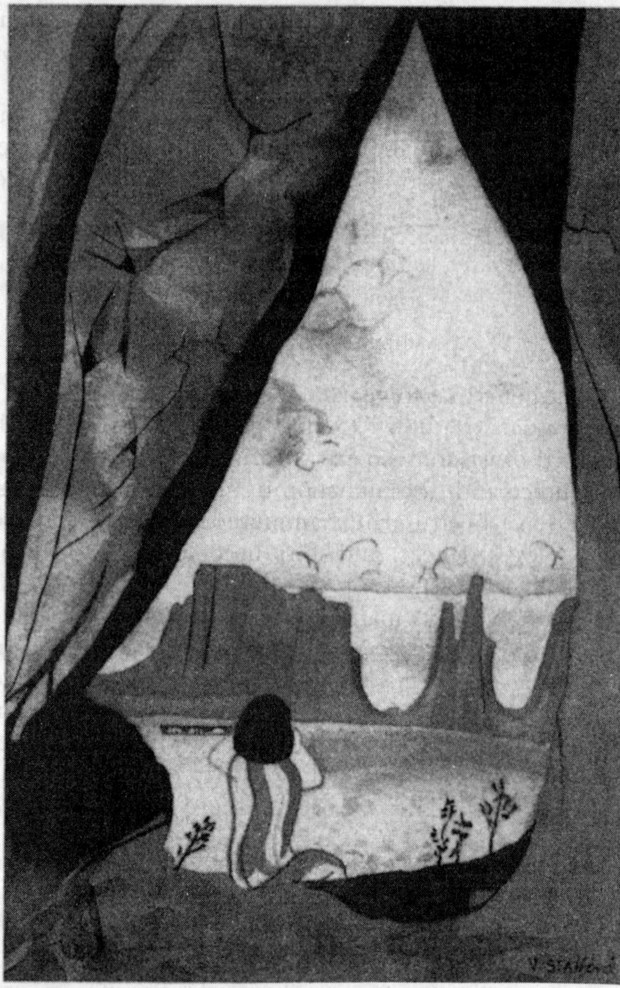

7

The Water Stage of Life Retirement & Rest

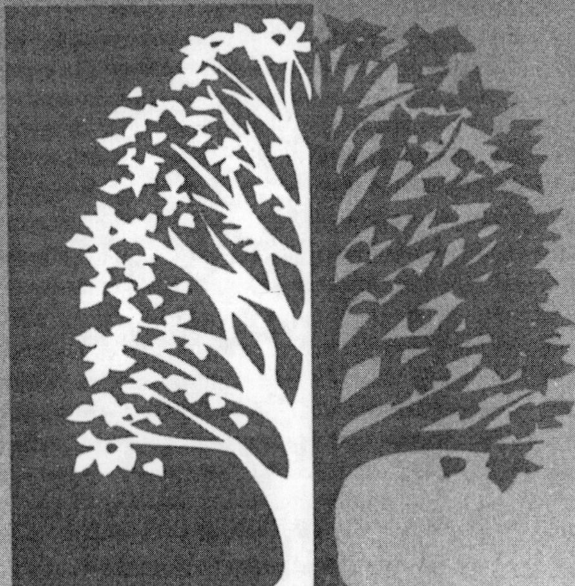

Wintertime/Water Element

BY GARY DOLOWICH, M.D., B.AC.

Inside the Great Mystery that is,
we don't really own anything.
What is this competition we feel then,
before we go one at a time, through the same gate?
RUMI

In the wintertime the downward direction in the life cycle, which began in the late summer, and continues in the autumn, moves to the next stage. The energy continues to contract, as life returns to the Source. The vegetative force is quiet now, the bears seek to hibernate, and everything descends into the stillness and darkness of winter. The ancient Chinese referred to the Water time as "the period of closing and storing." It is the completion of the circle, as nature comes to a rest, and yet also holds the seed for the activity to come. In this pause between the cycles, we sense the deep Mystery of life.

For humans, this Water phase, the winter of our lives, would correspond to old age. It is a time of rest, when we can allow ourselves to be still. Now it is imperative to withdraw attention from outside work and focus on the inner world, as one prepares for the inevitable passing. Lao Tzu, the founder of the mystical tradition of Taoism, offers this counsel:

Attain to utmost Emptiness.
Cling single-heartedly to interior peace.
While all things are stirring together,
I only contemplate the Return.
For flourishing as they do,
each of them will return to its root.

In the modern world, we face these tasks in the light of a dominant cultural bias, which values expansion and the qualities of youth. At this time nature dictates another set of priorities - learning to go inside, accepting our mortality, and finding the strength to face the fear of death. Again, understanding the natural rhythms provides support for the challenges of this stage. The Chinese concept of *yin-yang* teaches that there cannot be summer without winter, day without night. Indeed, being in touch with a deeper wisdom brings an acceptance of the wholeness of life. According to the Five Elements, the best preparation for being content in the wintertime is living fully in the earlier seasons. Only through planting the seeds in the time of Wood, experiencing the joys of the Fire element, completing the harvest of the Earth phase, and knowing the spiritual fulfillment of Metal, can we enter the Water stage without regrets. Towards the end of his life, Einstein once said: "I live in that solitude which is painful in youth, but delicious in the years of maturity." Clearly, different rules apply as one approaches the end of the journey.

I treated a woman in her 80's in my practice who had become frustrated and angry at the endless home repairs she was facing and at the irresponsibility of the contractor involved. When I reminded her that she might bring the wisdom of her years to this issue, she was able to immediately recover her sense of calmness. Through going inside, and being in touch with the richness of a life well lived, she was able to establish a perspective more appropriate to her stage of life. Once she reclaimed her balance she was also able to deal more effectively with these external demands. At this time of life her task was to hold a calm center that was deeper and more constant than the material level. Her attitude was now in harmony with the timeless wisdom of the Chinese poet Wang Wei, who said: "As the years go by, give me but peace, freedom from the ten thousand ensnarements."

D. H. Lawrence, in this poem entitled "Beautiful Old Age," describes the sense of fullness and completion that comes as we enter the wintertime of life:

It ought to be lovely to be old
to be full of the peace that comes of experience
and wrinkled ripe fulfillment.
The wrinkled smile of completeness that follows a life
lived undaunted and unsoured with accepted lies.
If people lived without accepting lies
they would ripen like apples, and be scented like pippins
in their old age.
Soothing, old people should be, like apples
when one is tired of love.
Fragrant like yellowing leaves, and dim with the soft
stillness and satisfaction of autumn.
And a girl should say:
It must be wonderful to live and grow old.
Look at my mother, how rich and still she is! -
And a young man should think: By Jove
my father has faced all weathers, but it's been a life!

D. H. LAWRENCE

In the winter, the time of stillness, we reach the end of the journey and accept the final letting go: death itself. However, when we live our lives with an awareness of the patterns in nature, it brings faith that this end is also a new beginning. By observing the natural world we know the life cycle to be recurrent, and realize that the rest of winter is essential for the whole. Only by allowing the reservoirs to fill up in winter, can there be the new growth of spring. And, just as the springtime follows the winter in nature, we sense that there are endless cycles to follow. To the degree that we can, in the later stages of life, be in touch with the Spirit and with qualities that are eternal, we can face death with dignity and grace. In experiencing ourselves to be part of the natural rhythm, we can accept that, on the deepest level, all is as it should be. The *I Ching* provides some reassurance here:

We learn by observing the beginnings and endings of life
that birth and death form one recurrent cycle.

Birth is the coming forth into the world of the visible;
death is the return into the regions of the invisible.
Neither of these signifies an absolute beginning
nor an absolute ending, any more than do
the changes of the seasons within the year.
Nor is it otherwise in the case of man.

The Calmness of the King

BY GARY DOLOWICH, M.D., B.AC.

On the archetypal level we can associate this stage with the King, largely because, in Jungian thinking, this archetype is the center of calmness. When the good king is on the throne then the entire realm is in order and there is a sense of great peace throughout the land. Essentially, the King holds the center. We can appreciate the connection to the time of retirement in the way the sovereign does not have to accomplish anything through his own activity. The ancient Chinese understood that the emperor rules from non-doing. All the other officials may have tasks to do, but it is the presence of "the Son of Heaven," on the thrown facing south, that provides order and purpose to their endeavors. This is because the true King does not rule based on his own ego, but provides a connection to the heavenly purpose, as witnessed by the crown pointing upward. When the King is ruling by Divine Will, it brings a blessing to all the subjects.

For both men and women, our world and the people who surround us can be viewed symbolically as our own individual kingdom, and it is the inner King that permits us to hold its center. Only when we have developed a relationship with this archetype can we look beyond ego needs and hold a genuine concern for the community at large. It is a connection to "the sovereign on the throne" that imbues our work with a sense of higher purpose. Through accessing the King archetype, a person can function with calmness. When a person is out of touch with this energy there may be feelings of anxiety, panic, and chaos.

Although we need this archetypal potential throughout life, it is in the later stages of our development that the King archetype becomes fully activated. This is the culmination of the development of the archetypal energies, the final piece in the jour-

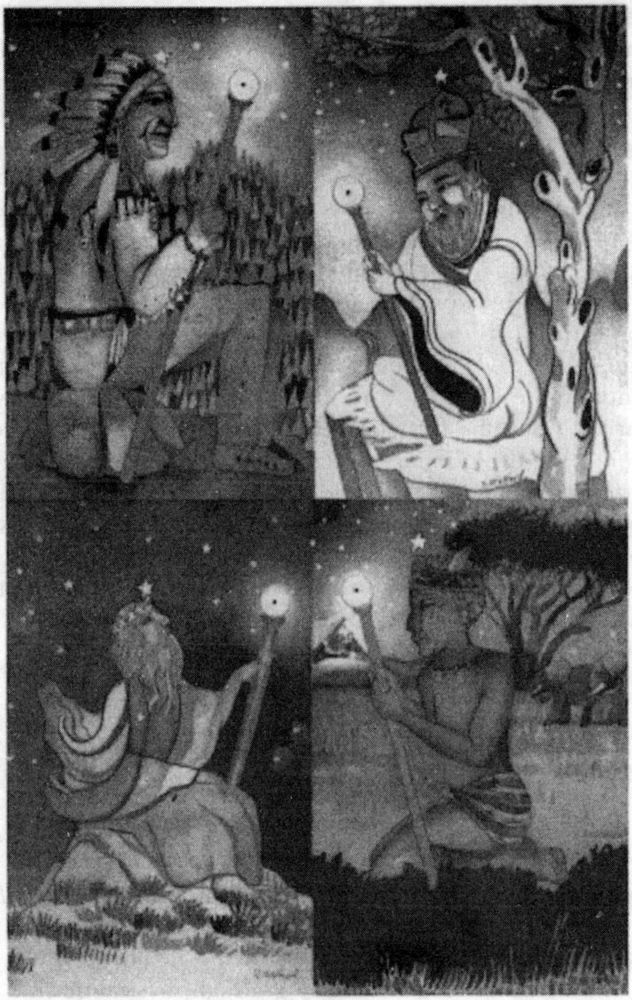

ney towards wholeness. It is only when we have completed the accomplishments of the Warrior, found the appreciation of the Lover, developed the compassion of the Queen, and cultivated the wisdom of the Sage, that we can rest in the calm centeredness of the King archetype. One can see why, in traditional cultures, it was only in the later years that a person was considered to have achieved the fullness of what it means to be a man or a woman. These societies valued their elders for holding these qualities for the tribe, recognizing the great contribution they brought to the common good by their mere presence.

Jung spoke of the goal of life as *individuation*, the process of becoming the unique individual that is our destiny. To fulfill this ideal requires the range of expressions provided by all these archetypal energies, without being taken over by any one of them. It is only through meeting the tasks of each stage in life's journey fully, with awareness, that we can approach this vision. Our map of the Five Elements offers the flexibility necessary to flow with life's changes so that we can express each phase appropriately. It is then possible to fulfill our potential and live our truth in the world, in touch with a constant core and yet responding to the ever-changing demands of the time. The image of the river comes to mind here - always different, yet essentially the same, flowing onward according to the laws of nature. To become fixated on one part of the cycle and refuse to honor the evolutionary process as life unfolds, would be akin to attempting to stop the river's flow and doomed to failure. The purpose of human life seems to be, instead, to express the wholeness of our unique self through the progression of life's stages. It is Jung's legacy to encourage us to embrace it all, as witnessed in his words: "I'd rather be whole than good."

Herbal Elixirs for Rejuvenation, Mental Clarity & Healthy Bones

The famous Greek philosopher Theophrastus,
left this world complaining that human life is too short,
it ends just when one is beginning to gain insight into its problems.

Today, more than ever, people are living healthfully and happily into their 80's and 90's. The gradual physical decline associated with graceful aging is more than compensated for by the development of wisdom. It is an inspiration to work with some of these extraordinary folks at the clinic and to have the privilege of being blessed by the experience of their years. My own grandma Lucy, a farming, Kansas prairie schoolteacher with twinkling blue eyes, kept active and alert until her last day. At 86 years old, Grandma was busy pruning her peach tree when she left this world. My uncle found her resting on a limb, with the saw still in hand and a peaceful smile on her face. Grandma always kept moving and I think that was one of the most important keys to her healthful elder years. May we all experience such a peaceful passing.

Some of the more common complaints of our elder citizens include fatigue, insomnia, incontinence, constipation, forgetfulness and brittle bones. A nutritious diet consisting of three solid meals daily with plenty of fresh fruit and vegetables and sufficient protein is essential. Also a good quality complex multi vitamin and mineral supplement is recommended. Now, let's simplify and use whole foods and some gentle, one herb aides to address those concerns associated with aging:

Rejuvenation

Please check the following tonifying herbs discussed in Chapter 6: **astragalus, codonopsis, Panax or American ginseng.** One or two of these will probably be suitable for your constitution. *Take two 250 mg tablets daily - one with breakfast and one with lunch. It is best to take these herbs only 6 days per week and rest from them for two weeks after a three month round - then repeat the round. In case of a cold, flu or infection, discontinue tonifying herbs until the imbalance has been resolved.*

Whole organic rolled oats is an excellent antidepressant tonic food that adds valuable fiber to the diet. A wholesome breakfast might include oatmeal cooked with half an apple, a dash of cinnamon and 4 or 5 walnut halves - stir in 1/2 cup of lowfat organic cottage cheese to boost protein and calcium. Once the mixture has been removed from the heat, mix in two tablespoons of freshly ground **organic flax seeds** *(for valuable Omega 3 fatty acids and to move stool)*, top the mixture with a couple of tablespoons of lowfat yogurt and a few strawberries, blueberries or slices of banana. *A dash of cardamom will antidote possible mucus producing qualities of the banana and dairy products.* Add a few drops of maple syrup or organic honey to taste. If weight or sugar sensitivity is a problem, stevia (an herbal sweetener discussed in Chapter 3) can be added to the mixture once it has been removed from the heat. If digestion of dairy products is a problem, try blending 4 to 5 ounces of organic tofu with half a banana and add it to the oatmeal instead of cottage cheese.

Mental Clarity

Medicinal usage of **ginkgo biloba** can be traced back nearly 5,000 years in Chinese medicine. In ages past it was used for memory loss in senior citizens as well as for respiratory tract ailments. Unique phytochemicals found in ginkgo increase circulation to the brain and other parts of the body. Recent animal research indicates that ginkgo may help regenerate damaged nerve cells. Ginkgo inhibits platelet stickiness and can help prevent atherosclerosis while regulating the tone and elasticity of blood vessels. Currently this herb is being used in the treatment of Alzheimer's, atherosclerosis, congestive heart failure, depression, diabetes, male impotence, migraine headaches, multiple sclerosis (to mention a few). *The dosage for seniors is generally 120 to 160 mg a day in capsule form divided into two or three doses. For severe cases of confusion and memory loss, up to 240 mg can be ingested. It may take 6 to 8 weeks before effects are noticed.*

As discussed in Chapter 6, gotu kola is often prescribed in conjunction with ginkgo biloba and you will find many herbal supplements in which the two are paired. In East Indian Ayurvedic medicine this herb is used to treat heart disease, water retention, bronchitis and as a poultice for many skin problems such as scleroderma, scars, minor burns, skin ulcers. Gotu kola boosts cognitive function and is useful in treating a number of systemic illnesses such as high blood pressure, rheumatism, varicose veins and nervous disorders. *Very few persons are allergic to gotu kola, however, it should be avoided during pregnancy and breast feeding. If taken in excessively high doses it can occasionally case nausea.*

Both gotu kola and ginkgo are considered to be extremely safe herbal medicines that can be taken indefinitely. *(However. it is always best to take any supplement only 6 days a week - rest from it the 7th. After a three month round, take two weeks off and repeat.)*

Healthy Bones

Comprehensive studies show that highly acidic substances common in our diet such as caffeine (found in coffee, tea, chocolate and cola drinks), excess animal protein, sugar and refined flour products force our body to buffer the acidity by leaching calcium and other valuable minerals from the bones. Try to moderate consumption of these products and concentrate on consuming more fresh fruits and vegetables and drinking healthful herbal teas that are packed with valuable bone-building minerals.

Nettles is rich in Vitamins A and C and is a treasure trove of those all-important bone-building minerals. In the springtime you can steam young stinging nettle leaves and consume them as a potherb. Nettle tea can be taken daily as a general tonic to relieve low energy and fatigue. At the same time, it is used to treat urinary problems (it has diuretic actions); hemorrhoids; mucous conditions of the lungs and colon; eczematous afflictions of the face, neck and ears; arthritis and rheumatism.

Chamomile tea contains highly assimible calcium. It is also effective in treating diarrhea, menstrual cramps, digestive disorders and, with ginger, for pain relief of back pain, sciatica or gout.

Regular weight bearing exercise is essential to maintain healthy bones. Since a total of 1500 mgm of calcium is generally recommended, a calcium carbonate and magnesium supplement (500 mg calcium carbonate/250 mg magnesium) 2 or 3 times daily may be beneficial (depending on the amount found in the diet). *Please see more information in Chapter 13 on sea vegetables (a valuable source of natural minerals) and on osteoporosis.*

Recognizing and Preventing Water Imbalances Through Life's Phases

The forces of winter create
cold in Heaven and water on Earth.
They create the kidney organ
and the bones within the body . . .
the emotion fear,
and the ability to make a groaning sound.

THE YELLOW EMPEROR'S CLASSIC OF INTERNAL MEDICINE

On a physical level, the Kidney/Adrenal complex is considered to be our body's battery pack (drawing on a Western metaphor). This organ system is the source of our energy, or Essence, as well as *yin* and *yang* energies. Deficiency of the Water element is therefore classified as either Deficient Kidney *Yin* or Deficient Kidney *Yang*. Because our *yin* and *yang* energies co-create each other, a prolonged deficiency in one will eventually lead to deficiency in the other.

Kidney *Yin* Deficiency is characterized by the following symptoms: insomnia, night sweats, pain in the lower back and knees, afternoon fevers, malar flush, sensation of heat in the palms of the hands and soles of the feet, scanty dark urine, dizziness, ringing in the ears, premature ejaculation, infertility, anxiety, feeling "wired but tired."

Deficient Kidney *Yin* conditions require an increase of full sweet Earth foods as well as moisturizing and cooling Water engendering foods such as apple, pear, banana, grapes, blueberries, melons, yam, cucumbers, eggplant, zucchini, winter squash, millet, barley, corn, amaranth, kamut, spelt, sweet rice, tofu, tempeh, black beans, low fat yogurt and cottage cheese, crab, clam, small portions of lean organic pork or beef, walnuts, black sesame seeds and mushrooms. Increase moisture by consuming more sea veggies; replace refined table salt with small amounts of sea salt, miso, soy sauce or tamari. Consume healthful oils such as ghee (clarified butter), olive oil and those found in nuts and seeds such as sunflower, pumpkin and flax seeds. Drink plenty of pure water.

Kidney *Yang* Deficiency is characterized by: weakness, fatigue, low back ache or pain, pale tongue, achy knees, cold extremities, fear of the cold, frequent urination, diarrhea, water retention, edema, poor appetite, impotence, infertility, wheezing, feelings of despair or paranoia - symptoms are worse in the morning.

Avoid ingesting cold and raw foods (such as salads, milk products, juices) and increase consumption of warming Metal foods and spices such as onions, garlic, fenugreek seed and ginger. Aduki beans, coix, celery, parsley, nettles, horsetail rush, as well as *ling zhi* and *fu ling* mushrooms can help resolve water retention and supply essential minerals. Daily, until the weakness and fatigue have improved, try to consume small portions of warming *yang* protein foods such as lean organic beef or pork. *(Note: Pork is thought to nourish the Kidney/Adrenals and considered to be of neutral energy in Chinese medicine).* Go easy on the sea salt, miso, soy sauce or tamari since they can increase water retention. Natural minerals found in sea veggies, walnuts, black sesame seeds and mushrooms are beneficial. *Consult a practitioner of Traditional Chinese Medicine - now might be the time to look into some tonifying herbs such as Panax ginseng. There are also a number of Chinese Patent herbal formulas that are extremely effective in treating Kidney Yin and Yang Deficiency.*

When our Water element is in balance we have the ability to flow through life's challenges in an alert state marked by gentle wisdom and quiet awareness. We easily move through feelings of fear to TRUST and have the strength to handle even the most difficult situations. We recognize how easy it is to become drowned in the endless tasks of our everyday lives and

realize that only by regularly seeking the tranquil depths of our inner self through rest and introspection can we rise again creatively to fulfill our vision and carry out commitments with calm compassion.

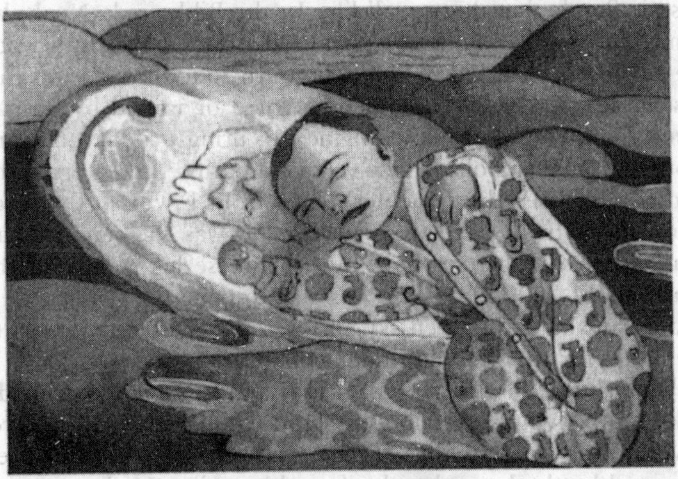

Yet the timeless in you
is aware of life's timelessness,
And know that
yesterday is but today's memory
and tomorrow is today's dream.
And that which sings and contemplates in you
is still dwelling, within the bounds
of that first moment
which scattered the stars into space . . .

KAHLIL GIBRAN

When entering the Water realm we dive deeply into the sacred inner sanctum of potentials . . . the very root of our being . . . the limitless domain of sleep, the subconscious, the emotions, procreation, creativity, archetypes, the ancestors, birth, death (or rebirth) and the Great Mystery.

From time's beginning, water has been a profound symbol for humankind. In many creation myths, water represents the womb or birthing place of the forefathers and mothers. It was along the Nile, Tigris and Euphrates, Indus and Yangtze rivers that the first great civilizations were born. In rituals that have been passed down from time immemorial, such as baptism, water

- the ultimate solvent - is used as a cleansing or purifying agent. Water possesses the power to sanctify or create but it can also annihilate.

Diverse cultures around the globe possess myths about cataclysmic floods that destroy all life. In the Bible, only Noah, his family and pairs of animals are spared from God's wrath when the earth was cleansed by the deluge. In spite of our most earnest endeavors, water cannot be formed or tamed by human hands - ultimately, only the Divine can bring order to the primordial chaos symbolized by water. God parted the waters of the Red Sea to assist the Israelites' flight from Egypt so that they could move from slavery to freedom. It was the semi-human dragon-like Great Yu, according to Chinese legends from the Xia Dynasty, 3000 BCE, who was able to tame the rising waters in a cosmic battle between sky and water to enable the earth to reemerge for the reestablishment of society.

Water is the dominion of magical creatures such as mermaids, selkies and nymphs. Symbols of fantasy, imagination and creativity, these water beings forfeit their ability to create when ensnared by the heavy bonds of earthly reality. In dreams, water symbolizes the unconscious. It is the realm of the unknown - terrifying sea monsters and creatures of the deep - most often, creations of our mind. Water serves as a bridge between worlds . . . between conscious and unconscious . . . waking and sleeping . . . birth and death or rebirth.

During periods of absolute rest tremendous transformative powers can build - giving us the vitality needed to fulfill our greatest potentials. Imagine the complete stillness experienced by a seed securely tucked under a soft, thick blanket of winter snow. By diving deeply into that utter peace and silence of the void we come to know ourselves, our hopes/our fears, our devils/our angels, our strengths/our weaknesses . . . and the archetypes by which we live. With the knowing comes integration of body/mind and spirit . . . and, ultimately, wholeness.

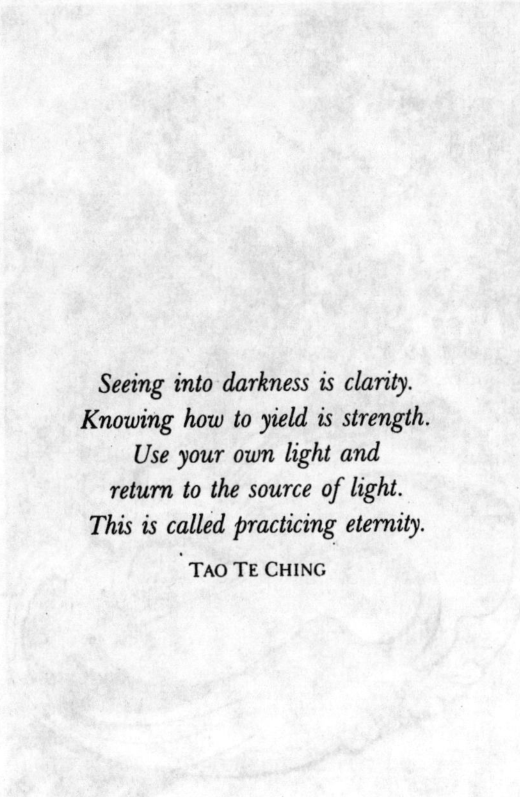

Seeing into darkness is clarity.
Knowing how to yield is strength.
Use your own light and
return to the source of light.
This is called practicing eternity.

TAO TE CHING

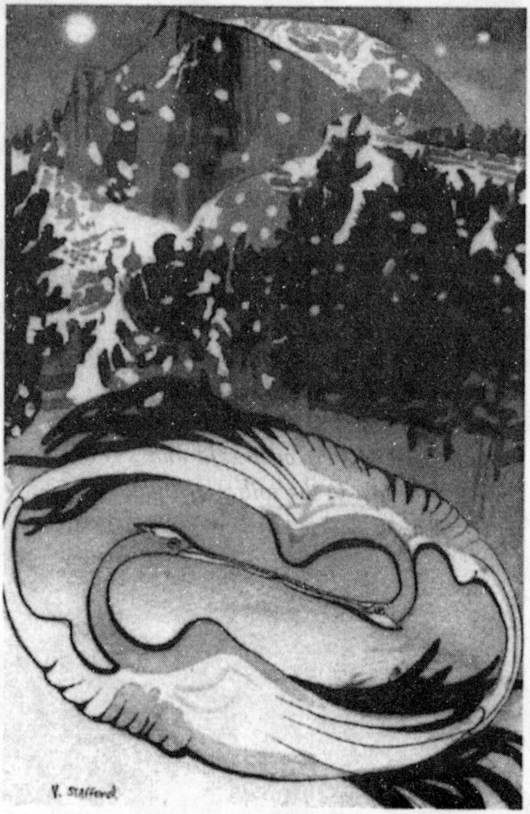

Ah, not to be cut off,
not through the slightest partition
shut out from the laws of the stars.
The inner - what is it?
If not intensified sky,
hurled through with birds
and deep with winds of homecoming.

RILKE

8

The Energetics of One

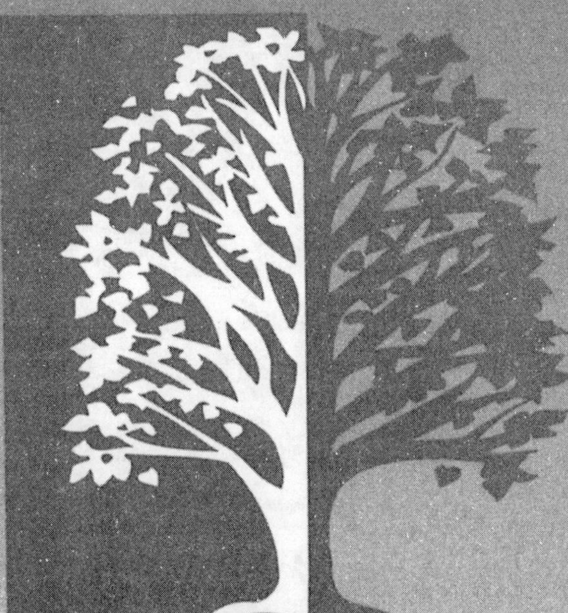

One instant is eternity.
Eternity is the now.
When you see through this one instant,
you see through the one who sees.

WU-MEN (1183-1260)

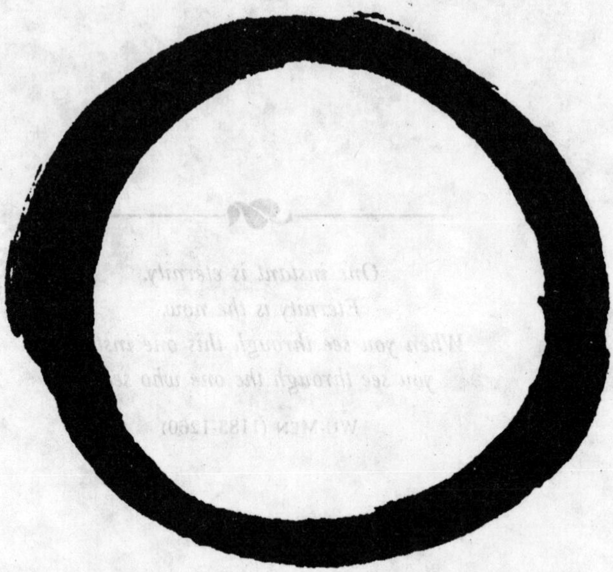

9

The Energetics of Two

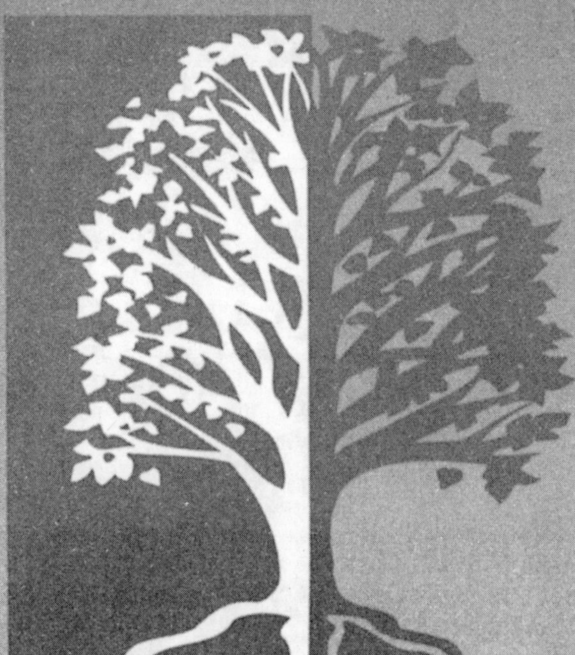

Hot and Cold Classification of Dis-Eases

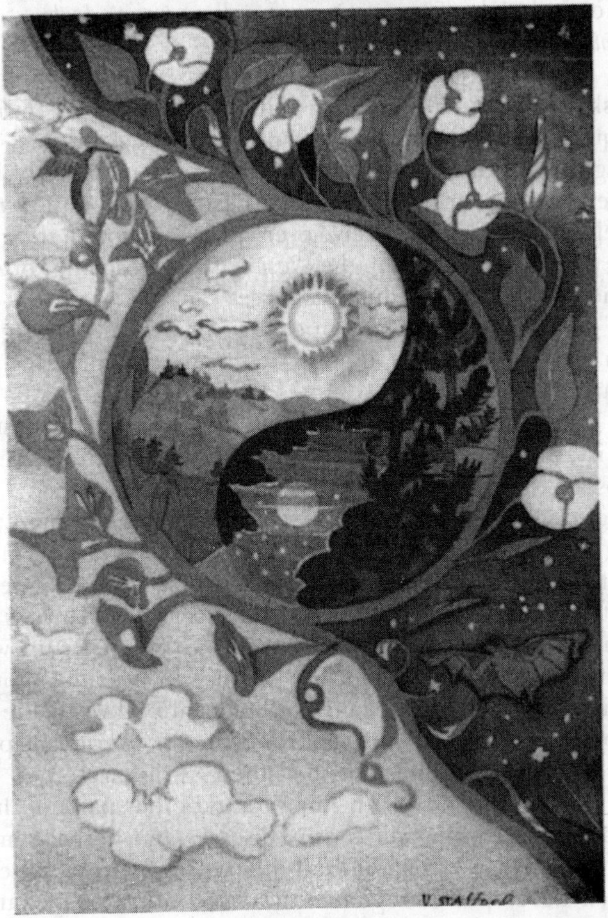

Yin/Yang in Nature

Let's take ourselves back in time some 5,000 years ago to ancient China. We live in a small settlement with six or seven other families on the eastern facing slopes of a low mountain range - a wide river cuts through the green valley below. We decided to build our hut on the eastern slope of the mountain in order to catch the warming rays of dawn's first light. In Chinese characters, the word *yang* represents the *sunny side of a mountain as well as sun, light, brightness, dryness, heat, activity and heaven.*

In the evening, when the sun disappears behind the mountain range we experience twilight cooling shade and then the cold still darkness of the night. It's time to rest when the moon and stars begin their journey across the sky and a foggy haze rises from the river below. *Yin*, in Chinese characters, refers to the *shady side of a mountain as well as moon, darkness, coolness, moisture, rest and earth.*

Our early forefathers and mothers, whether Olmec, Maya, Eskimo, Bushman, Viking, Celtic, Greek or East Indian, were equally aware of nature's two opposite stages in time - day and night. This dichotomy formed the very foundation of how they viewed the world. To this day, East or West, modern human beings continue to perceive every phenomenon in their universe in this way. However, in the West, with the teachings of Zoroaster and Aristotle, these dualistic forces came to be viewed as a pair of antagonistic bipolar opposites - black/white and good/bad. In our Western view, light is frequently considered superior to darkness.

In contrast, *yang* is not inherently better than *yin* just because it is associated with light in Asian thought. In a never-ending cosmic dance, *yin* and *yang* are constantly interacting, re-forming each other. Without day we could not have night; without light we could not have darkness; without rest we cannot have activity. The very nature of the universe is determined by the interaction of these two forces. However, the balance is dynamic and constantly changing from day to night; from winter to spring; from summer to fall. Balance in Oriental thought implies that there is a healthy relationship between the proportions of the cold *yin* principle and the hot *yang* principle; if the proportions are unequal, then there is disharmony.

In Central and South America and other parts of the world, traditional people still classify diseases and herbal remedies as "hot" or "cold". You will find differences between systems since each developed independently of the other. For example, an herb that is considered cooling in one healing system may be classified as warming in another. This is because, in some systems, the herb is classified by the energy of the disease it is used to treat - if it is used to treat a warm ailment, then the herb is classified as warm. So many misunderstandings are really a matter of semantics - it is important to delve deeply in order to thoroughly understand the unique perspective of each system of thought.

For our purposes, I prefer to present the tradition of hot/cold energetics that comes from China. This system of thought has survived, relatively untouched and in tact, for thousands of years. Shortly we are going to discover your hot and cold balance, but let's pause briefly to look at the basic theorems of this view. It is remarkable how much they sound like principles we learned in chemistry class - try substituting "positive charge" for *yang* and "negative charge" for *yin*.

Qualities of *Yin* and *Yang*

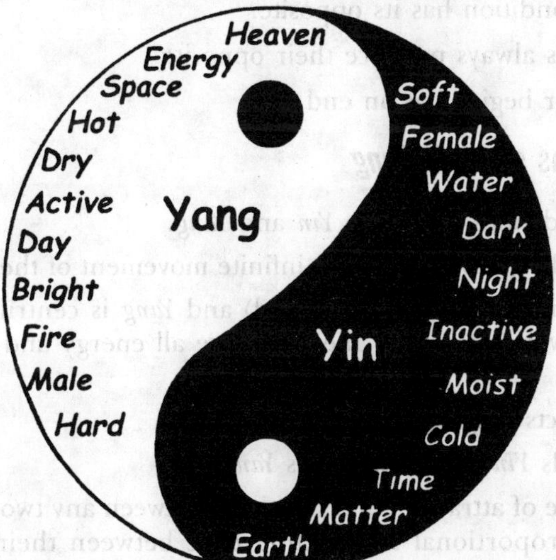

There are four principles that explain the dynamic, ever-changing relationship between *yin* and *yang*: 1) All phenomena contain two complementary aspects; 2) *yin* and *yang* are co-dependent; 3) *yin* and *yang* nurture each other; and 4) between *yin*

and *yang* there exists a transformative potential. At one of my workshops a participant asked, "If the sun represents *yang* energy, then what *yin* characteristics could possibly be attributed to it?" This is a really good question. Everything is composed of a combination of *yin* and *yang* characteristics. The sun is made of gaseous matter and while it is infinitely hot and light, it still has some substance - that substance is its *yin* nature. Everything is *yin* or *yang* relative to what it is being compared to. A rather calm, quiet, withdrawn man might be considered relatively *yin* when compared to a louder, assertive, talkative woman.

Laws Governing *Yin* & *Yang*

All things are the differentiated apparatus of One infinity. (In other words, all of creation comes from the Original Cause or God).

Everything changes.

All antagonisms are complementary.

No two things are identical.

Every condition has its opposite.

Extremes always produce their opposite.

Whatever begins has an end.

Theorems of *Yin* & *Yang*

Infinity divides itself into *Yin* and *Yang*.

Yin and *Yang* result from the infinite movement of the universe.

Yin is centripetal (spirals inward) and *Yang* is centrifugal (spirals outward); together they produce all energy and phenomena.

Yin attracts *Yang* and *Yang* attracts *Yin*.

Yin repels *Yin* and *Yang* repels *Yang*.

The force of attraction and repulsion between any two phenomena is proportional to the difference between their *Yin/Yang* constitution.

All things are ephemeral and changing their *Yin/Yang* constitution.

Nothing is neutral; either *Yin* or *Yang* is dominant.

Nothing is solely *Yin* or *Yang*; everything involves polarity.

Yin and *Yang* are relative; large *Yin* attracts small *Yin* and large *Yang* attracts small *Yang*.

At the extremes of manifestation, *Yin* produces *Yang* and *Yang* produces *Yin*.

All physical forms are *Yin* at the center and *Yang* on the surface.

Let's venture into the world of energetics. It all starts by trying to figure out the "hot and cold" or *yin* and *yang* of you and your loved ones. This is very important because, energetically speaking, we don't want to treat your dis-ease with hot or warm (*yang*) food and herbs *(like steak and Panax ginseng)* if you are basically a *yang* individual (active and assertive) or suffer from a *yang* disharmony (such as an acute, feverish condition or high blood pressure). In the interest of balance, we need to cool you down! The opposite is true if you tend to the cool *yin* side of the equation. Following is a simple test for you to take in order to determine your basic hot/cold constitutional type. *Simply circle the description that best describes your natural tendencies; then write the corresponding number that appears in the column above your selection (0, 3, 5, 8 or 10) on the blank line provided to the right. Total your score.* Review your answers with a friend or family member - often, we do not see ourselves the way others see us!

Cold or Hot

What's the Setting of Your Body's Thermostat?

	YIN			YANG		
	Cold	Cool	Neutral	Warm	Hot	
	0	3	5	8	10	TOTAL
Character	Withdrawn	Quiet	Somewhere In-Between	Assertive	Aggressive	____
Build	Emaciated or Heavy & Flabby	Slender	Medium	Muscular	Large & Stocky or Thin & Wiry	____
Activity	Lethargic	Little Movement	Normally Active	Animated	Hyperactive	____
Posture	Limp	Hunched Over	Relaxed	Erect	Rigid	____

	YIN			YANG		
	Cold	Cool	Neutral	Warm	Hot	
	0	3	5	8	10	TOTAL
Voice	Whisper	Soft	Average	Strong	Loud	____
Body Odors	Extremely Faint	Faint	Mild	Strong	Very Strong	____
Breathing	Soft Sighs	Light & Shallow	Normal	Stretching & Loud Sighing	Heavy & Loud	____
Mucus	Clear & Copious	Thin & Clear or White	White, Slight	Thick White, Yellow or Green	Thick Dark Yellow or Red	____
***Urine**	Clear	Very Pale Yellow	Golden	Dark Yellow	Very Dark Yellow or Red	____
Stool	Light Colored, Very Loose	Light & Slightly Formed	Medium	Firm & Slightly Dark	Dark & Hard	____
			Add to Determine TOTAL SCORE:			____

0 to 25: Holy Alaska, you're ready to go into hibernation! Concentrate on neutral to warm foods & herbs. Gradually introduce those of a "Hot" nature - they could present a shock to your system.

26 to 35: You are running a little on the cool side. Concentrate on neutral, warm and a few hot herbs & foods to bring yourself into balance.

36 to 65: You are basically in balance and can choose herbs and foods ranging from "Cold" to 'Hot" depending upon the climate and your state of health.

66 to 80: You are definitely running on the warm side. Concentrate on neutral to cold herbs & foods to bring yourself back into balance.

81 to 100: Hot chile peppers! It's time to schedule a cruise to the Antarctic! Consume neutral to cool foods & herbs; gradually introduce those of a "Cold" nature - they could present a shock to your system. Steer clear of contracting, icy or frozen foods; they will increase the heat by sealing it in!

**B Vitamins Color Your Urine Yellow - Discontinue Them for a Few Days to Verify the True Color.*

Balancing Hot & Cold
Choosing Herbs and Foods
That are Best for You

Now that you've arrived at your hot and cold balance in the ever-changing dance of life, following you will find pointers on how to arrive at correct decisions as to which herbs and foods will help bring you back into balance. It might have taken years for you to arrive at your present state of imbalance, so be patient. A general herbal rule of thumb is that you should count on one month of herbal and dietary therapy for each year you have had a condition.

Cold, cool or *yin* foods usually include those that grow and mature quickly like zucchini, cucumber, cantaloupe, watermelon, plums or peaches. Predominately *yin* foods tend to be large and soft. Most leafy vegetables, leaves, flowers, fruits, as well as fast-growing roots like carrot, turnip, or sweet potato are cooling. Do you tend to be warm or dry? **An herb or food that is considered *yin* cools and moistens the body and has a tranquilizing or relaxing effect.**

Warming foods and herbs, in contrast, are energizing and increase circulation. Most herbs in this category are smaller, more hard and compact than their *yin* counterparts. Hot or warming *yang* herbs are frequently slow-growing roots like ginseng, ginger, root bark or tree bark like cinnamon. *Yang* foods include most of the acid-forming foods like meat and dairy products, grains (with the exception of millet) and eggs.

Energetics of Balancing Hot and Cold

Nature provides the human body with exactly what it requires for the season of the year and the climate in which it lives. Often, herbs found thriving in warm climates (like the tropics and sub-tropics) are flowers and fruits that tend to be more cooling and eliminating in nature - like gardenia, hibiscus, bananas, papaya, mango and pineapple. People living in warmer climates need those cooling nutrients to help cool the body. On the other hand, people living in cool or cold climates require warming nutrients, and this is exactly where you find compact, warming *yang* roots and herbs like Panax ginseng (in Siberia) or nutri-

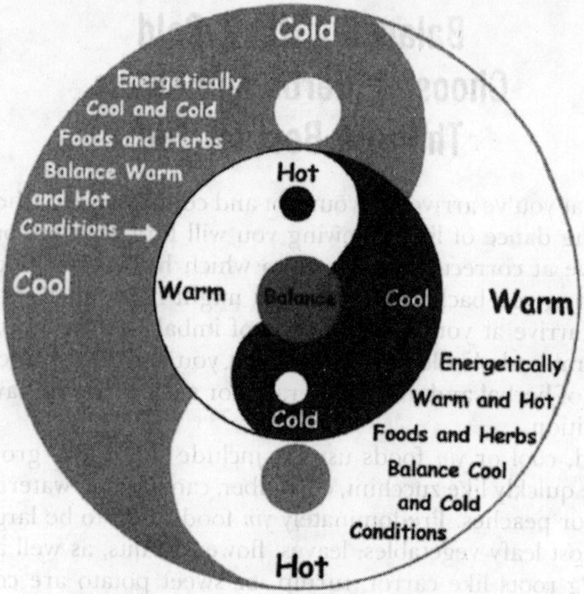

In the illustration above, the inner symbol represents your body's current condition based on *yin/yang* or hot/cold theory while the outer shaded symbol represents the balancing herbal and dietary changes needed to restore harmony.

ent-dense, heat-producing foods like seal, elk and caribou in Alaska.

Seasonally, nature offers us the herbs and foods that balance the energy of the season. For example, in spring and summer - the warm *yang* time of rapid expansion and growth - there are plenty of slightly sour and bitter fruits and vegetables that cool and contract - such as lemons, limes, apricots, strawberries and leafy greens. In the cool, *yin* autumn and winter season warming pungent root veggies and spices abound - like onions, garlic, turnips, parsnips, ginger, cinnamon and nutmeg.

Hot and Cold of Foods

On the following chart you will see foods with extreme energies at the top and bottom of the symbol. For example, refined table salt and coffee rank very high on the *yang* or heating side of the equation while sugar, alcohol and drugs can be considered very cold or *yin*. It is difficult to place these extreme items

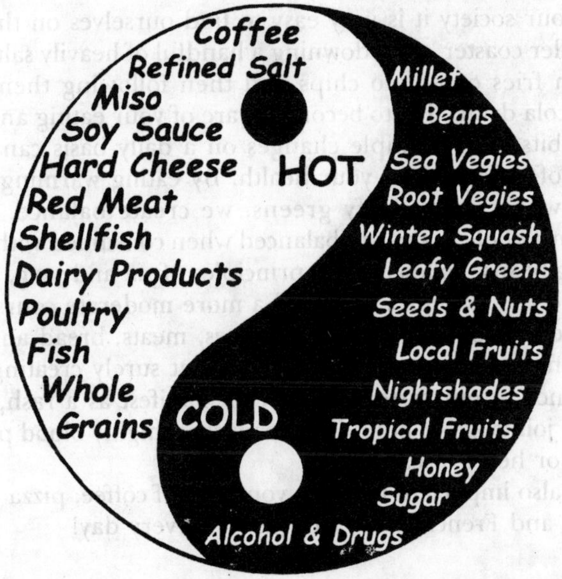

on any chart because they react differently with different body types. However, it's good to keep Theorem No. 11 in mind: At the extremes of manifestation, *yin* produces *yang* and *yang* produces *yin*. While a cup of coffee may be quite invigorating when you first drink it, your body's ultimate reaction is one of fatigue - you withdrew energy from your human battery pack (the adrenal glands) with a stimulating, empty substance that did not offer any building blocks of nutrition in return. Highly acidic foods and drinks like coffee, colas and excessive meat consumption induce the body to buffer the acidity with the release of valuable minerals, like calcium from the bones - contributing to osteoporosis and other disorders.

Thus, Knowing-How is the maintenance of life.
Do not fail to observe the Four Seasons
And to adapt to heat and cold,
To Harmonize elation and anger
And to be calm in activity as in rest,
To regulate the yin/yang
And to balance the hard and the soft.
In this way, having deflected the perverse energies,
There will be long life and everlasting vision.

THE YELLOW EMPEROR'S CLASSIC OF INTERNAL MEDICINE

In our society it is very easy to find ourselves on the sugar/ salt roller coaster - first downing a handful of heavily salted nuts, French fries or potato chips and then following them with a sweet cola drink. Try to become aware of your eating and drinking habits. A few simple changes on a daily basis can make a world of difference in your health. By eating warming protein foods with cooling leafy greens, we create balance. Slightly warming whole grains are balanced when consumed with slightly cooling beans. Following the principles of *yin* and *yang*, it is best to avoid the extremes and hold a more moderate course. If we consistently consume heating cheeses, meats, bread and coffee (ignoring the veggies) we are slowly but surely creating a heat imbalance in our system which can manifest as a rash, red inflamed joints, gout, pounding headaches, highly blood pressure, stroke or heart disease.

It's also important to enjoy your cup of coffee, pizza or hamburger and French fries - but just not every day!

In the history of human thinking
the most fruitful developments
frequently take place at those points
where two different lines of thought meet.

- Werner Heisenberg
one of the founders of quantum physics

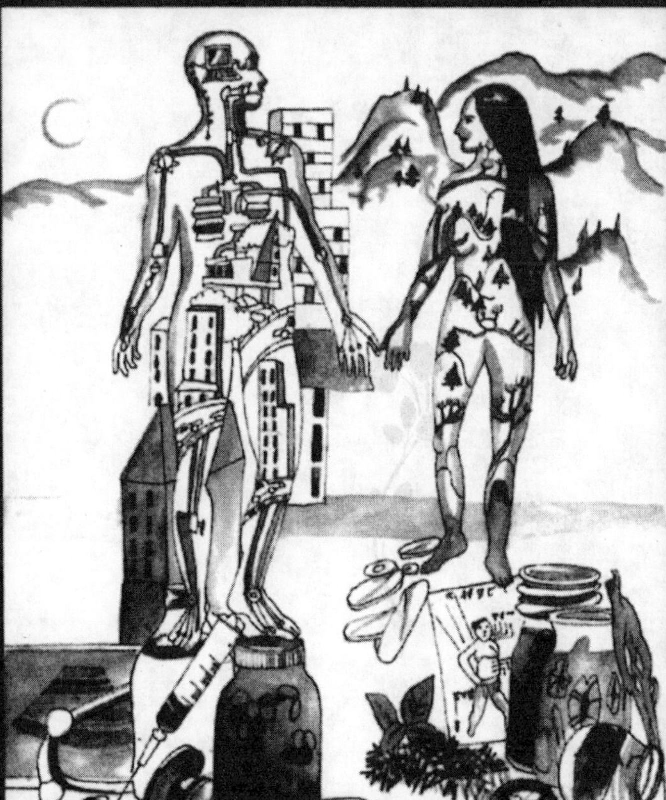

East Meets West

10

The Energetics of Three

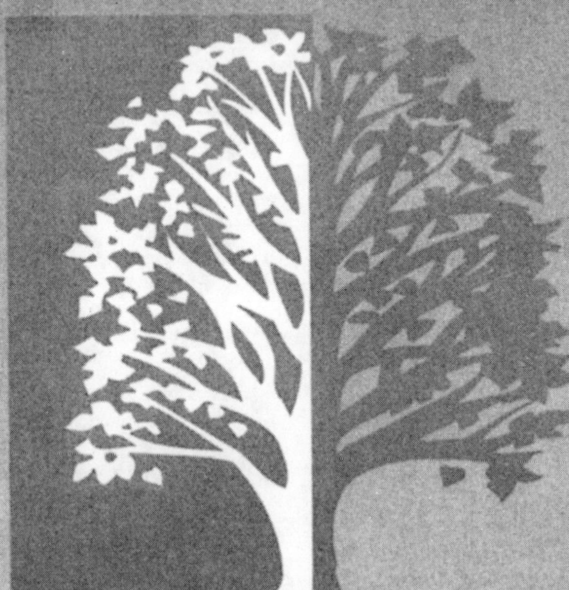

The Energetics of Three

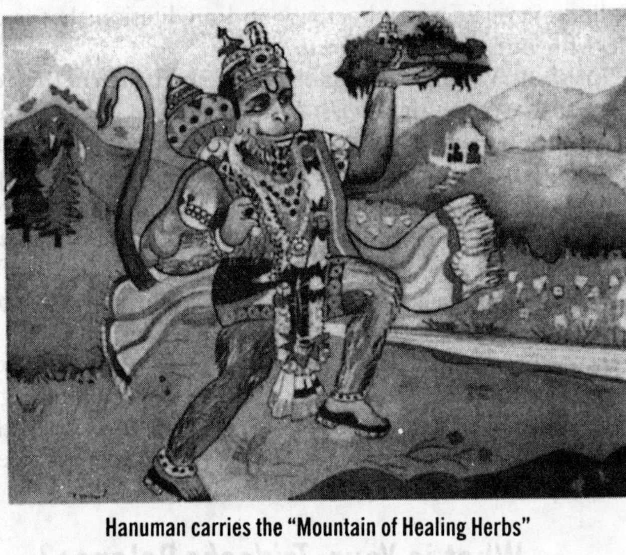

Hanuman carries the "Mountain of Healing Herbs"

If you let go of imperfection,
Perfection will appear by itself.

ANCIENT AYURVEDIC PROVERB

As discussed in Chapter 1, early East Indian people believed that the universe and our world were born from the union of two energies - male *(Purusha)* and female *(Prakriti)*. From this union sprang the five elements and all of creation as we know it. In varying degrees, the five basic elements are present in all matter, and since each human being is a microcosm of nature, these five basic elements also exist within each individual. Our personal characteristics, differences, preferences, moods, talents, tastes and even attractions to other people are dictated by the relative quantities of each element.

In Ayurvedic medicine the five elements combine to form three *doshas*: *vata dosha* is composed of the ether and air elements; *pitta dosha* - fire and water elements; and *kapha dosha* - water and earth elements. At the time of our conception, the three *doshas* united to form us - the unique body type and personality with which we were born, its inherent strengths and weaknesses - or basic nature (known as *prakruti*). According to Ayurvedic teachings, we can create balance by maintaining a certain regimen of diet, exercise, mental activity and meditation that is compatible with our original *prakruti*.

Just as the choices we make can create balance, they can also cause disharmony or illness. Each one of us, depending upon constitutional differences, reacts quite differently to the same stimuli - whether it's a bowl of chocolate ice cream, a piece of pizza, an argument with the boss or a card from a loved one. For example, if we are born with a predominantly *vata* constitution predisposed to anxiety, we would respond very differently to the caffeine in a cup of espresso as compared to a more placid *kapha* type.

Before continuing, let's find out which one or two *doshas* are predominant in your constitution. A few people are single *dosha* types while most persons have a predominant *dosha* with a secondary one that is not quite as strong. An equally balanced three *dosha* type is rare.

What is Your *Tridosha* Balance?

There are a total of 27 questions in the following test that will help determine your *tridosha* balance. Basic characteristics are listed in the first column. Decide which description most closely fit you at a time in your life when you felt healthy, happy and balanced (usually around 7 to 8 years of age or sometime dur-

Determine Your Tridosha Balance

Characteristics	Vata	V	Pitta	P	Kapha	K
Body Size	Small Slender Frame		Medium Frame		Large Heavy Bones	
Weight	Low or Underweight		Medium		Difficulty Losing Weight	
Hair	Dry, Fine, Brittle, Knots Easily		Straight, Red/Blond/Gray, Bald		Thick, Curly or Wavy, Oily	
Skin	Thin, Rough, Dry, Cold		Warm, Smooth, Shiny, Rosy		Thick, Oily, Pale, Cool	
Eye Shape and Size	Small, Active, Dark, Dry, Deep Set		Medium, Sharp, Bright, Light Sensitive		Large, Calm, Thick Lashes	
Eye Color	Brown or Black		Green, Gray, Copper, Pale Blue		Dark Blue or Brown	
Teeth	Large/Uneven/Protruding/Thin Gums		Medium/Yellow/Tender Gums/Cavities		Strong White Teeth&Gums/Few Cavities	
Lips	Thin, Dry, Chapped, Dark Tinge		Pink or Red, Inflamed, Yellowish Tinge		Pale, Moist, Smooth, Whitish Tinge	
Nose	Uneven Shape, Diviated Septem		Long, Pointed, Red Tip		Short, Rounded, Button Nose	
Chin	Thin, Angular		Tapering		Round, Double	
Neck	Long, Thin		Medium		Short, Thick	
Nails	Dry, Brittle, Break Easily		Flexible, Pink & Shiny		Thick, Smooth, Polished	
Chest	Flat		Moderate		Round & Expanded	
Stomach	Flat, Sunken		Moderate		Round or Potbelly	
Hips	Slender, Narrow		Moderate		Big, Broad, Heavy	
Joints	Dry, Cracking Sounds, Cold		Medium		Large, Well-Lubricated	
Appetite	Small, Irregular		Strong, Feelings of Being Famished		Regular, Slow and Steady	
Digestion & Elimination	Gas and/or Constipation		Fast, Loose Stools, Burning Sensation		Slow, Thick and Sluggish	
Thirst	Changeable		Craves Liquids		Very Little Thirst	
Physical Activity	Hyperactive		Moderate		Sedentary	
Emotions in Balance	Creative/Intuitive/Alert/Joyful/Loving		Bright/Disciplined/Intelligent/Altruistic		Calm/Kind/Loyal/Compassionate/Quiet	
Imbalanced Emotions	Restless/Anxious/Fearful/Lack Willpower		Critical/Competitive/Angry/Jealous		Envious/Greedy/Attached/Lethargic	
Memory	Good Short Term/Poor Long Term		Sharp		Excellent Long Term	
Speech	Rapid, Unclear		Sharp, Distinct		Soft, Slow Monotone	
Faith	Changeable		Intense, Extreme		Deep Consistent	
Sleep	Insomnia, Wakes Easily		Little but Sound		Prolonged and Deep	
Dreams	Many, Active, Fearful, Air		War, Fire, Violence		Romantic, Water	
Total	Vata		Pitta		Kapha	

ing youth) and then place a "3" in the column corresponding to *vata* (**V**), *pitta* (**P**) or *kapha* (**K**). ***Only*** if you have much difficulty in deciding between two descriptions, put a "1" in the column of the second description. Once you have completed the questionnaire, total the columns to find which *dosha* dominates your constitution. The possible total score ranges between 81 to 108 depending upon the number of 1's you used.

- The column with the highest score reveals your predominant *dosha*.
- If one of the columns is 40 or more points higher than the other two columns, then you are probably a single *dosha* type.
- If you scored 25 points or more on another column, then consider that to be your secondary *dosha*.
- Nearly equal scores on all three columns would indicate that you are a three *dosha* type.

Compare your results on the previous test to the following thumbnail sketches of the 10 basic body types in Ayurvedic medicine:

Vata: Endowed with a thin, sinewy, bony physique and a high-strung nature, people possessing a pure *vata* body type are extremely sensitive to their environment - they are intolerant of loud or sudden noises, physical discomfort and cold drafts. Joyful, creative, intuitive, quick moving, talkative and changeable, these hummingbird-like people can strike others as being unpredictable. Under duress they become anxious, excited or fearful.

Pitta: Bright, direct, focused eagle-like pitta people can strike others as being quite intense. Assertive and altruistic by nature, the orderly, decisive minds of *pitta* people love challenge and they aggressively strive to solve problems. Of medium build, warm-blooded *pitta* people cannot tolerate the heat. When under stress they become angry, critical or abrupt.

Kapha: This type is characterized by a solid, heavyset body and a calm, quiet, gentle manner. Naturally kind and compassionate by nature, they react to pressure by digging in their heels - becoming quite stubborn and silent. Their movements are slow, steady and graceful like a swan. Most people would describe the *kapha*-type as being "easy-going or relaxed".

Vata-Pitta: Similar to the pure *vata* type, *vata-pitta* people are quite thin, quick-moving and talkative but tend to be more focused and enterprising and less high-strung. Since *pitta* warmth improves circulation, they have greater tolerance for the cold.

Pitta-Vata: This type possesses the stronger medium build of the pure *pitta* person endowed with quick movement and good stamina. Most accurately described as the assertive "Type A" personality, these people are fond of a good challenge. However, in imbalance and under stress, they can become both fearful and angry as well as tense, insecure and hard-driven.

Pitta-Kapha: These people usually possess a solid *kapha* body with the intense, focused mannerisms characteristic of the *pitta* type. Naturally endowed with *pitta's* drive and energy and *kapha's* endurance, many good athletes are *pitta-kapha's*. They usually possess *pitta's* intense, critical nature with a tendency towards anger instead of *kapha* serenity and calmness.

Kapha-Pitta: These people have a strong musculature padded with a little more fat than the *pitta-kapha* types making them look rounder. Their energy level is steady and they tend to be more relaxed, easy-going and less active than *pitta-kapha* people.

Vata-Kapha: Endowed with the thin, wiry *vata* physique and *kapha's* calm, easy-going manner, this type usually has an even-temper but, when under stress, can react with anxiety. They can be quick and efficient when necessary but also have a tendency to procrastinate. Both *vata* and *kapha* doshas are cold, so these people can experience slow or irregular digestion as well as intolerance to cold weather.

Kapha-Vata: This type moves slower than the *vata-kapha* and is usually built more solidly. They are calmer and more relaxed than *vata-kaphas* with greater stamina and more athletic tendencies. They can also suffer from digestive complaints and cold intolerance.

Vata-Pitta-Kapha: There is good news and bad news regarding being a rare tridosha type. As long as balance is maintained, they tend to have good health, immunity and longevity. However, if imbalance does occur, it can become a juggling act to bring all three doshas back into balance.

Though we cannot change the ratio of the *doshas* with which we were born, to be a whole person, we need to learn the lessons that come from each of the *doshas* and live them fully. One *dosha* is not better than another - it is just different. *Vata* is related to spontaneity, sensitivity, imagination, creativity and intuition; *pitta* gives us the gifts of intelligence, confidence, discipline and drive; while from *kapha* comes our ability to be loyal, sympathetic, loving, forgiving, courageous and calm.

Making the Best Choices for Your Constitution

To balance our *doshas* does not mean that we try to change the ratio of *vata/pitta/kapha* with which we were born, *rather,* we strive to bring those natural tendencies back into balance. It is next to impossible for a round, padded *kapha* constitution to turn into a thin, wiry *vata* physique. Medium built *pitta*, round/solid *kapha* and small/slender *vata* are equally beautiful in nature's eyes; hopefully, one day we will all be able to see that beauty in each other and celebrate the differences. As Aristotle once said, "the perfect human being is all human beings put together." Each one of us, with our unique constitution and perspectives has so much to contribute to the betterment of this human experience.

While our basic body types do not change, the *doshas* are in continual flux. If we see a scary movie, listen to a waltz by Chopin or Santana's latest hit, go water skiing or eat a peanut - our *dosha* balance shifts. While we may possess an almost pure *kapha* constitution which is characterized by its calm nature, we can experience anger or fear (a *pitta* or *vata* reaction) depending on which *dosha* is moving in or out of balance. Each craving, each thought, each annoyance tells us something about the balance of our *doshas*. Ayurvedic medicine excels in its ability to detect these slight imbalances that later can turn into major disharmonies and illness if left unattended. Foods, herbs, exercises, meditation, breathing techniques and other activities help shift our *dosha* balance according to Ayurvedic wisdom.

- **Excess *kapha*** produces imbalances associated with heaviness, lethargy, depression, envy, greed, congestion, excess mucus (such as bronchitis, sinusitis, or pneumonia), diabetes, high cholesterol and edema.
- **Excess *pitta***, or heat, manifests as anger, irritability, resentment, self-criticism, fever, inflammation, hot flashes, heartburn, excessive hunger and thirst, stomach or duodonal ulcers, inflamed skin irritations, and allergies.
- **Excess *vata*** can contribute to worry, anxiety, pain, cramps, chills, spasms, high blood pressure, constipation, gas, dry skin, low stamina and other disorders of the nervous system.

Keys to Balancing Vata:

Vata dosha is considered the "king" of the *doshas* in that when it comes into balance, it pulls *pitta* and *kapha* along with it. **Regularity** in rest, meals, exercise and meditation is the key to success here. *Vata dosha* becomes imbalanced with overstimulation, mental strain, lack of sleep and subsequent exhaustion. Avoid alcohol, coffee, tea and tobacco. *Vata* is cold by nature, so *vata* predominant people should eat regular warm well-balanced meals; drink plenty of warm liquids; stay warm; massage their bodies in the morning with untoasted sesame oil before bathing; get plenty of rest and avoid loud music, violent movies as well as long hours of TV.

Keys to Balancing Pitta:

Pitta predominant people (the workaholics of the world) tend to push themselves to the limit, so the key to success in bringing this *dosha* into balance is **moderation**. *Pittas* need to schedule regular time for quiet and meditation. Coolness helps to sooth *pitta* - keep your bedroom temperature below 68 degrees and drink plenty of cool (not iced) fluids. *Pitta* people love nature - long, tranquil solitary walks beside the sea or in the mountains do wonders to calm their minds and bring balance. Pitta people tend to have runaway appetites - slowly decrease the size of your meals until you are consuming approximately two handfuls of food at each setting. *(This advice comes from Caraka, one of the founding fathers of Ayurvedic medicine).* Alcohol only further stimulates the *pitta* fire and should be avoided along with caffeine and tobacco.

Keys to Balancing Kapha:

Since *kapha dosha*, by nature, is heavy and lethargic, the key to balance is **stimulation.** Daily exercise is important to help reduce stagnation and avoid the build up of toxins. The *kapha* constitution is energy efficient - just the smell of a chocolate chip cookie can put weight on a predominately *kapha* physique. *Kapha* people need to reduce the sweet flavor in their diet - highly refined, sugary pastries, ice cream, white bread all wreak havoc with their system. *Kapha dosha* is cold with a tendency to dampness - therefore, it is important to avoid cold, damp conditions as well as cold foods and drinks. Sip on hot ginger tea between meals to promote digestion and warm the system.

Energetics of Food & Herbs According to Tridosha

In Chapter 12, the healing properties of the five flavors recognized by Chinese medicine will be discussed. Ayurvedic medicine recognizes six flavors: sweet, sour, salty, astringent, bitter and spicy. One of the major differences between the two systems is that astringency is coupled with the sour flavor in Asian medical thought. Let's take a moment to differentiate between the properties and effects of these two flavors:

According to Ayurveda, the **astringent taste** is found in foods like garbanzo beans, lentils, pears, apples, cauliflower, broccoli, cabbage and potatoes. The consistency of these foods tends to be dry and mealy (think of a grainy pear). Like the bitter flavor, the astringent taste is *vata* in nature; excess consumption contributes to gas and/or constipation. It's cooling constrictive qualities reduce the flow of body secretions such as tears, saliva or perspiration. If you are prone to anxiety, fear, gas and dryness, it will help to reduce the amount of astringent foods you are consuming. Eaten in excess, astringent foods contribute to coldness, shriveling and wrinkling. In the body, the astringent flavor decreases *pitta* and kapha *doshas* while increasing *vata dosha*.

The **sour flavor** in Ayurvedic thought is found in fermented or aged foods like alcohol, vinegar, yogurt, miso, sauerkraut and cheese. It is also found in predominately sour foods such as lemons, limes, grapes, tomatoes, plums and pineapple. This flavor aides digestion and adds savor to food but can contribute to water retention because it increases thirst. In general, fermented foods are considered to be toxic, and are associated with acidic conditions such as heartburn, ulcers and skin rashes. In the body, the sour flavor decreases *vata dosha* while increasing *pitta* and *kapha doshas*.

Each of the flavors, according to the Ayurvedic view, affects the *doshas* in a different manner (the flavor in **bold** print is the one that is most effective in reducing the ***dosha*** indicated):

Salty, sweet and sour flavors
as well as warm, heavy, oily foods balance ***vata.***

Bitter, sweet and astringent flavors
as well as heavy, cool, dry foods balance ***pitta.***

Spicy, bitter and astringent flavors
as well as light, dry, warm foods balance ***kapha***.

Each herb, food and spice has been assigned a taste profile in Ayurvedic medicine. Based on those characteristics, it increases or decreases the *doshas* - thus contributing to balance or imbalance depending upon the body type.

For example, cabbage is considered to be a sweet and astringent vegetable that dries and cools the body - therefore, it aggravates *vata* dosha which is naturally cool and dry. Ayurveda instructs us as to which herbs or foods can be eaten to counteract the affects of a particular food. For example, in the case of cabbage, someone might cook it with oil and fennel to counter any increase in *vata dosha*.

According to Ayurveda, *how* we eat affects our health just as much as *what* we eat. All our senses are equally alert during a meal - taste, sight, sound, touch and smell. Fresh fragrant food attractively served in a soothing setting appeals to those senses and enables our body to extract and process nutrients that bring balance and harmony to the body/mind/spirit. If we watch disturbing news on TV or exchange harsh words during dinner, we tense up, our stomachs knot up in distress and digestion is impaired. Food then has the potential of becoming poison instead of nourishment to our systems.

Ayurvedic wisdom recommends that we eat freshly cooked meals (seasoned with a little of each of the six flavors) at regular intervals in a pleasing environment; never eat when nervous or upset; eat at a moderate pace, thoroughly chewing each mouthful of food; minimize raw foods which are more difficult to digest; avoid consuming liquids with our meals (only a little warm water); leave the table slightly hungry (approximately 1/4 of the stomach should remain empty) to facilitate digestion; and that we allow time to sit quietly for a few minutes after eating to promote digestion.

From Darwin to Diet: Food Preferences, Intolerances and Taboos

It is important to keep in mind that all cultures have their food preferences and "taboos" For example, many Chinese people produce sufficient lactase enzyme to be able to consume dairy products without suffering from digestive disturbances. However, because milk and butter consumption was associated with the Mongolian people who invaded from the north, these food items were scorned and omitted from their diets. In contrast, milk products are an important source of protein in vegetarian East Indian cooking. To facilitate digestion, Ayurvedic practitioners recommend that milk be warmed before consumption (spices like cardamom or ginger may be added to counteract any mucus producing qualities).

For some individuals, particularly those of Dutch heritage, a reaction to gluten containing grains (wheat, rye, oats and barley) can result in digestive disturbances. In extreme cases, consumption of these grains can result in life-threatening conditions. Celiac disease, for example, is a severe degree of malabsorption of food due to gluten intolerance characterized by diarrhea, malnutrition and bleeding. The old adage, "One man's food is another's poison" is so true.

Our human ancestors evolved in entirely different geographic locations, exploiting the food sources available to them. Since it takes 20,000 to 30,000 years for minor genetic adaptations to occur, it is important to consider the foods consumed by our ancestors when constructing a diet for ourselves. Let's briefly review one example of this principle at work. Darwin found a total of fourteen species of finches on the Galapagos Islands. The ecology varies from island to island and over time, the various finch populations (though they share similar plumage, calls and nest-building techniques) evolved different feeding habits which is reflected in the size and shape of their beaks. The "cactus" finch, *Geospiza scandens*, developed a long, straight beak and forked tongue to extract nectar and pulp from cactus flowers; the "woodpecker" finch, *Camarhynchus pallidus*, uses its long, straight chisel-shaped beak to excavate insects from underneath the bark of trees; the "warbler" finch, *Certhidea olivacea*, consumes flying and ground-dwelling insects with its thin beak; the "ground" finch, *Geospiza fortis,* developed a shorter and thicker beak to feed on seeds; while the "vegetarian" finch, *Camarhynchus crassirostris*, has a short, thick, overlapping beak adapted to eating buds, leaves and fruit from tall trees.

As human populations evolved, we occupied diverse geological niches (such as Siberia, Alaska, Egypt and the rain forests of Brazil) and, depending upon our unique genetic code, we each are better adapted to consume certain foods. In the upcoming section on *vata, pitta* and *kapha* balancing diets, you will note that seafood and sea vegetables are not recommended for *pitta* or *kapha* constitutions because they are considered heavy, salty and oily in Ayurvedic thought. While refined salt, soy sauce and tamari are considered to be heating by Asian healthcare practitioners, sea veggies are believed to be cooling. If seafood was an important part of your ancestors' diet, it is quite possible that your body, to function optimally, requires these foods. In choosing the diet that is best for you, it is essential to experiment and see what works.

Energetics of Food & Herbs According to Ayurveda

Only the use of wholesome food
promotes the growth of a person,
and that of unwholesome food
is the cause of disorders.

CARAKA SAMHITA

As previously discussed, depending upon our unique constitution, we can greatly influence our health by choosing to ingest substances that either calm or aggravate our body's natural tendencies - bringing harmony or imbalance. Following are general guidelines to help balance the basic constitutional types. Each individual should make adjustments based on various considerations such as food allergies, genetic predispositions, seasons of the year, energy level, amount of exercise and their unique level of *dosha* predominance or current imbalance.

Vata-Balancing Diet

Salty, sweet and sour flavors as well as warm, heavy, oily foods BALANCE *vata*.

MINIMIZE foods, herbs & spices that are **cold, raw, light or dry** as well as **bitter, astringent or spicy in flavor.**

	Recommended	Minimize or Avoid
Oils	Read about fats on page 301. Consume healthful oils such as grape seed, ghee or canola oil for cooking. Sesame or olive oil to dress steamed veggies.	Flaxseed oil (however, freshly ground whole organic flaxseeds are recommended). Avoid margarine.
Vegetables	Emphasize moist sweet veggies such as asparagus, beets, carrots, cucumbers, green beans, okra, olives, parsnips, pumpkin, summer & winter squash, sweet potatoes, taro & zucchini. Cook cruciferous veggies (kale, broccoli, etc.) with oil & spices recommended below. Sea vegetables.	Avoid consuming raw vegetables and sprouts. Eggplant, peppers (sweet & hot), white potatoes & tomatoes.
Fruits	Enjoy sweet, heavy, sour fruits such as avocados, bananas, berries, coconut, dates, figs, grapes, kiwi, lemons, mangoes, melons, oranges, papaya, peaches, pineapple & plums.	Avoid dried fruit as well as fresh apples, pears, persimmons, pomegranates and unripe bananas.
Beans	Red lentils, mung dahl, fresh peas & small amounts of tofu.	Most beans should be avoided - they are drying & create gas in the vata constitution.

Grains	Amaranth, cooked oats, pancakes, quinoa, rice (all kinds), seitan (wheat meat), wheat.	Barley, buckwheat, corn, millet, dry oats, popcorn, rice cakes, rye, spelt, wheat bran.
Dairy	All dairy products recommended.	Avoid powdered milk and frozen yogurt.
Animal Protein	Duck, chicken, eggs, seafood, beef.	Most red meats & dry, white turkey breast.
Nuts and Seeds	Consume all nuts and seeds in moderation.	Psyllium.
Spices	Most herbs and spices can be used in moderation, emphasize the use of those that are sweet and/or heating such as allspice, anise, basil, bay leaf, cardamom, cilantro, cinnamon, clove, cumin, fennel, ginger, licorice root, marjoram, oregano, sage, tarragon, time.	Hot chilies, coriander, fenugreek, parsley, saffron & turmeric.
Sweeteners	In moderation, almost all.	White sugar, honey.

Recommended Ratio of Foods for Vata Constitutions

40 to 50% cooked, whole grains and cereals.

20 to 30% protein foods: mung dahl, red lentils, tofu, organic dairy (not non-fat), seafood, poultry & beef (if recovering from illness or surgery).

20 to 30% fresh vegetables: cooked with oil

10% fresh or stewed fruit.

Pitta-Pacifying Diet

Bitter, sweet and astringent flavors as well as heavy, cool, dry foods balance *pitta*.

MINIMIZE foods, herbs & spices that are **salty, sour or spicy in flavor** as well as those that are **steaming hot** from the stove. (Pitta predominant people require less added fat than vata predominant individuals).

	Recommended	Minimize or Avoid
Oils	Coconut, soy, sunflower, soy, grape seed, ghee or oil for cooking; olive oil is good for salads.	Almond, corn, safflower, and sesame as well as margarine.
Vegetables	Consume sweet and bitter veggies such as artichoke, asparagus, bell peppers, broccoli, cauliflower, celery, cucumber, dandelion greens, green beans, salad greens, mushrooms, black olives, cooked onion, peas, potatoes, sprouts, summer & winter squash.	Beets (raw), carrots, eggplant, garlic, leeks, hot peppers, green olives, onions, radishes, spinach, tomatoes, turnips.
Fruits	Fresh sweet fruits recommended such as sweet apples, apricots, avocado, berries, cherries, coconut, dates, figs, grapes, mangoes, sweet oranges, papayas, pears, raisins, watermelon.	Avoid sour fruits such as grapefruit, lemon, lime, pineapple, plums, rhubarb, strawberries. (If you find sweet varieties, they will be fine).
Beans	Almost all beans are fine.	Lentils, miso, soy sauce and soy sausages.
Grains	Amaranth, barley, cous-cous, granola, oats, whole	Buckwheat, corn, millet, quinoa, brown rice, rye.

Grains (cont'd)	grain pancakes, pasta, white rice, seitan (wheat meat), spelt, wheat.	Avoid breads made with yeast.
Dairy	Unsalted butter, soft cheese, cottage cheese, cow's milk, ghee, goat's milk, soft goat cheese, sweet lassi (diluted yogurt).	Buttermilk, hard cheese, sour cream, plain yogurt.
Other Protein Foods	Egg whites, chicken, turkey, pheasant, shrimp (all in small quantities).	Egg yolks, red meat & most seafood.
Nuts and Seeds	Almonds (soaked & peeled only), coconut, pumpkin seeds, sunflower seeds.	Avoid all others.
Spices	Sweet, bitter and astringent spices such as fresh basil, cardamom, cilantro, coriander, cumin, dill, fennel, fresh ginger, mint, saffron, turmeric.	Pungent, heating spices such as allspice, anise, cayenne, cloves, garlic, dry ginger, mustard seeds, nutmeg, oregano, pepper, sage, salt, thyme.
Sweeteners	Almost all sweeteners.	Honey, molasses - try to reduce the consumption of white sugar.

Recommended Ratio of Foods for Pitta Constitutions

40 to 50% cooked, whole grains & cereals

20 to 30% protein foods: Tofu, tempeh, all beans (except lentils), cottage cheese, egg whites, chicken, white turkey breast

20 to 30% fresh vegetables

10% fresh fruit

Kapha-Pacifying Diet

Spicy, bitter and astringent flavors as well as light, dry, warm foods BALANCE *kapha*.

MINIMIZE foods, herbs & spices that are **cold, oily and heavy** as well as sweet, sour or salty in flavor.

	Recommended	Minimize or Avoid
Oils	Minimize consumption: Use only small amounts of almond, ghee, grape seed & sunflower oils. Two to three tablespoons of freshly ground whole organic flaxseeds are recommended on a daily basis.	All except those listed. Avoid margarine.
Vegetables	All except the sweet, juicy ones listed.	Cucumber, olives, potatoes, winter squash, raw tomatoes & zucchini.
Fruits	Consume astringent fruits such as apples, apricots, berries, cherries, cranberries, peaches, pears, persimmons, pomegranates, strawberries. Unsulphured and unsweetened dried fruits such as apricots, figs, prunes.	Heavy, sweet & sour fruits such as avocados, bananas, coconut, dates, fresh figs, grapefruits, melons, papayas, pineapples and plums.
Beans	Almost all.	Kidney beans & tofu.
Grains	Amaranth, barley, buckwheat, corn, millet, oat bran, dry oats, quinoa, wild basmati rice, rye.	Breads made with yeast, cooked oats, pancakes, pasta, most rice, wheat.
Dairy	Small quantities of low-fat milk (preferably warmed with a pinch of	All except those listed.

Dairy (cont'd)	ginger), ghee, goat's cheese (unsalted & unaged), yogurt (diluted).	
Other Protein Foods	Eggs (not fried), chicken, turkey (white meat only), shrimp & freshwater fish.	Red meat, seafood in general.
Nuts and Seeds	Sunflower & pumpkin seeds.	All except those listed.
Spices	All except for salt.	Salt.
Sweeteners	All except for honey.	Raw, unheated honey.

Recommended Ratio of Foods for Kapha Constitutions

***20 to 30% cooked, whole grains** and cereals

20 to 30% protein foods: Most beans, seafood, chicken, white turkey breast, goat's milk, boiled or poached eggs

40 to 50% fresh vegetables

10% fresh or dried fruit

**In case of a serious imbalance such as excessive weight gain due to carbohydrate sensitivity (see pages 315 and 363) whole grain consumption may be reduced even more; see glycemic index, page 365.*

The preceding information has provided only a brief introduction to the ancient art of Ayurveda, which, translated from Sanskrit, means "the science of life and longevity." This holistic healing system empowers the individual by offering specific recommendations to enhance health through nutrition, exercise, breathing practices, meditation, rest and relaxation based on constitutional characteristics. Try to remember (or write down) your predominant *dosha* or *doshas* so that the suggestions provided in Chapter 13 will be more meaningful for you.

For recommended reading on Ayurvedic medicine, please see the Resources Section of this book.

11

The Energetics of Four

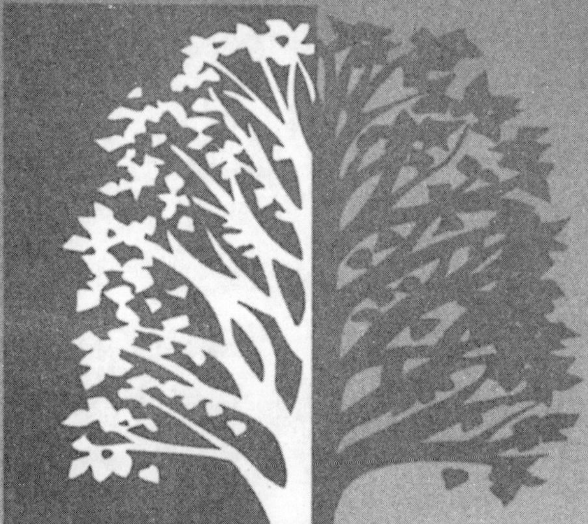

Four Directions and Four Humors

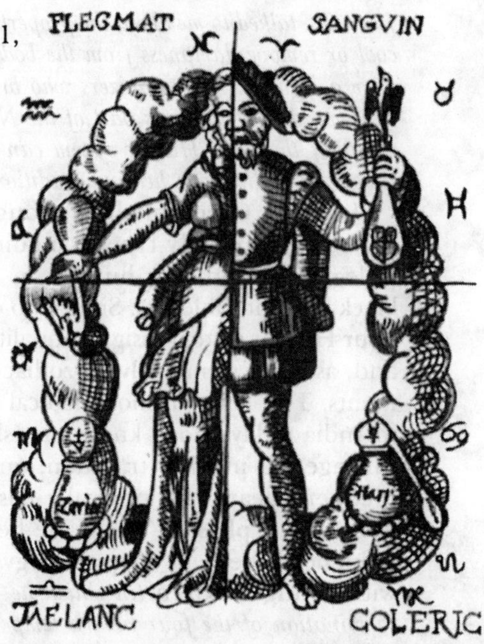

As discussed in Chapter 1, a history of thought systems based on the premise of four distinct energy patterns can be found in many cultures around the globe. Frequently, the *four directions* or *four seasons* served as the organizing principle for these complex systems of associations. For example, members of many Native American Plains tribes, in the medicine wheel tradition, categorized people according to directions: The East was associated with new ideas and imagination; North corresponded to innocence; South to wisdom; while introspection was the quality assigned to the Westerly direction.

Based on patterns of behavior, Plains Natives developed an elegant model of the human psyche. According to this tradition, each person is born with a *way* of perceiving the world that serves as a stepping off point into their life's journey - the ultimate goal being to understand others and the environment around them. Only after careful observation, tribal elders identified the path of each child: the *buffalo way* was logical and analytical; those on the *eagle way* saw patterns and tended to soar high above mundane details; the *bear way* was relational and connected to the environment; while the *mouse way* was grounded, close to the roots and details of every day life. Life's task was to master one's way of perception as well as to move around the medicine wheel in order to master each of the other views.

On the other side of the globe, the basic tenets of the Galenic Doctrine of Four Humors held that everything on earth was created from four elements: Air, Fire, Water and Earth. The cause of illness, linked to an imbalance in one of the elements, was due to an excess or deficiency in dryness, warmth, coldness, or dampness. *It is interesting to note that when I first started studying herbalism in South America over twenty-five years ago, my teacher, Juancito, talked to me about the properties of herbs that would dry, warm, cool or remove dampness from the body. I do not know if his teachings were a legacy of the colonizers who brought Four Humor theory to the new world or if this was part of the Native tradition. To this day, remnants of the Four Humor system can be found in Central and South American indigenous healing traditions.*

In early Greek medical thought, the four elements were linked to four body types (sanguine, choleric, melancholic and phlegmatic) and four humors in the body (blood, yellow bile, black bile and phlegm). Similar to other energetic traditions, the Four Humor system assigned qualities, seasons, personality traits, and, as the system evolved, zodiac signs to each of the four elements. The Four Humor medical system is still being practiced in India today and is known as Islamic Unani Medicine. While this age-old medical tradition, once practiced throughout the Mediterranean, has gradually passed out of existence in relationship to "physical" medicine here in the West, it has greatly influenced the field of psychology. From Rudolf Steiner's work with young children *(in which he maintained that each child is a combination of the four inborn temperaments with one of them being dominant)* to Carl Jung's work on psychological typology and on to the Myers-Briggs psychological profiling tests, the ancient roots of this thought system still survive and thrive. Since much of this book has already been devoted to "body and spirit", this chapter explores "mind" and the four different personality types defined by the ancient Greeks.

What is Your Four Humor Placement?

On the following page, you will find a simple test to help discover which of the Four Humors, according to Galenic thought, dominates your personal journey through life. In selecting answers to the questions, again, try not to allow cultural biases to enter the picture. Our youth-oriented society values extroversion, competition, success and endless activity. Try to answer the questions as honestly as possible - there are no right or wrong answers.

On this type of test, it is usually best to respond as quickly as possible, don't over think your answers. For each horizontal line, put a "4" in the column next to the word that most accurately describes you; if you are torn between two answers, put a "1" in the column that is the runner-up. Once you have finished, total the columns.

The element in which you scored 40 points or more is probably the one that best defines the way you live your life. A score of 25 or more on a second or third element indicates they are also significant contributors to your unique take on the world. Did you score 15 points or less on some of the humors? To create more balance in your life, could you benefit from calling on the energies of these humors?

Patterns of Behavior

Have you ever met someone that you instantly disliked or who "irked" you for no apparent reason? Do you have great difficulty in understanding or communicating with someone who you care about or must associate with - such as your spouse, child, parent, boss or co-worker? Or, are there times when you just "don't feel like yourself" and act in unexpected ways? Don't worry, it's all normal. Read on!

In this book we have discussed patterns in nature, patterns in cultures. and patterns of illness - all linked by traditional medical systems to patterns observed in nature. In this chapter we are going to explore patterns of "mind" or behavior that cut across time and through cultural, racial, religious and even family boundaries.

In his book **Psychological Types**, Swiss psychiatrist Carl Jung explored how ancient and modern cultures described human behavior. He offered his own insights about personality, which were inspired by the four humoral types, defining certain nor-

Determine Your Four Humor Placement

Air: Sanguine		Fire: Choleric		Earth: Melancholic		Water: Phlegmatic	
Carefree		Impulsive		Pessimistic		Reserved	
Lively		Restless		Withdrawn		Unhurried	
Easy-Going		Quick Tempered		Moody		Even-Tempered	
Vivacious		A Leader		Introspective		Shy	
Social Butterfly		Pioneer		Intellectual		Wise	
Talkative		Boisterous		Observer		Placid	
Workaholic		Competitive		Unsatisfied		Dreamy	
Friendly		Aggressive		Thoughtful		Obstinate	
Unreliable		Domineering		Demanding		Perservering	
Flexible		Obstinate		Resigned		Controlled	
Adaptable		Practical		Nervous		Methodical	
Responsive		Impatient		Easily Hurt		Peaceful	
Sociable		Sportive		Reader		Enjoys Routine	
Superficial		Dramatic		Quiet		Passive	
Happy		Angry		Brooding		Calm	
Chatterer		Initiator		Gloomy		Comfortable	
Colorful		Active		Sober		Slow	
Irresponsible		Intolerant		Inconsolable		Indifferent	
Eloquent		Heroic		Self-Sacrificing		Untroubled	
Total:		Total:		Total:		Total:	

mal aspects of conduct. The first distinction has to do with how human beings view the world and assimilate information: How is it we *know or perceive* things? This facet of personality is referred to as ***perception.*** Jung's second assessment dealt with the way in which people make *decisions or judgments* about things. This dimension of personality is referred to as ***judgment.*** The third overlying question that Jung defined takes into consideration the manner in which people *get and expend their energy* and their relative interest in the *inner* versus *outer world*. This aspect of the human psyche is referred to as *introverted or extraverted* ***orientation***.

Later, in the 1940's, an American mother/daughter team, Katharine Briggs and Isabel Myers expanded Jung's work by adding a fourth category that defines a person's preferred ***attitude*** when relating to the outer world. They went on to develop an invaluable counseling resource known as the *Myers-Briggs Type Indicator.* This popular personality inventory can help us better understand ourselves and others - the ways in which we form social relationships and handle interactions with our peers or family; activities that we seek and avoid; as well as types of careers to which we gravitate and in which we will feel most happy and fulfilled.

Each of the four aspects of temperament discussed above (perception, judgment, orientation and attitude) are sub-divided into pairs of opposites which ultimately combine to form sixteen distinct personality types. Each of us is born with a personality preference for functioning with one of each pair of opposites. According to Jung, our first goal along life's path is to fully develop the four aspects of the personality type with which we come into this world *(similar to the Native American medicine wheel system of thought)*. However, just when we get comfortable with ourselves, it is time to change! Later, especially in mid-life, our unconscious goal becomes one of completing our personality - bringing the dormant qualities of our psyche to the forefront. This means that the quiet introvert might find themselves reaching out to others in an extraverted way. Life is forever changing and even in our middle years and beyond, if we do not become rigid, amazingly . . . we are still growing!

Forty is the old age of youth;
fifty the youth of old age.

VICTOR HUGO

Each of the different styles of relating to the world discussed below are all normal and equally valid - one is not better or worse than the other - just different.

Perception: *Sensing* versus *Intuitive*

Sensing types are generally contented; they tend to focus on the present and on concrete information they get from their five senses. Intensely aware of their external environment, this type craves enjoyment, recreation, comfort and luxury. Sensing types are imitative and desire to do what other people do and have what other people have. Unless balanced by the judging process, Sensing types can be frivolous, sacrificing achievement to live in the moment.

Intuitive types are generally restless; living life expectantly, they pay little attention to living in the present and can be imaginative at the expense of observation. Original and inventive, they are quite indifferent to what other people have and do. Intuitive types use their initiative and enterprise in every direction of human interest. Unless balanced by the judging process, this type can be changeable and lack persistence.

Judgment: *Thinking* versus *Feeling*

Thinking types value logic above sentiment and base their decisions on objective analysis of cause and effect. Impersonal thinking types are more interested in things than in people. Having stronger executive abilities than social skills, this type will be truthful rather than tactful. Without knowing it, brief and businesslike Thinking types seem to lack friendliness and sociability. They will ignore or suppress feelings that are not compatible with their thinking judgments.

Feeling types, in contrast, value sentiment above logic and base their decisions on deeply held personal values, focusing on people-oriented considerations. People are more important to them than things. Having stronger social skills than executive abilities, this type, will usually be tactful rather than truthful. Naturally friendly Feeling types find it difficult to be brief and businesslike. They will ignore or suppress thinking that is not compatible with their feeling judgments.

Orientation: *Extraversion* versus *Introversion*

The mind of the **extraverted person** is directed towards the outer world of people and things. Their attitude is confident and relaxed - they get energized through social interactions. Extraverts can't understand life until they have lived it and are eager to plunge into new experiences. Action and achievement oriented, the extravert tends to unload any emotional baggage as they move along. A typical weakness of the extraverted personality is a tendency to intellectual superficiality. As they move through life, health and balance depend upon their ability to develop latent introverted characteristics.

Famous Extraverts

Darwin	Theodore Roosevelt
Freud	Franklin Delano Roosevelt

The mind of the **introverted person** is directed towards the inner world of impressions and ideas. Their attitude is questioning, shy and reserved - they frequently feel drained by social gatherings and require time alone to recharge. Introverts can't live life until they understand it. People of abstract invention and ideas, the passionate and intense introvert tends to bottle up emotions and carefully guard them. A typical weakness of the introverted personality is a tendency towards impracticality. As they move through life, health and balance depend upon their ability to develop latent extraverted characteristics.

Famous Introverts

Jung	Lincoln
Einstein	

In family situations alone, you can see how these two polar opposite personality types could potentially experience much conflict. The extraverted partner, who becomes energized by social gatherings, might find it extremely difficult to understand their introverted mate who desperately needs time to recharge their batteries by withdrawing from the world.

Attitude: *Judging* versus *Perceiving*

Purposeful, exacting **Judging** types live their lives in an organized fashion - their plans, standards and customs are not lightly set aside. They take pleasure in completing projects and like to get matters settled as soon as possible. Judging types believe they know what is best for other people and are not reluctant to tell them. They tend to view Perceiving types as "aimless drifters."

Tolerant and adaptable **Perceiving** types live their lives in a flexible manner - adapting to the situation of the moment. They enjoy starting new endeavors - but tend to leave them unfinished once the newness wears off. Perceiving types know what other people are doing and enjoy observing how it turns out without interfering or offering advice. They tend to view Judging types as being "only half alive."

Were you able to distinguish some of your behavior patterns in the descriptions above? Now, it is time to meet the other you - the one that lurks in your subconscious - the one referred to by Jung as the unconscious **inferior function!**

You/Me - and My Shadow

We meet ourselves in
a thousand different disguises.

CARL JUNG

When over-extended, tired or confronted by very stressful circumstances, do your own reactions sometimes come as a big surprise to you? It happens to all of us. It is as if someone we don't even know comes in and takes over our personality. For example, an introvert might find themselves suddenly seeking company at a party while an extravert may need to isolate themselves. Or, a sensitive Feeling type might find themselves being tactless. That different "you" represents the opposite side of your personality that has not.yet had an opportunity to fully develop. When things just aren't working the way we feel they should our **inferior function** or "shadow" steps in and takes over. While the experience may be unsettling for us, Jung felt such out-of-character experiences actually play a crucial role in restoring balance to the mind. **Compensation** is the term Jung coined to refer to this mechanism for correcting one-sidedness.

That shadow part of our psyche can be a great mystery to us and when we meet it in the outside world in the form of another person, it is only natural for our fears as well as fantasies or dreams to get **projected** upon them. In the process of projection we attribute qualities to other people that are actually an unacknowledged part of ourselves. We identify and magnify a certain quality that we perceive in another person and we see them as more lazy, dishonest, hostile, brilliant, talented or admirable than is really the case.

Without projection life would be a very lonely experience because this process enables us to relate to others by recognizing shared interests and values. Just as we feel secure and comfortable when we see aspects of our dominant personality characteristics in other people, we tend to feel suspicious and distrustful of persons who are very different from us. According to Jung, this process of projection is responsible for our initial feelings of attraction to, or rejection of others.

Often, when we have strong negative feelings toward another, that person is showing us our shadow - the part of ourselves we have disowned. If we stay unconscious about the process, this psychological mechanism can lead to hatred, confrontation and even, on a national scale, war. If we are able to contain these reactions, and use the situation as an opportunity for self awareness, there is tremendous potential for growth and wholeness. Likewise, powerful positive feelings often reflect an unconscious recognition of aspects of ourselves. For example, falling in love stems from finding the mysterious feminine or masculine within another. Our interest in the guru is due to the fact that this wise person holds the archetype of the sage. Ultimately, projections need to be withdrawn and these qualities found within. This opens the way for independence, self development, and, ultimately individuation. Again, most people tend to stay unconscious and depend on another person to carry these aspects for them. As the poet Robert Bly has said, "it is easier to marry these archetypes than develop them ourselves." - *Dr. Gary*

12

The Energetics of Five

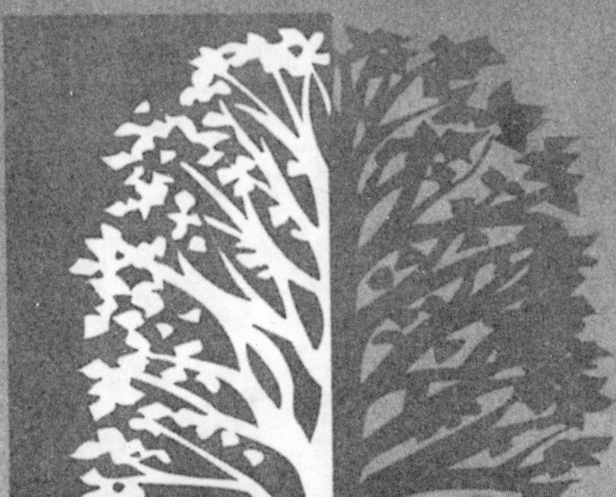

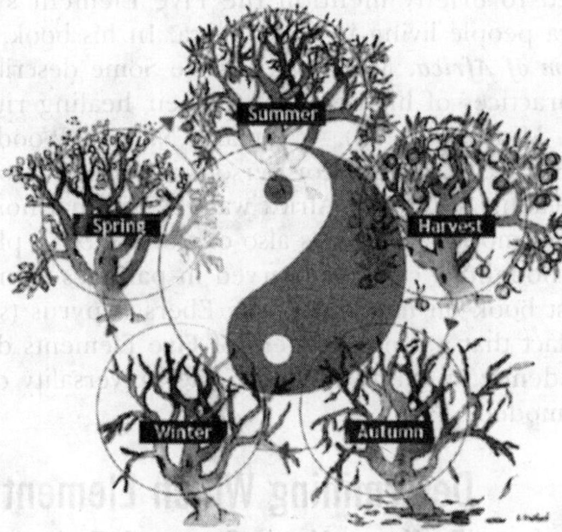

Collected together,
the ethers of the universe constitute
a Unity;
divided, they constitute
Yin and Yang;
quartered, they constitute
the Four Seasons;
still further
sundered, they constitute
the Five Elements.
These Elements represent
movement.

TUNG CHUNG-SHU

By now, you have had quite an introduction to energetic thinking! Hopefully, you have a good idea if your tendency is to "run to hot or cold" as well as your Ayurvedic and Four

Humor typology. Though each system is unique, you should see at least a couple of central themes emerging. You might find it helpful at this time to briefly review the information given by Dr. Gary in Chapter 1 on the Chinese Five Element system of thought (see page 26).

Before continuing with the Asian Five Element model, I wanted to briefly mention the Five Element system of the Dagara people living in West Africa. In his book, ***The Healing Wisdom of Africa,*** Malidoma Patrice Some describes the spiritual practices of his people and their healing rituals of Fire, Earth, Mineral (Metal), Water and Nature (Wood). This book is highly recommended for persons interested in other cultures and healing traditions. Africa was the original homeland of us all - and most likely, it was also one of the birth places of energetic thought as can be observed in passages from the world's earliest book on medicine - the Ebers Papyrus (see page 18). That fact that a similar system of Five Elements developed independently in China speaks to the universality of this archetypal model.

Determining Which Element Defines Your Central Focus

As we pass through life's stages each one of us gets countless opportunities to learn the lessons of each of the five elements - the focus of the Warrior (Wood); the delight of the Lover (Fire); the nurturance of the Mother (Earth); the spiritual quest of the Sage (Metal); and the calm serenity of the King (Water).

The Five Element System of Acupuncture teaches that each of us is governed by a single element which is the source of both our greatest strengths and our weaknesses. Professor J. R. Worsley, who brought the Five Element system to the West from China, coined the term "Causative Factor" to denote this primary imbalance that is the key to addressing a vast array of symptoms. In this book, we have chosen to use "Central Focus" to express this idea, since it has more of a Chinese flavor and avoids the implication of Western cause and effect thinking. This allows us to share the same acronym as other practitioners. The

"CF" describes the underlying pattern that becomes the organizing principle for acupuncture therapy. As we address the issues that involve this fundamental energetic, problems related to other elements tend to come into balance and health is restored. - *Dr. Gary*

On the following page, you will find a simple test to help discover which of the elements seem to be dominating your journey through life. In selecting answers to the questions, try to take yourself back to a point in time when you felt balanced - healthy and happy. Keep in mind that our cultural biases should not enter the picture here. Our society values youth, extroversion, competition, success, endless activity - these are the qualities of the Wood and Fire elements. Women are also expected to take on the nurturing qualities of Earth - but perhaps that is not you. It is possible that you have always been happiest when quietly absorbed in research or a good book; leading a dance aerobics class or attending a church service. Try to answer the questions as honestly as possible remembering there are no right or wrong answers.

On this type of test, it is usually best to respond as quickly as possible, don't over think your answers. Put a "5" in the column next to the word that most accurately describes you; if you are torn between two answers, put a "2" in the column that is the runner-up. Once you have finished, total the columns.

The element in which you scored 45 points or more is probably the one that most greatly influences the way you live your life. A score of 25 or more on a second or third element indicates they are also significant contributors to your unique take on the world; in many cases, several elements may enter into our personal Five Element equation. Did you score 15 points or less on some of the elements? Perhaps, to create more balance in your life, you could benefit from calling on the energies of these archetypes. For example, if your highest score was in Wood warrior energy, would it help you to take on some of the qualities of the Sage to temper that drive with wisdom? Remember the Control *(K'o)* Cycle of the Elements as described by Dr. Gary in Chapter 1 - a Metal ax chops Wood that is growing out of control. The *K'o* Cycle relationship allows each element to function in harmony and balance. Applying the archetypal associations of the elements, the Control Cycle brings the reserve and spirituality of the Sage to the activity of the Warrior. The vision and plan of our Wood now has quality, balanced

What is Your Five Element Focus?

Characteristics	Wood	Fire	Earth	Metal	Water
Friends describe me	as competitive	as playful	as thoughtful	as reserved	as quiet
For fun I prefer	physical activity	to go to a party	to host a family dinner	to do an art project	read a good book
I am	goal oriented	fun oriented	family oriented	spiritually oriented	security oriented
When angry I	am critical or forceful	joke or explode	am quiet & stubborn	can be cold & cutting	become sarcastic
I love	a challenge	excitement	peace & harmony	beauty & refinement	knowledge
When pushed I tend	to get impatient	become anxious	to worry	distance myself	to be inaccessible
Image I project	the first & best	bright & intuitive	friendly & loyal	discreet & disciplined	clever & articulate
I do best when I	am under pressure	am in a relationship	am needed	live a structured life	absorbed in research
I am a born	leader	optimist	nurturer	judge	critic
My body is naturally	muscular	lithe & willowy	soft & round	small & compact	lean & large boned
A health concern is	tight muscles	insomnia	difficult weight loss	dry skin & hair	backache
Sometimes I can be	perfectionistic	hypersensitive	overprotective	ungrounded	fearful
Friends say I need to	be more flexible	be more reserved	to express myself	be spontaneous	be more open
I like to be thought of	as a warrior	as a lover	as a peacemaker	as a sage	as a philosopher
I am criticized for	being too bold	too dramatic	too involved	too strict	too blunt
When tired I become	ineffectual	giddy	wishy-washy	sloppy	absentminded
I seek	adventure	romance	togetherness	meaning	wisdom
I have a tendency	to anger easily	laugh a lot	become obsessive	to feel depressed	to feel frightened
It is difficult for me	to forgive	to really relax	to take care of myself	find companionship	have faith
One of my best qualities	enthusiasm	compassion	nurturance	fairness	modesty
I know	my plan will work	love is all there is	peace can happen	life is a spiritual quest	knowledge is strength
I strongly like or dislike	the green color	the red color	the yellow color	the white color	the black color
I greatly like or dislike	the sour flavor	the bitter flavor	the sweet flavor	the spicy flavor	the salty flavor
Totals	**Wood:**	**Fire:**	**Earth:**	**Metal:**	**Water:**

by Metal's principles of connection and respect for other living beings. Similarly, just as planting trees can keep a hillside from eroding in the natural world, Earth nurturer's might find it helpful to call on Wood energy to form the boundaries so crucial for creating the time and space that care-givers need to nourish themselves.

The Five Elements dance through our lives every second of every day. When you see a child giggling in merriment - that is the Fire element. Have you heard the groan of fatigue in your friend's voice after a long day at work? That is the Water Element calling out for rest. On the following page is a Five Element Chart of Correspondences that allows us to understand each element as it is associated with a wide range of energetic expressions. Even after years of working with this model, the beauty of the Five Element system is that everyday it can be discovered anew.

Healing With the Five Flavors: Choosing the Herbs & Foods Best Suited for Your Constitution

In the preceding chart, you probably noticed that each element has a flavor assigned to it. Each of the five flavors has the ability to heal or create imbalance depending upon our unique constitution. With a knowledge of the characteristics of a substance, an experienced herbalist can discern the healing properties of its unique chemical constituents and how it will react in the human body. This is how it works:

Foods and Herbs that Build the Wood Element

Are you ready to become a real herbalist? Close observation can reveal so much information about the healing properties of an herb or vegetable and, for that matter, all the foods we ingest. For example, does the plant grow straight and tall like a corn stalk or does it cling to the earth like moss? Does its leaf feel soft and downy like that of mullein or is it smooth and ribbed like that of plantain? What is the fragrance and taste of the plant? Place a few drops of lemon or lime juice on your tongue and experience it for a few minutes as you really taste the **sour flavor**. In herbal jargon we say that lemon juice has cooling, drying and astringent properties. Notice what happens whenever you eat or drink something sour - this flavor has a drawing effect on the tissues of your mouth - you pucker up. The sour flavor affects all body tissues in the same way. *(Note: As dis-*

Chart of 5 Element Correspondences

	Wood	Fire	Earth	Metal	Water
Season	Spring	Summer	Late Summer	Fall	Winter
Color	Green	Red	Yellow	White	Blue/Black
Taste	Sour	Bitter	Sweet	Spicy	Salty
Direction	East	South	Center	West	North
Climate	Wind	Heat	Damp	Dryness	Cold
Sound	Shouting	Laughing	Singing	Weeping	Groaning
Emotion	Anger	Joy/Sorrow	Worry/Sympathy	Grief/Depression	Fear
Smell	Rancid	Scorched	Fragrant	Rotten	Putrid
Sense Organ	Eyes/Sight	Tongue/Speech	Mouth/Taste	Nose/Smell	Ears/Hearing
Body Fluid	Tears	Perspiration	Saliva/Lymph	Mucus	Urine
Body Tissue	Tendons	Blood Vessels	Flesh/Muscles	Skin/Hair	Bones
External Indicator	Nails	Complexion	Lips	Body Hair	Hair on Head
Animal	Chicken	Lamb	Cow	Horse	Pig
Grain	Wheat	Corn	Millet	Rice	Bean
Fruit	Plum	Apricot	Date	Peach	Black Cherry
Cooking Mode	Steam	Raw	Stew	Bake	Saute
Activity	Seeing	Walking	Sitting	Reclining	Standing
Quality	Growth	Ripening	Transition/Harvest	Spirit	Storage
Mother of	Fire	Earth	Metal	Water	Wood
Child of	Water	Wood	Fire	Earth	Metal
Controls	Earth	Metal	Water	Wood	Fire
Controlled by	Metal	Water	Wood	Fire	Earth
Spiritual Quality	Soul	Spirit	Thought	Instinct	Will
Positive Aspect	Focus	Love	Thoughtfulness	Spirituality	Courage
Task	Creativity	Compassion	Caring	Find Meaning	Find Inner Strength
Resolution for Emotional Imbalance	Forgiveness	Stillness	Service/Boundaries	Companionship	Faith
Yin Organ	Liver	Heart	Spleen/Pancreas	Lungs	Kidney/Adrenals
Yin Organ Time	1 a.m. to 3 a.m.	11 a.m. to 1 p.m.	9 a.m. to 11 a.m.	3 a.m. to 5 a.m.	5 p.m. to 7 p.m.
Yang Organ	Gall Bladder	Small Intestine	Stomach	Large Intestine	Urinary Bladder
Yang Organ Time	11 p.m. to 1 a.m.	1 p.m. to 3 p.m.	7 a.m. to 9 a.m.	5 a.m. to 7 a.m.	3 p.m. to 5 p.m.
Note: The Fire Element has two paired sets of organ systems - the Heart/Small Intestine & Pericardium/Triple Warmer					
Yin Organ		Pericardium			
Yin Organ Time		7 p.m. to 9 p.m.			
Yang Organ		Triple Warmer			
Yang Organ Time		9 p.m. to 11 p.m.			

cussed in Chapter 10, Ayurvedic practitioners view "astringency" as the sixth flavor. Please see page 256.)

Sour is the flavor that was assigned to the Wood element by Chinese sages and it is the flavor that helps us to keep our personal Wood element in balance. Interestingly, the energy of the sour flavor is cool, drying and contracting - exactly opposite to the warm, moist rising energy of springtime. In spring, the winter snows have melted, the days are gradually getting warmer and gentle rains encourage dormant seeds to swell, sending out tender young shoots that reach for the sun. It is precisely in springtime and early summer that Mother Nature offers an abundance of fresh fruits and vegetables with sour properties to clear our Wood element. Green is the color assigned to springtime and all green plants have a natural affinity with Wood energy. Slightly sour foods cleanse the liver of toxins accumulated over the cold winter season due to lack of exercise, and heavy foods associated with holiday celebrations. The acids in these herbs and foods (lactic, citric, malic and oxalic) act as solvents that enable the liver to eliminate fats, hormones and other chemicals from the system. Vegetables that rapidly shoot upwards on stems and stalks (the energy of spring) also have a strong correlation to the Wood element - celery, fennel, asparagus, bok choy, horsetail rush, bamboo.

Sour substances are astringent and detoxifying with diuretic and anti-microbial properties; Vitamin C contained in naturally sour foods helps build immunity to protect against spring colds and flu. Some examples of slightly sour herbs and foods would include: lemon, lime, grapefruit, blackberry, boysenberry, kiwi, quince, raspberry, sour plum, strawberry, grape, star fruit (carambola), purslane, schisandra, lemon balm, hibiscus, hawthorn berry and rose hips. *(In Ayurveda and Chinese medicine we are taught that all foods and herbs actually have two or three predominate flavors. For example, the sour flavor is found in conjunction with the sweet flavor in fruits like cherry, apple, apricot, and tomato - but let's keep it simple for now).*

Foods & Herbs That Fuel the Fire Element

One of the oldest medical texts in Traditional Chinese Medicine, the *Nei Ching* states that "the bitter flavor drains and drys". This is the flavor associated with summertime, the Fire element, and the Heart/Small Intestine and Pericardium/Triple Warmer Meridian Systems. Herbal bitters aid digestion and have anti-inflammatory, antispasmodic and antimicrobial effects. Major plant constituents that impart the bitter flavor are alkaloids (some glycosides and sesquiterpenes); in energetic thought, most of these phytochemicals are Cooling or Cold in nature while a few are Warming. The Cold bitter flavor treats Excess Fire element imbalances by draining Heat.

It's important to remember that the flavor of a food or herb tells you exactly how it is going to affect the body. In order to get a true sense of what is meant by the "bitter flavor", take a piece of endive or dandelion leaf and slowly chew on it. You might find this flavor less than appealing at first, and, indeed Americans rarely consume bitter greens. Interestingly, it grows on you and one day you might actually look forward to eating some of those steamed bitter greens for dinner. To boost your immune system, consume plenty of nature's greens (which act as natural antibiotics) during the spring and summer months. Without them you might have to rely on bitter synthetic pharmaceutical drugs to fight off autumn and winter infections. Several important bitter herbal medicines influence the heart. Most people are familiar with foxglove which contains digitoxin - a bitter cardiac glycoside.

Part of the appeal of coffee is its bitter flavor. I wonder if our love of coffee, beer and chocolate, with their bitter constituents, is not due to a call from nature to add more of this flavor to our diets. Unfortunately, coffee diminishes our natural mineral stores. It gives us a false start in the morning and picks us up in the afternoon when our energy begins to sag. In Asian medical thought, we are drawing valuable resources from our Kidney/Adrenal "battery-pack". Scandinavian research has demonstrated that 435 mg of calcium is excreted in the urine immediately after drinking one cup of coffee (we ingest approximately 435 mg of calcium daily in the foods we eat). You can see how easy it would be to run up a calcium deficit! More extensive research is needed to identify the exact role that excess caffeine plays in osteoporosis. Try to limit coffee intake to three or four cups a week.

Foods & Herbs That Nurture the Earth Element

If you want to come on this next taste adventure, you are going to have to take me up on a challenge. To truly taste the *full sweet flavor* of whole, natural foods, it will be necessary for you to completely eliminate *empty* refined sugars, pastries and processed foods containing sweeteners as well as concentrated sweet foods such as fruit juices, honey, cane sugar, brown sugar and maple syrup from your diet for a week or two. Earth foods are *full* of nutrients as compared to the *empty* sweet calories, devoid of any nutritional value, supplied by refined sugars and starches. The *full sweet flavor* associated with the Earth element is found in beans, whole grains, root veggies, winter squash, nuts and seeds, low fat dairy products, fish, poultry, lean organic meats, and tonifying herbs. Once your palate has been cleared you will be amazed at the natural sweetness so many of these foods possess; the great side benefit is that you will now be able to taste the subtle rich flavors of different foods you have been missing!

Are you ready? Slowly chew on a spoonful of butternut squash or black beans, a bite of sweet potato, an almond, a piece of baked chicken or halibut, or a few grains of cooked brown rice - this is the full sweet flavor of nutritious, life-giving, body-building food. Earth's flavor nurtures all body tissues which require protein to rebuild and glucose as their fuel. In Chinese Medical thought, the energy of these nutrients can range from slightly Cool to Hot (see the Food and Herb Chart in Chapter 9). *(Note: Classically, all foods which promote growth are identified with the Earth element; however, because of its yang or heating nature, I have opted to associate animal protein with the Fire element. Vegetable protein from beans and grains is less heating and therefore, more neutral, which is characteristic of the Earth element.)*

The Spleen/Pancreas and Stomach meridians (as they relate to our body's digestive system) were assigned to the Earth Element in ancient Chinese medicine; as was the sweet flavor, harvest-time of the year, and yellow color (notice how most earth foods range from cream color, to yellow, to orange, to brown). The Earth element is associated with **nourishment** and **rhythmic movement** - just think of how the earth sustains and feeds us all as it moves through space and cycles through the seasons. Our choices - *what* we eat and *how* we eat it - directly affect our health and the health of our planet. Are you able to gather energy from the foods you ingest? If you consume poor quality foods, you will continue functioning, but poor eating habits will ultimately take their toll, creating disorder and disease in the body.

Sweet Earth foods are meant to be eaten with a balance of the other four flavors - the sour and bitter flavors help fight off infections, stimulate digestion and have drying effects. The spicy flavor disperses congestion and stagnation - the salty flavor cools and moistens while providing essential mineral salts.

Important immune-enhancing herbs that belong to the sweet Earth category include astragalus, ginseng, codonopsis, dioscorea, licorice, and jujube dates. Most full sweet foods of the Earth element increase moisture in the human body. If your human garden is too Damp (bloating or edema), look at the types of sweet foods you are ingesting. If you are over-doing it on the empty sweet side of the equation (candies, doughnuts, cookies, ice cream), that would be aggravating the situation. Since Earth has a natural tendency to accumulate dampness - certain drying foods and herbs can help: aduki beans, coix, fu ling and zhu ling. If you are experiencing Dryness (dry skin and hair, or constipation), this can be balanced by consuming more full sweet foods that moisten - like walnuts, black sesame seeds, figs, dates, mangoes, carrots, yogurt, oysters and clams.

Remember that sugar cravings can indicate protein and/or mood-enhancing hormonal deficiencies. If you are well-nourished, cravings of all kinds tend to disappear.

Foods & Herbs That Strengthen the Metal Element

Spicy, pungent or acrid was the flavor assigned to the autumn season, the Metal Element and Lung/Colon meridians by Chinese sages. To experience this flavor, bite into a clove of garlic or place a tiny bit of horseradish, Chinese mustard or cayenne pepper on your tongue - it is not subtle. If you try Chinese mustard, your nostrils will clear immediately and your ears might even turn red. Like the rapidly expanding energy of springtime, the spicy flavor is usually warm or *yang* - it mimics the actions of Wood and Fire by rapidly penetrating, rising and expanding outward. Now, think of the energy of autumn - exactly the opposite is happening. Nature is contracting; the temperature is cool or *yin*, leaves are drying and the sap is sinking into the roots of the trees. Right on cue, Mother Nature offers us an abundance of roots and vegetables (like onions, garlic, leeks, ginger, horseradish, turnips and parsnips) to help balance the contracting energy of the season. These spicy roots are harvested in late summer and fall, just in time to help build our immunity to avoid those going-back-to-school colds and flu. Many pungent foods like garlic, leeks and onions are also rich in sulfur - a natural antibiotic.

An imbalance in our Metal element can set the stage for excess phlegm or dryness, colds, flu, bronchitis, pneumonia, constipation and other bowel irregularities. The nose opens into the Lungs and our sense of smell is related to Metal - as is mucus, the body fluid associated with this element. The spicy flavor contains essential oils and resins that irritate and dry the mucus membranes, increasing the circulation of blood and lymph while counteracting phlegm production.

White is the color assigned to autumn and many of Metal's roots and vegetables are white or pale in color: onions, garlic, leeks, scallions, parsnips, turnips, daikon radish, potatoes, cauliflower, cabbage, white pepper. *The correspondence between the appearance of an herb and its energetic affect is known as "the doctrine of signatures."* Pungent foods are divided into two categories - those that are cooling (like mint, marjoram, turnips, cauliflower and parsnips) and those that are warming (like anise, black pepper, cayenne pepper, cardamom, cinnamon, clove, ginger, mustard seed, nutmeg, garlic and onions).

Flowers possessing four petals are referred to as "cruciferous" in botany because of their resemblance to a cross. The cross has different meanings in other cultures, but here in the West it is frequently associated with a spiritual quest. How about starting your own personal health crusade? Studies from Harvard have shown that these plants contain phytochemicals that significantly protect against heart disease and stroke as well as oral, esophageal, lung, stomach and colon cancers. Following is a list of fifteen pungent or spicy life-enhancing cruciferous vegetables to nourish your Metal element: bok choy, broccoli, Brussels sprouts, cabbage, Chinese cabbage, cauliflower, daikon radish, horseradish, kale, kohlrabi, mustard greens, radish, rutabaga, turnip and watercress.

Foods & Herbs that Support the Water Element

The salty flavor was assigned to the winter season, the Water element and Kidney/Urinary Bladder meridians by the Chinese sages. While the true salty flavor is most often *yin* or cooling in nature (with the exception of Kidney *yang* tonics), refined table salt is considered to be extremely heating - with excess consumption ultimately contributing to edema, urinary difficulties, high blood pressure and heart disease.

The American diet tends to be heavily flavored with refined salt and sugar, therefore, it is difficult to experience the true salty flavor in its subtle form unless we have cleansed our taste buds for a few weeks as described in the previous section on the sweet flavor. Once you have cleared your palate, chew on a piece of dulse seaweed - this is the true flavor of mineral salts that your body requires for optimum balance. Like the contracting energy of winter, the salty flavor is usually cold or *yin* - it mimics the actions of Earth and Water by centering and settling inward and downward. While the other flavors work opposite to the energy of the season to balance it, the true natural salty flavor works in the same direction. There is a good reason for this - you can never have too much *ch'i* or essence and . . . it is all too easy to burn the candle on both ends. In Chapter 7, Kidney *Yin* and *Yang* energies were discussed: the foods and herbs that nourish Kidney *Yin* generally cool and moisten, those that nourish Kidney *Yang* are warming tonics. Even though these tonics are heating, their heavy, mineral-laden energy still settles inward and downward - stoking the slow burning coals of our body's battery pack - the Kidney/Adrenal complex.

The salty flavor stimulates the appetite, moistens dryness, softens lumps, improves digestion and provides important minerals to support the growth and maintenance of healthy teeth and bones.

Black or dark blue is the color assigned to winter - many foods and herbs that support our Water element have this coloration: black beans, black sesame seeds, black walnuts, blackberries, blueberries, eggplant, purple grapes, reishi mushrooms, sea veggies, wild rice. Mineral laden mushrooms such as shiitake, portabello and crimini thrive in dark, damp, cool conditions characteristic of the Water element.

In my practice, I often see patients who experience tremendous cravings for salty foods. Most frequently these cravings are a sign that the person is deficient in mineral salts and highly refined table salt does not supply these required nutrients. Purchase real unadulterated sea salt or earth salt at your health food store - but use it sparingly. Miso and Bragg Liquid Amino Acids are good products that supply the salty flavor along with essential nutrients.

> *Sandy, a petite 38-year-old artist consulted me a few years ago regarding two breast lumps and a number of lymph-node enlargements on her neck, under her armpits and on the soles of her feet. She consumed a typical American fast-food diet plus a can or two of salted nuts on a daily basis "just to get at the salt". Sandy's gynecologist consented to a month of acupuncture and herbal therapy before scheduling a biopsy. Sandy was able to change her diet as directed - consuming only fresh veggies, grains, beans and lots of seaweed. At the end of three weeks, the lymph-node swell-*

ings in her armpits, neck and soles were gone and the breast lumps had diminished in size. At the end of six weeks all lumps had disappeared as well as her salt cravings.

Five Element Journey

Will you come on a Five Element journey with me? Many of my patients enjoy this meditation (the inspiration for it comes directly from classes with Dr. Gary). Let your body relax into a comfortable position as you release the stresses of the day. This is your time to rebuild and recharge. If any troublesome thoughts come to mind, mentally place them in a drawer or on the kitchen table and tell them that you'll address them latter. Hopefully, they will just disappear. With all this taken care of, check in on your body. If you notice any tension, shift your awareness to that part of your body, send healing energy to the area and feel it begin to warm and relax.

You are now ready to embark on a gentle, healing journey through the Five Elements. Each one of us is a part of nature; we just need to relearn how to flow as nature does - through the five seasons. As you read through the following paragraphs, pause briefly between sentences and try to create an image in your mind of the word picture you have just read.

Let's start with the **WATER Element**, the season is **Winter** - the energy is one of complete stillness - of inward gathering. This Element holds and IS our ESSENCE. The deep water aspect of our being is centered in the area of the **Kidneys**. Locate this area in the lower back, letting go of any tension; feel the muscles relax. Surround your body in a deep blue color - indigo blue - the color of aspiration . . . the vault of the midnight sky. The quality of water is one of gentleness, humility and compassion. It relates to our very essence and is the direct link to our ancestors.

Feel the deep blue darkness. Life here is present but hidden - as it is in the Winter Season. Water is the place of beginnings - the mysterious place of THAT which is not yet known. This energy within us is the root of our being and the potential for all that will follow in the seasons to come. Winter is the season when we seek shelter as we go within to do quiet tasks while regenerating ourselves. It is the time to recharge and rebuild - the time to move through fear to TRUST. The water element calls us to renew our trust in the divine plan, the unfolding of our universe. Water is the holder of knowledge of all that is - of wisdom and the willingness to be in the state of not-knowing - a state of inquiry.

Water supports the understanding of our inner depths and exploration of the unknown. It replenishes resources and helps us flow through life. The Water Element in harmony, when not blocked by fear, is gentle - like a deep, calm sapphire blue lake inviting you to dive into its depths. Our reservoirs can then be filled as a result of rest and as the Water Element generates energy, it very naturally expands into the **WOOD Element . . .**

Notice how the dark blue color slowly transforms, surrounding your body in mists of **Green** - the green of a lush forest, a jungle, or the green of verdant hillsides in **SPRING**time. The air is fresh and crisp. This is the energy of rebirth. The creative time of new beginnings - the time of clarity, vision and intention.

Sense within yourself the power of vision and purpose, of knowing the direction of your life. Feel the power of new possibilities growing. A force, that when impeded, will manifest and be experienced as frustration and anger. Perhaps a thought comes, reminding you of when this has happened in your life - acknowledge it and then let it go. The Wood Element creates your future and gives clarity to plans and ideas.

Find the area of the **Liver** and **Gallbladder** in your body and fill it with healing spring green light. When there is tenseness in this element, our energy is not moving and feelings of impatience and frustration are experienced. When harmonious and relaxed, we can allow all things to unfold at their own pace and are not judgmental. Often, anger is a signal that calls us to forgiveness and acceptance of ourselves and others. Take a moment to enhance this quality of forgiveness and acceptance within you - and let it grow. As it expands notice how the light surrounding your body begins to take on a rosy glow - the color of sunrise. We are entering the next phase, that of the **FIRE Element . . .**

The Fire Element represents the full expression of energy as all of nature bursts forth into its maturity. In the **Summer** season - this energy is at its apex and with it comes action, enthusiasm, vitality and great joy - joy that is to be expressed and shared. Perhaps you remember such a time in your life - a time filled with carefree laughter, passion and play.

Let the brilliant flame colors of a desert sunset sweep through your body - cleansing and rejuvenating. This is the energy of sunshine, warmth and radiance. The Fire Element represents activity, intuition and motion - it gives us the force required to bring to fruition the "idea or vision" that originated with the Wood Element.

Imagine the color of a beautiful bright red velvety rose - bring the color of that light to the area of the **Heart**. Feel it pulsing and radiating out from the chest area. Greet this area and see what resides there. Take a look and ask yourself - "How is my heart?" . . .

Though you might discover some pain there, allow the warm red radiating energy of prosperity and abundance flood your chest with exuberant FIRE. This is the warmth that opens the heart and, in joy, calls us to companionship and honest friendship that is inclusive of others. Perhaps you can hear the inner sound of your own laughter bubbling up . . . feel, for a few moments, the joy that resides in your heart.

However, like all fires, this one must begin to subside . . . it can't burn this brightly forever. As it does, let the image of the field surrounding your body begin to transform in to shades of peach, then golden yellow . . . the colors of the **EARTH Element** . . .

The Earth, your Mother, nourishes you, understands you. . . the season is that of Late Summer - of **Harvest**. This is the time when fruits and vegetables, if not gathered, will rot and return to the Earth. The food that is collected during this time is meant to be distributed to others in the spirit of service, caring, sympathy and sharing. This season may hold special memories for you - mild days when all of nature seems to pause; the fragrance of honeysuckle; fields filled with golden grains drenched in sunshine - the Earth gives back for the goodness put into it. The air is fragrant; the taste of nature's ripe bounty is sweet.

Bring that golden light of Earth energy in to your solar plexus - the area of the **Stomach** and **Spleen**. Feel these organs of nourishment as they begin to relax. When there is an imbalance here, there may be tension - such as feelings of worry or anxiety - feelings due to excess thoughtfulness. You may feel off-center or have obsessive tendencies when the Earth Element is working too hard to create stability and nurturance. On the other hand, consider the quality of feeling well-nourished in all ways. You are filled with a quality of openness, fairness and sympathy for others. You are harmonious, centered and stable in your being and in your sense of HOME.

As you rest here notice that the seasons once again inevitably change and we must let go and move on. The harvest is past, the sap is sinking back into the roots, leaves are drifting to the ground, the days are becoming cooler and shorter - we are moving into the Fall Season, the time of the **Metal Element**...

In Metal, the energy of Nature is moving downward and inward. To allow this, a letting go must occur, but we are called upon to acknowledge that which has taken place, what has come before . . . with gratitude and respect.

The color of Metal is white, like the first frost shimmering opalescent in the morning light. Breathe in deeply, focusing this white healing light in the area of the **Lungs** and **Large Intestine.** Both of these organs have important functions related to letting go - letting go of the old, clearing out the waste of what has already been used. When there is imbalance in this element we may feel GRIEF or sadness about having to release - but come it must. Once we are empty, the Lungs allow us to take in the new breath. And with it comes the fresh and pure ch'i, and we are filled with quality and Spirit.

...and, as we remember the peace that comes with sweet surrender, let's relax once again into Winter, into the **Water Element**. Go deeply within yourself, glide gently into the deep blue depths to reflect, recharge and rebuild.

You have completed a journey through the 5-Elements. Each one of us is an extension of nature, and the cycles of the elements, so apparent in the world outside are inseparable from the currents that flow within our inner being. The end of one cycle marks a new beginning. Reflect on any images, words, feelings, symbols, or experiences that seemed significant to you. Review these for a moment in your mind as you remain relaxed and empty. Were any of the elements easier or more difficult to experience? Which element did you enjoy the most... the least?

13

Support for Chronic Imbalances

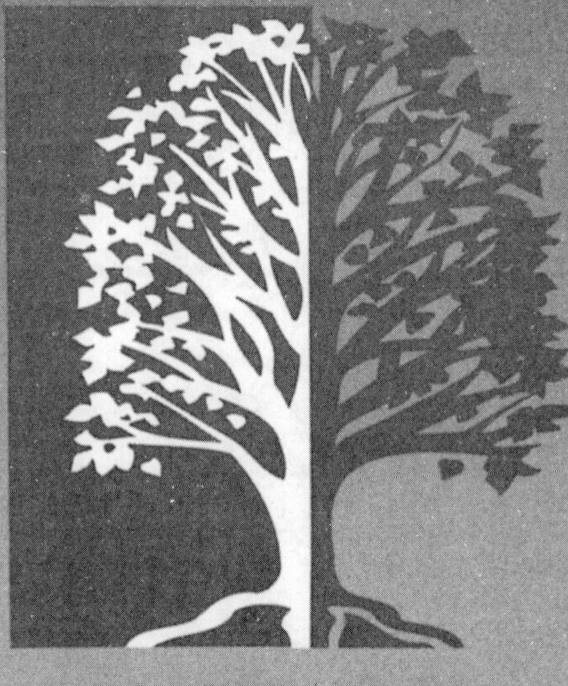

Longevity has changed little,
and the major illnesses
such as malignancy and cardiovascular disease
remain unimpeded . . .
Illnesses disproportionately affect the poor,
major environmental and occupational causes of illnesses
receive little attention and less action . . .
clearly, there is a crisis in health care,
Both in its effects upon health and in its cost . . .
Some medical outcomes are inadequate not because
appropriate technical interventions are lacking,
but because our conceptual thinking is inadequate.

H. R. HOLMAN, M.D., STANFORD UNIVERSITY

Food Allies: The First Line of Defense in Overcoming Dis-Ease

Our home,
the human body,
is miraculously constructed from
water, food, oxygen and light!

Our bodies are not solid, unchanging forms constructed from iron, steel and concrete, but constantly shifting energy systems composed of millions of living creatures - our cells. A cell from the stomach's lining lives only a few days; a skin cell lives two to three weeks and a red blood cell for two to three months. Our skin is replaced every five weeks and our seemingly solid skeletal system is replenished every three months. Radioisotope studies conducted by Oak Ridge Laboratories in California confirmed that 98 percent of the atoms in our bodies are completely replaced every year. In 1988, a San Francisco cardiologist Dr. Dean Ornish, proved that heart disease can be reversed with lifestyle changes. One group of patients in Dr. Ornish's study successfully relied on a healthful diet, yoga exercises and meditation instead of conventional surgical and pharmaceutical drug interventions to shrink the fatty deposits that blocked their coronary arteries.

The frequent occurrence of chronic degenerative diseases is relatively recent in the evolution of humankind. Over the past 100 years we have witnessed an epidemic increase in such illnesses as cancer, heart disease, AIDS, chronic fatigue, rheumatoid arthritis and auto-immune disorders. There are a number of studies demonstrating that almost 20 years "to the day" after refined, highly processed food products have been introduced to a traditional culture, the first cases of chronic illness start surfacing in the form of cancer, diabetes or immune disorders. It's sad that in this nation of plenty, far too many of us are nutritionally bankrupt but calorically over-extended and are not even aware of it - we just become accustomed to feeling under the weather. The first step in achieving wellness is to eliminate as many of these *false foods* from our daily diet as possible.

Each cell in our body is created from the food we ingest. If we are reconstructing our bodies every day, then, by simply giving them the best building blocks available - fat, protein, carbohydrates, minerals, water and oxygen in the correct proportions for our unique constitution - we can build new arteries or healthy bones. Day by day, slowly but surely, molecule by molecule - we can rebuild our health. In the naturalistic thought process, whole foods along with exercise and a healthy lifestyle form our first line of defense in maintaining health and combating chronic disorders, herbal remedies compose the second line of defense, while vitamin and mineral supplements would be the third consideration.

Wood Element: Fats and Their Role in Defending Our Human Garden

The Liver and Gall Bladder organ systems correspond to the Wood element in the Asian Medical tradition. A few pages back you read about common symptoms or patterns of dis-ease associated with Wood Imbalances in traditional Asian thought. But, for now, let's try to bridge worlds. As mentioned in Chapter 2, in my mind, I like to link each of the Five Elements with a specific essential nutrient or substance (fat, protein, carbohydrates, oxygen, water and minerals) required for life as we know it to exist. In workshops and lectures, FAT is the substance I link to the Wood element, since, in Western thought it is the liver/gall-bladder organ system that is responsible for the breakdown and assimilation of fat. Healthful fat is an essential building block used by each of our cells to create its outer boundary or membrane - its first-line of defense against microbial attacks.

Dietary fat has gotten a bad rap over the past decade as low-fat diets became the fad. Unfortunately, serious imbalances have been the result of our prolonged flirtation with fat-free fare. Are you a fat addict? Do you find yourself constantly craving fatty foods like cheese, ice cream, French fries, potato chips, peanuts? It is probable that you are so deficient in good, life-promoting fats (known as essential fatty acids) that your body is virtually screaming for them, causing you to swallow anything that is oily in the hopes it will eventually get what it needs.

Researcher Artemis Simopoulos, M.D.,
author of The Omega Plan,
has found that most Americans are consuming
only about 1/10th of the good fats they require,

and that 20 percent of the population have such low levels of essential fatty acids "as to be undetectable."

What does this mean in the life of just one of your cells? Every cell constructs its outer "wall" (to be scientifically correct, we should say cellular "membrane") from fat. This boundary of fat serves as the barrier that keeps harmful microbes from entering the cell, otherwise unfriendly invaders would happily set up housekeeping. Special attention needs to be paid to the kinds and proportions of oils we give our cells so they can construct a strong cellular membrane. Saturated fats (like those found in butter, cheese, flesh foods, and coconut oil) help firm up cell membranes while the omega oils keep them flexible. For now, let's talk about defending boundaries and the role that essential fatty acids play in helping each of our cell's protect its perimeter - a function of the Wood element at the microscopic level.

A hundred years ago, before the advent of highly refined convenience foods we probably would not even have had to worry about this. We naturally would have munched on a handful of pumpkin, sunflower, flax or sesame seeds, an avocado, almonds or walnuts, as well as organic dairy, fish or game, fulfilling our body's requirement for essential fats. This in not the case in our modern world of high-tech food. Nutrient-deficient convenience foods are laced with highly refined oils, to help insure a shelf life of "forever"; however, these oils are chemically closer to plastic than anything remotely edible. Margarine and other solid vegetable oils are created through a chemical process in which hydrogen is combined with highly heated vegetable oils. The Dutch government outlawed the sale of margarine and solid vegetable oils years ago due to their adverse effects on human health, yet in the United States they are still freely consumed by an unsuspecting public who actually believe that they are good for the heart. Why are they still in our food chain? Unfortunately, once again, advertising works. While hydrogenated oils do not elevate cholesterol, the American Heart Association recognizes that they are detrimental to our wellbeing. They have negative effects on our nervous system, lower immunity and cause cell membrane irregularities. Let's take an up-close look at the membrane of a cell just to see what happens when it is forced to build its boundaries with hydrogenated oils. Ultimately, wellbeing depends upon the health of each and every one of the billions of cells that compose our human body.

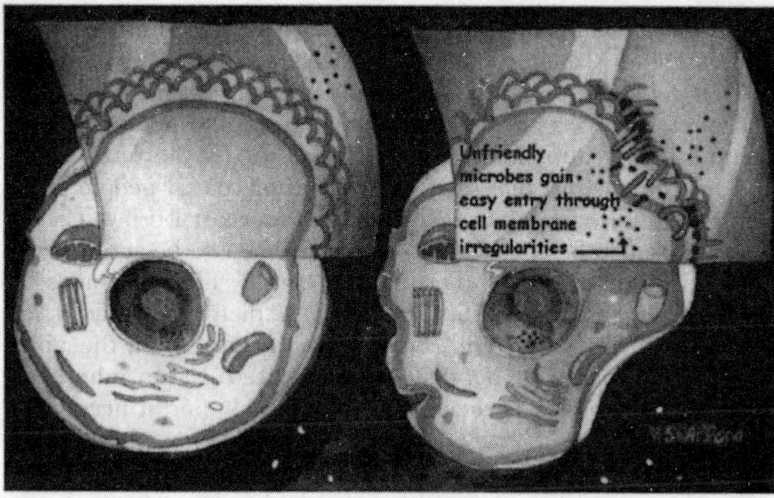

The two cells in the illustration following look similar except the one on the left has had an ample supply of cis-shaped fatty acids with which to construct its membrane. Cis-fatty acid molecules are shaped like the letter "**C**"; they link neatly together, in a lock and key fashion, to form a strong barrier. The cell on the right, unfortunately, has been forced to construct its membrane with oils that have been highly heated and processed. When subjected to high temperatures, the "cis" molecule formation of healthy fats straightens out and becomes a villain - a "trans-" fatty acid. The molecule is then shaped like a rod "**I**" which still fits into one side of the lock and key formation - leaving the other side open, unprotected and vulnerable to entry by unfriendly microbes.

Let's talk about healthy fats - the good guys! Fresh cold-water fish, flax and hemp seeds contain high levels of omega-3 oils while vegetable oils like safflower; sunflower and soy bean oil are naturally high in omega-6 fatty acids; however,

our bodies require omega-6 fats
in a balanced proportion to omega-3's.
The best ratio of omega-6 to omega-3 fats
is somewhere between 1 to 1 and 2 to 1.
The current ratio of omega-6 to omega-3 fat
consumption in the average U.S. diet is 20 to 1.

The imbalanced ingestion of omega-6 to omega-3 fats contributes to many inflammatory and auto-immune disorders such as asthma, rheumatoid arthritis, cancer, osteoporosis, Chrohn's disease and Alzheimer's disease. Studies also find a strong correlation between essential fatty acid deficiency and cravings for alcohol, fat, sugar and other carbohydrates. Descendants of certain ethnic groups have a greater need for oils found in cold water fish. If your ancestors were island or coastal people (like the Scandinavians, Native North American coastal tribes, Celtic Irish, Scottish or Welsh) your genetic code could be adapted to a cold water fish-based diet that is naturally high in omega 3 oils. When researchers supplemented the diets of chronic alcoholics with fish oil or GLA-rich evening primrose oil, their interest in alcohol and depression disappeared. If you inherited genes from coastal dwellers, you will probably find it necessary to supplement your daily diet with fish oil, GLA-rich black currant seed oil or evening primrose oil capsules to get the quantity of omega-3 fats required by your body.

A serious lack of omega-3 essential fatty acids, and an excess of omega-6 fats is affecting the health of virtually everyone in our nation. Omega-3 fats actually raise our metabolic rate; they are like sparks that ignite our body's ability to burn fat. They also have diuretic properties and aid in flushing excess dampness from our tissues.

Don't you think it's time we made friends with fat?

- The protective membrane surrounding each one of our cells is constructed from fat that acts as a barrier against harmful microbial invaders.
- Essential fatty acids are required for normal growth and reproduction. Prostaglandins, constructed from fats, regulate many body functions and play an important role in blood clotting, blood pressure, tumor growth, inflammation, allergic reactions, water and sodium balance - to mention a few.
- Suffering from depression or insomnia? Fat is needed by the body to produce serotonin (our body's natural mood elevator) which is later converted into melatonin to promote good sleep.
- Our human garden requires healthful fats for the fabrication of all hormones, including reproductive hormones like estrogen, testosterone and progesterone.
- Our human brain is composed of 60 percent fat.
- The correct answer to the ideal percentage of fat in our diet continues to elude us. Some nutritionists recommend 10 per-

cent while others recommend 20 or 30 percent. Healthy Italians average about 40 percent fat while healthy Eskimos require a diet containing 75 percent. Ultimately, the answer is probably answered by the unique genetic code that each one of us possesses and has to do with the locale in which our ancient ancestors evolved.

What to do? Daily, adults should be ingesting approximately 125 calories of essential fatty acids, in addition to other healthful fats. Ideally, one-third to one-half of those calories will be from omega-3 oils while the other one-half to two-thirds will come from omega-6's. Sources rich in omega-3's include cold-water fish like salmon, sardines, tuna, sea bass, flax seeds, walnuts and leafy greens, particularly purslane (a vegetable that is eaten in soups and salads in Greece and other parts of the Mediterranean). Omega-6's are much easier to come by and most of us are overdoing it on that front - or at least creating a substantial imbalance. In fact, Dr. John Kinsella, a lipid biochemist at Cornell University has found that **high levels of omega-6 fatty acids in the diet may foster the growth of tumors in laboratory test animals**. While several large clinical studies indicated that diets high in omega-6 oils decreased rates heart attack rates, death rates due to cancer and other causes actually *increased*.

Patients frequently ask about olive oil. Virgin, cold-pressed olive oil has many health promoting qualities and can be used on a daily basis; however, olive oil is very low in essential fatty acids - so it is important to realize that olive oil alone is not going to supply these life-promoting nutrients. Patients also frequently ask about butter. Unfortunately, butter got a bad rap over the past few decades when advertisers were trying to promote the sale of margarine. Composed of over 500 different elements - none of which are harmful, some of the properties of butter are health promoting, others are neutral. Remember that our body needs saturated as well as unsaturated fats to build healthy cell membranes. Saturated fats are solid at room temperature and help give firmness to the cell membrane while the omega oils keep them flexible. To that extent, all of us require some saturated fats; they can be found in animal products like cheese, milk, butter or in non-hydrogenated coconut or cocoa oil. If you consume red meat or poultry it is still best to trim off all the extra fat. Excess saturated fat can interfere with our body's ability to absorb beneficial fatty acids. Also, unless you purchase organically produced dairy and meat products, animal fat tends to store antibiotics and pesticides. Annually, over 20 million pounds of antibiotics are given to animals in the United States; many countries refuse to import our meat and dairy products for this reason.

Here are a few simple pointers to help you get on the right fat track:

- Purchase an inexpensive coffee grinder that you can use for flax seeds. Daily, grind 2 tablespoons of organic flax seeds and add them to your cereal, salad or any dish that seems appropriate. They have a delicious nutty flavor and will help supply omega-3 oils. It is important to grind them at the time you are going to ingest them because good oils go bad very quickly when exposed to light, oxygen or warm temperatures. If an oil can sit on your kitchen shelf for months without going rancid, then question its life promoting qualities! Discard any oil or nuts that have a bitter or biting flavor.
- Cook with small amounts of cold-pressed, organic grape seed oil, or clarified butter (also known as ghee); olive oil should not be subjected to high temperatures. Olive or sesame oils are great for salads *(according to Dr. Peter D'Adamo, sesame seeds and oil are contraindicated for B blood types)*. Grape seed oil has a light nutty flavor and can be heated to temperatures up to 485 degrees Fahrenheit without breaking down (producing dangerous free radicals).
- Read labels. Products that list "vegetable oils" as an ingredient should be left on the grocer's shelf. Convenience food manufacturers frequently use cottonseed oil, labeling their package "vegetable oil". It contains cyclopropene fatty acid which has a toxic effect on the liver and gallbladder. Cottonseed oil also has the highest content of pesticide residues.
- Try to eat cold water fish two to three times a week. If you are a vegetarian, algae oil capsules may prove beneficial.

Fire Element: Protein Sources to Ignite the Spark of Life

In traditional Asian medical thought, animal proteins are some of the most fiery, *yang* or heating substances in our diet. Energetically, if we tend to go out of balance to the cool *yin* side of the equation, symptoms might include cold hands and feet, lethargy, fatigue, spaciness, a soft voice and passive behavior. This is where heating *yang* protein foods come to the rescue. Protein (fresh fish, poultry, lean meat, low fat dairy products, and/or a balance of whole grains and beans for those who thrive on plant protein) provide fundamental building blocks essential to all forms of life. In the human body, proteins comprise about 75 percent of the body's solid materials. Like carbohydrates and fats, proteins are composed of carbon, hydrogen, and oxygen; however, they are unique in that they also contain approximately 16 percent nitrogen - an element required for life to exist.

Generally, the American diet is overabundant in protein - especially highly processed protein. Nitrates and nitrites, which form cancer-causing compounds, are used as preservatives in many fish and meat products. However, with the advent of low fat diets, many healthy, life-promoting protein foods are now being avoided because of their fat content. Do you forgo consuming foods like fresh eggs, fish, chicken, lean red meat, cheese, nuts and seeds due to their seemingly high percentages of fat? Far too frequently dieters restrict these foods rationalizing that they would prefer to *enjoy* their fat calories by consuming ice cream, cookies, pastries or similar foods. Protein deficiency can be signaled by cravings for highly refined sugar-laden foods - this is particularly true for vegans or vegetarians who do not balance their nutrients. Other symptoms of protein deficiency can include spaciness or an inability to concentrate, anxiety, depression, irritability, and/or obsessiveness.

Isn't it time we made friends with protein?

- All of the body's tissues need healthful protein for growth, reproduction, maintenance and repair; it is the only food that can be used to build new muscle fibers.
- Protein is required for the manufacture of important enzymes and hormones that regulate body processes like digestion, ovulation and stress reduction. Even our moods are dictated by four brain chemicals that are produced from the amino acids that are the building blocks of protein foods.
- Protein carriers transport oxygen, vitamins and minerals to cells.
- The body utilizes protein as a fuel source during periods of fasting or extended physical exertion; it is required for blood clotting as well as to maintain a proper fluid balance.
- Growth is impaired in infants and children who do not con-

sume sufficient protein.

- Protein sustains life - a dietary deficiency effects the body in profound ways including low immunity, weakness, loss of vigor, wasting of body tissues, fatty liver - as well as a host of other metabolic and physiologic consequences.

Over the past decade, a debate has raged regarding daily protein requirements and whether animal or vegetable protein is superior. As a person who spent approximately 20 years on a vegetarian diet (12 years on a poorly planned diet highlighted by extreme fasting; and about 8 years using the best macrobiotic principles); I have studied and experienced both sides of this issue. Over eight years I gained 70 pounds and my cholesterol sky-rocketed on an excellent, well-planned low-calorie vegetarian diet composed of whole organic foods. While this is the diet I favor (due to ethical and ecological reasons as well as taste preferences), it proved disastrous for me. My cholesterol dropped dramatically within six weeks after reducing consumption of whole grains and integrating animal protein into my meal plan. At the same time, in my clinic I regularly see vegetarians who thrive on whole grains, beans, fruits and veggies. I believe many genetic factors are at play regarding which foods best nourish our bodies - one of which is blood type. Dr. Peter D'Adamo, in his book, ***Eat Right for Your Type***, uses blood types as an indicator of which foods can best nourish us - as well as those which can create allergic responses.

According to D'Adamo, our Cro-Magnon ancestors (who lived approximately 40,000 years ago) possessed Blood Type O - it was the only Blood Type around. They were skilled hunters who thrived on the big game that inhabited their hunting range. Due to a rapid increase in population, competition for sources of food and changing climactic conditions, by 20,000 BCE populations had moved into Europe and Asia. Every major land mass on our planet (with the exception of Antarctica) had been populated by 10,000 BCE.

Sometime between 25,000 to 15,000 BCE early humans were forced to exploit other food resources such as roots, nuts, berries, grubs and small animals - it was then that Blood Type A appeared. Type A's seem to flourish on a vegetarian diet. In fact, the Blood Type A's who visit my clinic invariably do poorly with a diet based on high quantities of animal protein. Today, many Blood Type A people inhabit areas around the Adriatic, Mediterranean and Aegean seas - particularly Spain, Turkey, Corsica,

Sardinia and the Balkans - precisely where archaeologists have found evidence of the beginnings of our planet's first agricultural societies.

Sometime between 10,000 and 15,000 BCE, pastoral nomadic people pushed into Asia and Eastern Europe and the highly adaptable B Blood Type came into existence. Most B Blood Types usually can consume either animal or plant protein foods as well as dairy products.

The rare but modern Blood Type AB evolved only ten or twelve centuries ago. Type AB's seem to fare best on a semi-vegetarian diet supplemented by minor amounts of animal protein.

While one of the arguments for vegetarianism is that humankind has been practicing agriculture for 10,000 to 12,000 years and is, therefore, best-suited to consume a plant-based diet, archaeological studies demonstrate that 10,000 to 15,000 years is but a brief lapse in time when one considers evolutionary history. Humankind's genetic structure has actually changed very little over the past 100,000 years. In fact, the most minor genetic adaptation takes 20,000 to 30,000 years to become established . . . it would seem that Blood Types A, B and AB are nature's evolutive response to a grain and dairy-based diet . . . and that change has just begun.

Blood Type Percentages in Some Human Populations

Population	0	A	B	AB
Armenians	0.29	.05	0.13	0.08
Austrians	0.43	0.39	0.12	0.06
Brahmin East Indians	0.55	0.25	0.2	0.05
Chinese	0.44	0.27	0.23	0.06
English	0.7	0.25	0.05	0
Eskimos	0.47	0.45	0.06	0.02
Fench	0.42	0.45	0.09	0.04
Irish	0.54	0.32	0.11	0.03
Navajo Native Americans	0.87	0.13	0	0
U.S. Caucasians Living in St. Louis, MS	0.45	0.41	0.1	0.04
U.S. African Americans Living in Iowa	0.49	0.27	0.2	0.04

Do you know your Blood Type? Roughly, according to Blood Bank statistics, 44% of the population has Type O, 42% Type A, 10% Type B and 4% Type AB. Below is a chart based on studies conducted on various populations:

Studies demonstrate that the "ideal" protein intake varies greatly from individual to individual depending upon age, health, activity level, lean body (muscle) mass, the type of protein ingested (animal or vegetable) and other genetic factors. The current established *minimum* daily adult requirement for protein in the U.S. is 0.8 grams per 2.2 pounds of body weight. For a 135 pound adult this would equal approximately 49 grams of animal protein daily. Since one ounce of lean meat or poultry contains 7 grams of protein, this translates into 49 grams divided by 7 grams to come up with 7 ounces of animal protein daily. *(Note: 3-1/2 ounces of animal protein is about the size of a deck of cards).* With most fish, you can calculate 1.5 ounces per 7 grams, or 10.5 ounces daily for a 135 pound adult *(calculate tuna like lean meat or poultry).* Not all protein is alike - it requires 3 ounces of soft tofu (soybean) protein for each ounce of animal protein. In other words, a 135 pound vegetarian would need to consume 21 ounces of tofu daily to meet their *minimum* daily protein requirement. Below is a chart to help you with calculations based on weight - roughly, you can add one ounce of lean meat or poultry protein, **or** one 1.5 ounces of fish **or** 3 ounces of tofu for each additional 15 pounds of body weight. Whole grains, beans and many plant foods also contain varying amounts of protein. Keep in mind that it is best to consume protein from various sources:

Minimum Daily Protein Requirement

Body Weight	Minimum Daily Protein	Meat/Poultry	Fish	Tofu
120 pounds	44 grams	6 oz.	9 oz.	18 oz.
135 pounds	49 grams	7 oz.	10.5 oz.	21 oz.
150 pounds	55 grams	8 oz.	12 oz.	24 oz.
165 pounds	60 grams	9 oz.	13 oz.	27 oz.
180 pounds	65 grams	10 oz.	14 oz.	30 oz.
195 pounds	71 grams	11 oz.	15 oz.	33 oz.
210 pounds	76 grams	12 oz.	16 oz.	36 oz.

NOTE: Persons who are recovering from illness or surgery, children, athletes, mothers who are breast-feeding, frequent dieters, the elderly or persons subjected to constant stress may require more protein than indicated above. Some persons suffering from kidney disease or other disorders may find it necessary to drastically reduce protein consumption - consult with your healthcare professional.

As a vegetarian at heart, I find myself in a very difficult ideological position - forced to argue in favor of the consumption of animal foods. I think it is extremely important for the health of our planet to eat foods as low on the food chain as possible - for this reason, cold-water fish seems to be a good solution to my particular problem (one of carbohydrate sensitivity, affecting up to 50 to 75% of the population, see page 363). If you prefer small amounts of poultry and/or red meat, try to purchase animal products that have been organically grown. Also, trim off as much of the fat as possible - animal fat stores toxins and estrogens found in growth hormones, chemical fertilizers and pesticides.

If you are a vegetarian, be certain to combine sufficient quantities of whole grains and beans, nuts and seeds in the proper ratio to supply your body with essential amino acids found in protein foods (the ones your body cannot make) to match the needs of your body's tissues. Though not difficult, it takes time and planning to construct a nourishing vegetarian diet. For persons willing to ingest some animal products, eggs and low fat dairy products such as yogurt and cottage cheese can offer a boost to protein nutrition. It is important to note that the only time-tested vegetarian culture is that of East India - and they rely on dairy products. During special times such as pregnancy, illness or surgery Ayurvedic practitioners may recommend consumption of meat to facilitate a speedy recovery.

Dairy products have gotten somewhat of a bad rap over the past few decades - in compliance with the advice of a health professional I removed them from my diet for over 25 years. Interestingly, my system processes organic low-fat yogurt or cottage cheese very well and does not produce any mucus. In some individuals they lead to mucus production - this may be remedied by ingesting them with a dash of cardamom powder or 4 or 5 whole cardamom seeds (an East Indian Ayurvedic remedy). On the other hand, many people are lactose intolerant - studies show that 85 percent of Hispanic persons and over 90 percent of African Americans cannot digest dairy. A lactase supplement, available at most health food stores, could help eliminate this problem. The best advice is to experiment in order to discover what works best for you. Always be alert to cravings - they are usually an indication that you are allergic to the food you are craving or that you are deficient in some essential nutrient. *(Note: It is always wisest to purchase low-fat dairy products since some studies indicate that arteriosclerosis is more prevalent in societies that consume large amounts of dairy).*

Frequently, in my practice, I meet people who have switched to a vegetarian diet - for the first two or three years they felt wonderful and their health improved. However, as time progressed they lacked energy, mental clarity and had become much more susceptible to colds and flus. It can take a long while for any dietary deficiency to make itself apparent - so please practice prevention by becoming fully knowledgeable about your body's food requirements. With a simple lesson in the hot/cold or *yin/yang* energetics of food many of my vegetarian patients were able to understand that their bodies now required more heating foods and herbs. *Please see Chapter 9 for helpful tips in understanding energetics of foods and herbs.*

On the other side of the equation is excess consumption of poor quality highly processed animal products which certainly contributes to ill-health. If you ingest too much animal protein you might feel over-heated, anxious, and suffer from insomnia, hyperactivity, high blood pressure and/or heart disease. In Chapter 9 you will find recommendations to help balance that excess *yang* condition.

What is the final answer on the quantity and types of protein best suited for you? On one hand we have the John Robbins, Drs. Ornish, MacDougall and Whittaker debate in which plant protein is considered superior to animal protein. On the other hand we have Drs. Atkins, Rachel and Richard Heller who advocate more animal protein in order to control excess insulin production (the hormone that ultimately controls fat storage). As a frustrated lifelong dieter trying to get to the bottom of the truth, I have come to the conclusion that the argument of each of these scientists is equally valid - for about 50 percent of the population. Did you notice that approximately 44% of us have Blood Type O while 46% percent of the population possesses Blood Types A or AB; and 10% has Blood Type B? Dr D'Adamo argues that Blood Type O requires animal protein while Blood Types A and AB do better with more plant protein - that's almost a 50/50 split! No wonder the debate rages on. Meanwhile, the versatile Blood Type B (who thrives on both types of protein) looks on questioningly, wondering what the argument is all about.

If we add the opinion of yet another researcher, we have Dr. Barry Sears who considers the ideal ratio of carbohydrate to protein to fat to be 40/30/30 (again, in order to control insulin). This ratio became the basis for the only diet that has ever worked well for me and I am still in the process of trying to fine-tune it for my particular constitution based on Dr. D'Adamo's work as well as my own knowledge of Chinese, Ayurvedic and Macrobiotic food and herbal energetics.

Five Element Professor J. R. Worsley considers it "barbaric to prescribe one diet for everyone" and, indeed, traditional medical systems teach us that each food has a different energy that affects various body types in distinct ways. At the same time, the ancient masters of these healing traditions did not have to deal with the added confusion of highly processed, nutrient-deficient, chemically-enhanced refined foods that fill our supermarkets. In Macrobiotic, Ayurvedic and Chinese Medicine we try to prescribe the diet that fits the individual's constitution. However, it is important to keep in mind that all three traditions use rice as a major part of the diet and for carbohydrate sensitive individuals this triggers weight gain. One of my teachers found a passage in an ancient Ayurvedic or Chinese medical text (he cannot recall which one) with an illustration of a large pot-bellied individual. The condition of this person was referred to as "grain belly" and the text recommended elimination of grains from the diet. It seems this condition was recognized hundreds of years ago in at least one traditional medical system.

D'Adamo's Blood Type work might be just the starting point in determining which foods are best suited for you. The ultimate answer will have to do with many genetic factors. For example, you might outwardly look like your Italian ancestors, but perhaps genes inherited from Irish ancestors require you to consume more cold water fish, high in Omega 3 oils.

Fish oil reduces depression and alcohol cravings
in persons descended from Irish,
Scandinavian and Native American stock.

In the upcoming section on the Earth element, the debate will rage on as we discuss carbohydrate foods. But before moving on, we can't talk about Blood Type without mentioning how this red river of life connects us to each other - cutting across all boundaries - sizes, shapes, skin colors, races, religions, cultures and nationalities. Actually, an African, an Hispanic, an Asian and a Caucasian possessing Blood Type A have far more biological similarities to each other than someone from their same race with Blood Type O, B or AB. A blood transfusion or donated organ from an African or Caucasian person can save the life of an Asian or Hispanic sharing the same Blood Type (and vice versa).

We are all truly brothers and sisters!
According to one tale told by Native
Americans living in Florida,
"In the beginning, human beings were created in
in five colors: red, black, white, yellow and blue.
At one point in time, our blue brothers - the dolphins -
decided to return to the sea."

Earth Element: Carbohydrates that Promote a Peaceful Feeling

Everyday you are rebuilding your body with the water, protein, fat, vitamins and minerals you ingest - your bones, muscles, blood, lymph and hormones are all constructed from these materials. Your body cannot reconstruct itself from simple carbohydrates - though they serve as a valuable source of energy for many people and play a key role in the production of important mood altering hormones. High quality *complex* carbohydrates are found in such foods as beans, lentils, vegetables, rolled oats and brown rice (these foods also contain varying quantities of vegetable fat and protein). *(To increase the amount of protein contained in whole grains and beans by up to 70 percent, soak them for 24 hours prior to cooking. Protein surges in these foods during the first stages of sprouting but diminishes rapidly after 24 hours of soaking for grains and 36 hours for beans).*

Serotonin

Over fifteen years of dedicated research at MIT and other facilities has begun to shed light on why many of us feel an uncontrollable urge to eat carbohydrate foods when under stress. Carbohydrates (in conjunction with the amino acid tryptophan) are essential for the production of serotonin - that all important brain chemical which helps us feel calm, peaceful, focused, energetic but relaxed.

In fact, the mood-enhancing drugs Prozac, Zoloft, Effexor and Paxil were developed to activate serotonin. This is how it works: Normally our blood contains all amino acids in fairly regular proportions. The smaller amino acid tryptophan has to compete with larger amino acids to make its way to the brain where serotonin is produced. When a person consumes carbohydrate foods, the body releases insulin which immediately goes to work, pushing glucose into the cells as well as amino acids, ***with the exception of tryptophan***, into the muscle cells. The way is now clear for the freely circulating tryptophan to enter the brain; serotonin synthesis starts up quickly and unpleasant emotional states are relieved. Serotonin is later converted into melatonin - our natural sleeping pill. You can see why mood disorders such as anxiety and depression as well as sleeping disorders are so closely connected to what we ingest - most specifically foods that are high in tryptophan as well as carbohydrates to activate insulin. *Note: If protein is consumed along with the carbohydrates, serotonin production does not increase since tryptophan is still competing with the other larger amino acids to gain entry into the brain.*

This explains why many carbohydrate-intolerant, overweight people are stuck between a rock and a hard place - between insulin over-production and serotonin under-production. If they follow a high protein diet, insulin is controlled and weight drops, but serotonin production is impaired. The resulting depression, irritability and/or anxiety pushes them to self-medicate by reaching for that candy bar or bagel. With this in mind, drug manufacturers developed Redux and fen/phen. Unfortunately 30% of persons using these drugs developed abnormalities in the shape of their heart valves - side-effects that can lead to serious cardiac weakness and even death.

Beta endorphin

While the scientific community has been studying beta endorphin for nearly twenty-five years, most of us have very limited knowledge about its effects. Beta endorphin is our body's incredibly powerful natural painkiller - it is responsible for the euphoria known as "runner's high". It also reduces feelings of anger and fear, controls anxiety, relieves certain types of depression and boosts feelings of self-esteem. This brain chemical is an endogenous opioid meaning that its effects are opium like, such as those of morphine, heroin and codeine. Beta endorphin works like a narcotic because its molecules are shaped identically and it fits into the same brain receptor sites.

Some individuals have naturally low levels of beta endorphin in their bodies and more receptor sites in the brain to receive whatever is there. For this reason, these people are extremely sensitive to the instantaneous blood sugar spiking and beta endorphin releasing effects of alcohol, sugar and other refined carbohydrates. While eating sugar may affect some people by reducing physical and emotional pain, for the sugar sensitive individual, sugar can have the same effect as drinking alcohol or taking a narcotic drug.

Back in the 1980's, Dr. Elliott Blass, researcher at Cornell University was interested in the possibility of using sugar as a safe painkiller for infants. In an experiment with mice, he demonstrated that it normally takes 10 seconds for them to lift their front paws off a hot plate; however, after drinking an 11.5 percent sugar solution, the average went up to 20 seconds before paws were lifted. Dr. Blass then gave the mice Naltrexone, a substance that blocks brain receptor sites for opiates and beta endorphin - the mice lifted their paws in 8 seconds. In 1986 Dr. Blass went on to demonstrate the painkilling effects of sugar on emotional pain. When separated from their mothers, baby mice cried over 300 times in a six-minute period; when given sugar water, they cried only 75 times in six minutes; when given Naltrexone, the little pups cried as often as those who did not have sugar. Since then, scientists have continued to study the ability of sugar and alcohol to evoke a beta endorphin response.

Sugar sensitive people are drawn to alcohol, sugar or refined starchy carbohydrates *(like those found in white bread, rice cakes or even a baked potato, see the glycemic index on page 365)* as if they were a narcotic - but the drug-like induced "happiness" is short-lived and sets up unbearable cravings. Like alcoholics, the sugar sensitive person may give up eating foods containing sugar and highly refined carbohydrates - however, all it takes is one slip - an innocent bite of birthday cake - and they are back in to the vicious cycle. Needless to say, this devastating condition can lead to weight gain.

Isn't it time to become more discriminating about the types of carbohydrates that we ingest and give our youngsters?

Our grocery stores, restaurants, offices and homes are virtually filled with poor quality carbohydrate convenience foods -

we can't escape from them.

During childhood and early adulthood most people seem to be able to get by ingesting relatively large quantities of simple carbohydrates that abound in highly processed foods like cakes, cookies, candy bars, soft drinks and white bread. *(According to Dr. Sears, about 25 percent of the population has a blunt insulimic reaction - meaning that they only produce a limited amount of insulin. They are the lucky ones in, our society, who will never have a weight problem regardless of caloric intake. Others, again about 25 percent of the population, are extremely carbohydrate sensitive with a tendency towards weight gain early in life).* As we get older, the blood sugar spiking effect these foods possess ultimately takes its toll on the adrenals and insulin producing pancreas - the organs that are responsible for controlling blood sugar levels.

After childbirth or during midlife many people (another 25% of the population) find they just do not have the metabolism they once had and weight loss becomes a real struggle. The problem with highly refined carbohydrates and other foods that rank high on the glycemic index is that they trick the brain into believing it is getting exactly what it needs - that's because the human brain is a glucose hog. The only fuel the brain uses is sugar! This is one of the major reasons why we are so attracted to the sweet flavor. Unfortunately, by the time we reach midlife, our food preferences and eating habits are firmly established and we may find it extremely difficult to alter our diets.

However, if we can get off the refined carbohydrate track and supply our bodies with good quality complex carbohydrates at regular intervals, in the quantity that our unique constitution requires, our brain receives the sugar it needs in a slow, steady stream and we feel happy, peaceful and centered.

Metal Element:
Oxygen - Essential for Life and a Link to Spirit

Without water we can survive for a few days, without food - for a few weeks, but without oxygen we cannot survive for more than a few minutes. Life itself can be looked upon as the mingling of our Earthly form (or material body) with activating Celestial *ch'i* - or oxygen. The breath of Heaven, in the form of oxygen, ignites every cell in our body with the Fire of Being. The metabolic process that results is the energy of life. With each inspiration, we fill our lungs with this pure essence - reuniting with the pulsating energy of Creation. With each expiration we eliminate waste and metabolic byproducts into the atmosphere where they are once again purified by members of the plant kingdom - they breathe in what we breathe out and we breathe in what they breathe out. Inhalation/exhalation, expansion/contraction - this is the primal heartbeat of our Universe.

Thousands of years ago, ancient sages recognized that the mind and emotions are intimately tied to our breathing patterns. Have you ever noticed how rapid and shallow your breathe becomes when you are excited or agitated? Try checking in on your breathing at various times throughout the day - observe how it changes when you are relaxed or sleepy, calm or agitated, angry or afraid, happy or depressed.

Becoming aware of breathing patterns is the first step toward meditation practices. At first, you will be amazed at how quickly your mind will attempt to run away to any other topic . . . watch your thoughts and where they take you. Observing the mind can be a fascinating experience. Like a monkey in a tree jumping from limb to limb, our minds leap from topic to topic. You might want to try sitting in a comfortable position to become acquainted with your whole breathing process. First exhale completely, then slowly inhale, notice how the oxygen enters the nostrils . . . how your diaphragm sinks . . . and the stomach muscles expand to draw in the new breath. In the beginning, do not try to hold your breathe, simply be aware of the breathing process. Is is smooth or rough? loud or soft? deep or shallow? It reveals so much about your state of mind.

Many types of breathing practices are taught in Yoga or *Ch'i Gong* classes - different kinds of breathing patterns are used to regulate and direct the body's energy (*prana* in Yoga and *ch'i* in *Ch'i Gong*). When regularly practiced over a period of time, such breathing practices help attune us with the natural rhythms of our universe - soothing the mind and healing the body. Abdominal breathing, a technique in which the breath is smoothly and gently pulled deep into the lungs and slowly exhaled, brings more oxygen into the body. Our body's cells, tissues and organs are nourished, the heartbeat becomes slow and steady and the mind and spirit become quiet and tranquil.

There is an unspoken language.

It comes from the silence

and can't be heard by the ears,
only by the heart.

BABA HARI DASS AUTHOR OF ***SILENCE SPEAKS***

In the West we use prayer as a means to "communicate" with God but we are not commonly taught methods (in conventional religious practice) to quiet the mind so we can "listen" to the Creator. What if the Prime Source, G-d, Allah, Purusha, Taiowa, the Great Spirit or Heavenly Father (same energy, different names) actually has a message for us but we are so busy talking that we have no time to listen? Meditation can be viewed as the "passive" counterpart of "active" prayer in our efforts to communicate with the Sublime - it is actually a form of "quiet prayer". And assuredly, if our minds are truly tranquil, any message or "inspiration" we receive will be one of love, peace and compassion for ourselves and others.

Water Element: Pure Water & Natural Minerals - The Foundation of Life

Water . . . flows on and on, and merely
fills up all the places through which it flows,
it does not shrink from any dangerous spot
nor from any plunge,
and nothing can make it lose its own essential nature.
It remains true to itself under all conditions.

I CHING

Pure Water

Water is the most abundant element on the face of our planet (covering over two-thirds of its surface). It is also the most plentiful element in our body - approximately 70 percent is composed of water as is 90 percent of our brain. The human body is actually a miniature saltwater ecosystem that continually struggles to self-regulate as we down artificially colored and flavored sodas, fruit drinks or alcoholic beverages. While many of us do our best to consume wholesome foods, we seldom give thought to the liquids we ingest. Our body requires an abundant supply of pure, clean water on a daily basis to replenish its stores and to cleanse toxins from the cells and interstitial tissues. If the water we drink is polluted with chemicals or other waste products, its life-giving energy is diminished.

Today, well water, if in close proximity to agricultural zones, is polluted with herbicides, pesticides, defoliants and soil fumigants. Nitrates found in these farm chemicals convert to toxic carcinogenic nitrites when exposed to heat, certain microbes or metals. Toxicology researchers tell us that free radicals formed by these nitrites neutralize enzymes in our bodies - contributing to degenerative diseases.

It is estimated that at least 40 percent of all recycled city water has passed through someone's sewer or was the by-product of industrial waste. It is questionable how well this water is purified before coming through our tap. To disinfect water, most cities add chlorine (as well as sodium fluoride to prevent tooth-decay). While chlorine will evaporate if we let the water stand for about thirty minutes - chloroform, a toxic cancer-producing chemical does not evaporate. Chlorine combines with organic substances found in water to produce chloroform. Studies indicate that regular ingestion of chlorine destroys vitamin E in the body, kills beneficial intestinal microbes, and is closely associated with vascular disease. The Environmental Protection Agency warns that prolonged exposure to chlorinated water through bathing or swimming can contribute to skin cancer. Why would we want to ingest something that has been determined to be harmful to the outside of our bodies?

Studies conducted in Europe on the effects of sodium fluoride have resulted in its usage being banned by the governments of Holland, Sweden and Denmark. The original tests to determine fluoride's value in the prevention of tooth decay were performed with *calcium* fluoride. However, the chemical added to city water supplies is *sodium* fluoride - an extremely toxic by-product of the aluminum industry. The price of sodium fluoride, most commonly used as rat poison, went up 1,000% almost overnight when it was approved as an additive to city water supplies.

Natural fluorine is available in goat's milk, avocados, seaweed, parsley, cabbage, black-eyed peas, juniper berries, licorice, lemon grass, bancha tea twigs. *Fluorine evaporates during cooking so try to consume most of these foods as near to the raw state as possible.*

Today many effective, reasonably-priced water filters are found on the market. Filters leave all minerals while removing other impurities; however, they do not remove water-soluble toxins like nitrites and sodium fluoride. To remove sodium fluoride from filtered water, briskly stir one teaspoon of calcium powder into each gallon of water. *(Call your water supplier to determine if sodium fluoride is added to your drinking water).*

Many factors influence the amount of fresh pure water each of us needs to drink daily. Somewhere between six to twelve 8-ounce glasses will probably be appropriate for you depending on the following: If you are a vegetarian, or consume lots of fresh fruit and vegetables, have a tendency to feel cold, live in a cold or damp climate and lead a relatively sedentary lifestyle you will need less water than someone who consumes more animal products and salty foods, or exercises vigorously, suffers from heat conditions or lives in a hot, dry or windy climate.

Natural Minerals

The human body, to function optimally, must receive the nutrients it needs on a daily basis. The body manufactures some vitamins, however, it cannot make minerals - they must come to us though the food we consume. While minerals do not contain calories, they assist the body in producing energy. Mineral deficiencies can be responsible for any number of minor and major disorders, for example: calcium deficiency is related to osteoporosis; low levels of magnesium are associated with nerve-related pain, muscular spasms and acute heart attacks; immune function is lowered when zinc intake is inadequate; chromium is essential for metabolism of carbohydrates and regulation of blood sugar levels; selenium assists heart and immune function and helps prevent cancer. The list goes on.

Natural minerals come to us from the earth - from the food we eat. If the foods we consume are grown in nutrient-poor soil, our body is not getting what it requires. Fertilizers are used in the agricultural industry, however, they contain only three minerals - potassium, nitrogen and phosphorus (used to stimulate plant growth). But there are over 56 minerals that have been identified as *essential* nutrients. Unfortunately, during food processing many essential trace minerals are lost. For example, raw cane sugar loses the following percentages of minerals during the refining process: 99% magnesium, 98% zinc, 93% chromium, 93% manganese, etc. When wheat is milled, mineral loss is as follows: 88% manganese, 87% chromium, 80% magnesium, 78% sodium, 77% potassium, 76% iron and 72% zinc. The same holds true of corn, oats and other refined commodities.

The best way to obtain optimum mineral levels is through the consumption of whole organic foods. As previously discussed, a number of herbs offer valuable minerals including nettles, horsetail rush, chamomile, red clover blossoms and many more. However, considering the depleted condition of most of our nation's top soil, it seems wise to look to the oceans for valuable minerals.

The Resource of Sea Vegetables

Sea veggies contain all 56 minerals and *essential* trace elements *critical* for life to exist. Constantly bathed in the ocean's nutrient-rich broth, sea veggies naturally offer our human cells important building blocks in the exact proportion they inherently understand. Marine animals, such as whales, whose diets contain the broadest range of minerals found in sea vegetables and algae, show no obvious signs of cellular aging. Adult whales have the identical cellular structure as their newborns in comparison to adult humans who suffer from massive cellular degeneration when compared to infants. The water in the human body is *nearly* identical to that found in our oceans today *(but identical to the water in pre Ice Age oceans in which life evolved)*.

Sea veggies assist the body in eliminating common radioactive contaminants and heavy toxic metals such as lead, barium, radium, plutonium, and cadmium. According to studies conducted at McGill University in Montreal, Canada, a compound found in members of the kelp family, called sodium alginate, binds with heavy metals in the intestinal tract, forming an insoluble gel-like salt that is excreted in the feces. These same studies showed that sea veggies reduced the absorption of radioactive strontium from 50 to 80 percent. Sea veggies also possess the ability to lower serum cholesterol, aid digestion and stimulate metabolism. Ancient Chinese and Egyptians used seaweed to treat cancer, and, to this day, practitioners of Traditional Chinese Medicine use it therapeutically to soften and dissolve growths.

An important source of nutrients, sea veggies have been consumed by human beings around the globe since antiquity. From members of South Pacific island cultures to native people living in the high Andes - throughout Northern Europe, Russia and the Arctic, sea veggies have always found a place in the human diet. Remains found in ten-thousand year-old Japanese burial mounds reveal seaweed consumption, while Iceland's oldest book of laws from 981 BCE, defines rights for harvesting dulse on your neighbor's property.

Most varieties of seaweed contain less than two percent fat while offering a high mineral content. A half-cup of cooked hijiki seaweed has more iron than two eggs and approximately the same amount of calcium as a half-cup of milk. Nori seaweed is composed of nearly 30 percent protein while other varieties range from 12 to 18 percent.

Sea vegetables are delicious once you become accustomed to their unique flavors which range from extremely mild to a strong sea tang - and they come in a variety of rich flavors, textures and colors. Sprinkle them on popcorn or add them to your favorite soups, stews, casseroles, stir fries, grain dishes and salads. Some are also used as thickeners for desserts. Sea veggies can be purchased in most health food stores and many supermarkets.

Responsible harvesters gather sea vegetables in clean ocean water; frequent tests are performed to detect the presence of chemical pollutants. While sea veggies cannot be considered a panacea to cure all ailments, ideally, they should form a part of our daily diet, just like broccoli, cabbage, cauliflower or kale.

Please remember that our home,
the human body
is miraculously constructed from
water, food, oxygen and light!
Every day, with each molecule you ingest,
you are rebuilding
and recreating your home!

Herbal Allies - Our Second Line of Defense in Overcoming Dis-ease

Hopefully, the preceding chapters have enabled you to form a new view of your body, based on energetics, and its special needs to achieve optimum balance. Following are chronic disorders that plague many of us with insights from diverse healing tra-

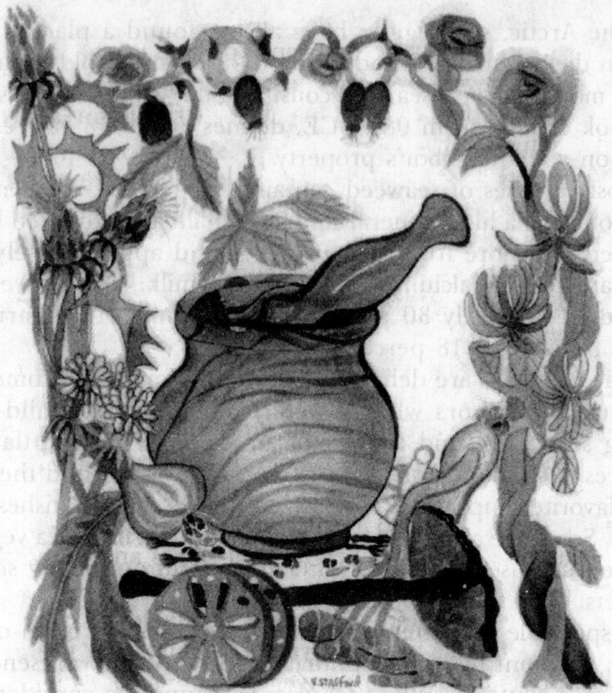

ditions around the globe. While this section is primarily devoted to presenting herbal treatments for these imbalances, other healing modalities (including dietary, vitamin and mineral recommendations) may be discussed as well.

Wisdom From Around the World in Treating Imbalances Associated with the Wood Element

Allergies

Maladies, melodies
Allergies to dust and grain
Maladies, remedies
Still these allergies remain . . .
Allergies, allergies
Something's living on my skin

Doctor please, doctor please
Open up it's me again
I go to a famous physician
I sleep in the local hotel
From what I can see of the people like me
We get better, but we never get well . . .

"ALLERGIES" BY PAUL SIMON

Allergies can plague us during any stage of life. They are associated with the Wood element in Chinese Medicine, since it is an overly sensitive immune-system (our body's internal warrior) that battles with "perceived" harmful invaders.

In allergies the body attacks proteins that, in themselves, are not harmful, such as pollens, dust, foods and poison oak resin. It is the inflammatory reaction around this response that creates the wide range of symptoms we label as allergies. - *Dr. Gary*

Let's see how allergic reactions have been handled in different healing systems.

A Few Folk Remedies for Allergies from Around the World

Ancient Egyptians drank a cup of fenugreek seed tea prior to each meal to clear and stimulate their senses of taste and smell. You might find this popular herb, which is packed full of calcium and other minerals, right on your spice rack. Some hay fever sufferers find relief by drinking a cup of fenugreek seed tea daily.

Greeks, Hungarians, Asians and Italians have long used honey to help prevent hay fever. Be sure to purchase raw organic honey that has been gathered in your area and ingest a small amount daily (one to two teaspoons). It contains minuscule amounts of pollen from local flowers that help desensitize you to these specific allergens. *(Note: Children under two years of age should not ingest raw honey - see page 118).*

Inhalation of eucalyptus vapors to ease congestion comes to us from the land down under. Favorite food of koalas, this soothing Australian herb offers prompt relief. Simply bring a large pot filled with water to a boil; drop in 5 to 10 eucalyptus leaves; cover, reduce heat and simmer for 10 minutes; remove the pot from the heat and with a towel draped over your head breathe in the fragrant steam being careful not to burn your face. You can also add a few drops of chamomile or lemon balm oil to the pot once you have removed it from the heat to help soothe mucous membranes. *(Note: Never take eucalyptus internally - it could be fatal to humans).*

For prevention, Japanese hay fever sufferers ingest a small spoonful of washabi (a potent form of horseradish well-known to sushi lovers) daily. Washabi in sufficient quantity can make you gasp for breath, your eyes will water and your sinuses clear immediately. Most grocery stores carry washabi now but you can also substitute regular horseradish.

Singing the Kansas Wheatfield Blues

Having been born in Kansas (literally in the middle of a wheat field) and suffering from wheat, grass and pollen allergies my entire life, Paul Simon's song takes on special meaning for me! My allergies have improved dramatically over the years with herbal therapy (down from five months to four weeks per year). However, I find that my diet (refraining from wheat products and other refined foods) throughout the year has a major effect on just "how bad" the month of June is going to be for me. This was not a particularly good year (time for true confessions). Quercetin plus bromelain, nettles and a homeopathic allergy formula worked well for the first two weeks. Then the grass pollen count sky-rocketed, making life miserable. We were away on vacation, at my brother's Oregon beach summer home that was surrounded by tall pollen-laden grasses. I didn't have access to all of my herbal supplies, so, taking a walk on the wild side (for an herbalist), I decided to try various pharmaceutical drugs for the next two weeks; in general, one worked but made me feel extremely groggy, nauseous and caused edema; another didn't work at all and I became a zombie. At that point, I wondered if just living with the allergy symptoms wouldn't be better - it wasn't. Allergies are very personal in nature. Together, let's see if we can make some sense of it all.

Allergies are one of those great medical mysteries - biomedicine tells us that virtually anyone can react to a substance for unknown reasons. Before reaching middle age, it is estimated that at least half of the U.S. population experiences allergic reactions of one type or another. Basically, there's good news and bad news. The good news is that allergy sufferers have a really strong immune system, albeit, one that is over-responsive. *Russell Roby, LL.B., M.D. reports that in over 18 years of experience as an allergist he has had only one patient who also had cançer; it would be interesting to find more data on the subject.* Our immune system was designed to defend us against unfriendly invaders like virus, bacteria, cancer cells and toxins. However, sometimes it gets overprotective and reacts to common substances like orange juice, strawberries, tomatoes, chocolate, milk, eggs, peanuts, wheat, corn, pollens, molds, dust, animal hair or dander, penicillin, sulfites, MSG, other chemicals, detergent - potentially anything can be an allergen to any given individual. Some allergic reactions can be extremely dangerous - in some people a certain food or bee or wasp sting can trigger severe swelling which constricts the upper airway, resulting in an inability to breathe.

It's probably important to differentiate between food intolerances and food allergies at this point. Due to the lack of a certain enzyme or enzymes, persons suffering from a food intolerance cannot digest or process the food in question. For example, it is estimated that 82 to 85% of the members of our North and Central Native American/Hispanic population; and up to 95% of the African American population cannot digest lactose found in unfermented milk products. A fair percentage of persons with a Northern European ancestry also become lactose intolerant as they age. Lactase, the enzyme required to digest lactose, is produced in abundance in intestinal cells during infancy in almost all mammals. However, its production decreases rapidly during weaning and is at minimal levels during adulthood. Shortly after ingesting milk, a lactose intolerant individual will experience annoying digestive disturbances such as intestinal cramping, bloating, gas and diarrhea. *(Note: Some lactose intolerant people find that they can consume small amounts of yogurt or cottage cheese without a problem; in the case of these fermented foods, the lactose is already predigested by microorganisms.)*

An allergic reaction differs in that your immune system responds to the ingested food, pollen or other allergen and combats the "invader", triggering a chain of chemical reactions. The substances released (including histamine) create an inflammatory response that actually can do more damage to the body than the protein particle itself, with such common symptoms as itching, hives, rashes, coughing, wheezing, asthma, nasal congestion, sore throat, headache, migraines and fatigue. A memory of the incident is imprinted in sensitized lymph tissues that are ready to produce antibodies every time the same allergen is encountered.

Now comes the part about food allergies that is most difficult to contend with, much less understand. The very foods that we love the most and tend to consume everyday are most frequently the culprits for creating allergic responses. You actually become addicted to the very foods that are causing your problems. This is the way it works: The body releases hormone-like substances in response to a food allergy; these substances give you a "lift"; once the hormonal pick-me-up has worn off, the unpleasant allergy symptoms set in; you unconsciously will reach for the very food that created the problem, trying to recreate the "lift" you experienced a few hours earlier. Sounds like a cruel plot on the part of the gods and nature - doesn't it? Frequently, when interviewing patients, we stumble into the truth regarding which substance or substances are responsible for their allergenic woes with the simple question, "Which foods do you love the very most and tend to consume on a daily basis?" I have seen so many cases in which this proved to be the simple yet effective key to discovering the culprit behind years of allergic reactions. Here's one such example:

Liz Beck, a bright, focused professional woman, was referred to me in June 1999. She had been on Prednisone the previous year to control severe rashes and itching from eczema that covered most of her body. She was currently taking other prescription drugs to control the symptoms. In asking Liz if there were any foods she consumed on a daily basis, her immediate answer was, "orange juice." I asked Liz to refrain from drinking orange juice - to switch to other organic, non acidic juices like apple, pear or peach and to increase her consumption of leafy green veggies. She was given Triphala (please see upcoming section on Ayurvedic herbs for allergies); as well as other Chinese and Western herbs to help clear the "heat" from her system. This was Liz's first experience with complementary medicine; here is her assessment: "Within 2-1/2 months after starting treatment with herbs, acupuncture and dietary changes, 98 percent of my eczema was gone and I was off prescription drugs. I was surprised and thrilled with the results."

In the 1960's, three percent of America's children were diagnosed with allergic dermatitis; in the 1990's, it has increased to ten percent.

You can actually conduct a simple test to determine if you are allergic to a specific food. Most foods are a combination of many ingredients, so it is important to obtain the purest form of the food that you think might be responsible for your allergic reactions. For example, if you feel you are allergic to tomatoes, conduct your experiment with a nice fresh tomato. Now sit down and relax, taking your pulse at the wrist for a 60 second period. It will probably be somewhere between 60 to 90 beats per minute. Ingest 3 to 4 tablespoons of the food that you are testing; remain seated and relaxed for fifteen to twenty minutes and recheck your pulse. If you find that your pulse rate went up 10 beats or more per minute, eliminate this food from your diet for four to six weeks and then retest yourself.

In East Indian **Ayurvedic** medicine, allergies are classified as being of the *vata, pitta,* or *kapha* type: Allergies of the *vata* type usually involve gastric discomfort with bloating, gas and sometimes intestinal colic. Other *vata* reactions include sneezing, wheezing, insomnia, headache or ringing in the ears. *Pitta* allergies usually manifest as an itchy rash, hives, eczema, or allergic dermatitis. Most *kapha* allergies are experienced during the spring season as a reaction to pollens in the air with such reactions as congestion, hay fever, cough, colds, sinus infections and, in severe cases, asthma.

For *vata*-type allergies affecting the gastric tract, an enema of *dashamoola* tea is recommended: Simply bring one pint of water to a boil; add one tablespoon of *dashamoola* and let it boil for five minutes; cool and strain, using the liquid as an enema. Following is an herbal formula that can be ingested three times daily with warm water: Mix 1/4 teaspoon of each of the following three herbal powders: *ashwagandha, bala* and *vidari.* Either licorice or ginger tea will help ease wheezing: Simply boil 1 teaspoon of licorice or ginger root in one cup of water for 3 minutes; add 1/2 teaspoon of plain ghee or *mahanarayan* oil.

Pitta allergies respond to blood purification methods: Mix equal parts of *neem* and *manjistha* herbal powders; take 1/2 teaspoon three times daily after meals with water. To help cool the *pitta* imbalance, in India, it is recommended that the person donate blood to the blood bank.

For *kapha* conditions, the following herbal formula is recommended: Mix 4 parts of *sitopaladi* and *yashti madhu* powders with 1/8 parts *abrak bhasma*. Take 1/4 teaspoon of this mixture with raw organic honey three times daily. *Virechana*, or purgation therapy, is also recommended. Take one teaspoon of organic cold-pressed flax seed oil three times daily for two or three days.

Ayurvedic medicine emphasizes the importance of eliminating foods that increase or aggravate the *dosha* that is out of balance - be sure to see Chapter 10. Other helpful hints from Ayurveda include: 1) Lubricating nostril passages with ghee to protect the mucous membrane from airborne allergens. 2) Triphala is an effective Ayurvedic remedy consisting of three fruits - *amalaki, bibbitaki* and *haritaki*, that treats all three doshas *(vata, pitta and kapha)*. Take 2 to 3 tablets or 1/2 to 1 teaspoon of the powder prior to bedtime. 3) The series of yoga postures known as the Sun Salutation is recommended for those suffering from *vata* or *kapha* allergies while the Moon Salutation is used to pacify *pitta* allergies. 4) Alternate Nostril Breathing can help with allergies affecting the respiratory system with such symptoms as sneezing, wheezing and hay fever. For congestive, *kapha*-type allergies use the Breath of Fire (also known as *Bhastrika*).

Like East Indian Ayurveda, Traditional **Chinese** medicine treats the whole person, and different herbal remedies will be prescribed for each individual, depending upon one's constitution and particular allergic reactions. The idea of Wind in Chinese thought can be compared to our Western concept of allergens. An allergy attack, caused by the inhalation of pollen, dust, dander or other irritants would be called an "invasion of Wind" in the Chinese medical system. The Chinese pictogram for Wind actually includes the radical for "insect" which is translated as "germ or allergenic substance carried by the wind". Wind is the climactic condition which is assigned to the Wood element in Asian thought (just think of the March "winds" that bring April showers). The immune system is the Wood warrior aspect of our bodies that defends our boundaries from external invaders. In the case of allergies and many auto-immune disorders, this warrior aspect is over-vigilant.

For allergies affecting the respiratory tract, and/or intestinal tract, herbal and acupuncture treatment will often be directed toward balancing the Metal or Water elements, which include the Lung/Colon or Kidney acupuncture meridians. In the case of allergic rashes, insomnia, chronic irritability and/or emotional overactivity, practitioners of Chinese medicine will frequently treat the Wood element or Liver acupuncture meridian. If food allergies are the major complaint, accompanied with digestive disturbances, joint pain, chronic sinusitis, and/or itchy, irritated eyes, special attention will be directed to balancing the Earth element or Stomach/Spleen acupuncture meridians.

Effective Chinese Patent Remedies that can be purchased at most health food stores include *Hsiao Yao Wan* (also known as Relaxed Wanderer Pills) which helps treat constrained Liver *ch'i* that interferes with proper digestion (usually accompanied with irritability and/or allergic rashes); *Bi Yan Pian* is traditionally used to treat acute and chronic sinusitis but is effective for hay fever as well; *Pe Min Kan Wan* specifically treats post nasal drip; sneezing, itchy, watery eyes, rhinitis, acute or chronic sinusitis and hay fever. For allergy symptoms affecting the digestive system, *Bu Zhong Yi Qi Wan* helps balance the Earth element, relieving such symptoms as abdominal bloating, pain, gas and irregular bowels.

There are a great number of individual Chinese herbs, as well as traditional formulas, that are beneficial for allergy prevention and symptomatic relief. For a program designed to fit your unique constitution, please consult with a licensed acupuncturist/herbalist.

Western herbal helpers for allergy symptoms are many and varied. Spicy, drying foods like black pepper, cayenne pepper, garlic, onions and Quercetin (wild onion) are used to help dry runny noses and congested respiratory tracts. Studies have shown that some herbs help reduce inflammation by reducing the body's production of histamines - these include chamomile, licorice, garlic and onions. One German study shows that chamomile may actually stimulate natural cortisone production in the body. Marshmallow root is another effective Western herb (found growing along the banks of streams and in marshes) that reduces inflammation and allergic responses while improving digestion. Yarrow and elder flowers help relieve congestion and stop sneezing while ginger, peppermint, anise, feverfew and chamomile supply natural antihistamines.

One of my favorite herbs is stinging nettles - a 1990 study demonstrated that freeze-dried nettle tablets reduced symptoms in hay fever sufferers. This herb tastes something like spinach and was once a popular addition to soups and stews. Gather it in the springtime (be sure to wear gloves); you can dry it for later use, brew a tea of the leaves, or add it to your steamed veggies. Farmers hate nettles because they say it leeches all of the minerals out of the soil; herbalists love it for the same reason - it is packed full of nutrients that help replenish our body's mineral stores. Once cooked, nettle leaves lose their sting.

Other Western herbs that can be beneficial for allergy sufferers include burdock root and dandelion root.

Interestingly, I was unable to locate **Native American** herbs or herbal formulas specific for allergies. Because of their natural lifestyle and diet, it is doubtful that allergies were a problem for most native people. However, numerous herbal remedies have been used by Native Americans for disorders such as coughs, wheezing and sinus congestion and you will find these herbs mentioned in the appropriate sections of the book.

From **Western Nutritional studies** we are learning that our ancestry, as well as blood type can be indicators regarding allergic sensitivities. If you continuously suffer from some of the symptoms listed earlier and the cause remains a mystery to you and your physician, you might want to look into a very interesting book by Dr. Peter J. D'Adamo entitled ***Eat Right For Your Type***. This book outlines specific diets for each of the four blood types: O, A, B and AB. Depending upon your blood type, you may be intolerant or allergic to any number of common foods.

Within the last 50 years, our diets have changed dramatically with the advent of frozen, canned, preserved and other convenience and fast foods. Many people have developed sensitivities to sulfites which are common food additives used to preserve food and prevent its discoloration. Symptoms can include abdominal pain, severe headaches, diarrhea, irritability or feelings of anger, hot flashes, stuffy and/or runny nose. If you are allergic to sulfa drugs, be on the alert, more than likely you suffer from sulfite sensitivity. It can be quite difficult to know if a food product contains sulfites - they may be found on food ingredient labels in a number of different chemical forms, such as: Sodium sulfite, sodium bisulfite, sodium metabisulfite, sulfur dioxide, potassium bisulfite, and potassium sulfite. For a number of asthma patients in my practice, the ultimate answer was simply to eliminate all sulfite containing foods from their diet.

Alicia Albertson, a 38 year old professional woman, head of a busy marketing department in the computer industry, started treatment in 1997 for severe, debilitating asthma, allergies and depression (at her first visit she described it this way, "I haven't been able to crawl out of bed to get to work for two weeks"). Alicia was taking a number of prescription drugs for allergies, two inhalers for the asthma, and an anti-depressant; nothing seemed to work. Her medical history form indicated she was allergic to sulfa drugs. When questioned, Alicia said she always enjoyed drinking a glass of red wine with dinner to unwind. Her case was relatively simple to solve. I asked Alicia to refrain from drinking commercial red wine (grapes are a crop that are heavily sprayed with sulfur containing chemicals). Instead, she substituted organic red wine and refrained from other foods known to contain sulfur products. Even without ingesting herbs for the first two weeks, Alicia's improvement was immediate. Within the first week most of her symptoms were subsiding and she returned to work. Two years later she is doing well; she still has dust and mold allergies but now manages to keep her reactions under control with herbal formulas.

Following is a partial list of foods that contain or are sprayed with sulfites: Fresh grapes, bell peppers, peaches, cherries, mushrooms, iceberg lettuce and potatoes; canned seafoods, dried fish, fresh shrimp, clams, crabs, lobster, scallops and oysters; frozen, canned or dried fruits and vegetables; cornstarch, brown sugar, hard candies, olives, jams and jellies, potato chips, trail mixes, baked goods, colas, gelatin, instant tea mixes. The best advice is to buy organic when possible; eat fresh veggies and fruits; wash your foods well; and always read labels.

Another piece of helpful advice for allergy sufferers is to rotate your foods. Basically you can eat as many foods as you want on a specific day, however, it is essential that none of those foods be repeated more often than every four days. Avoid food products containing artificial coloring as well as other food additives such as benzyldehyde, eucayptol, vanillin, BHT-BHA, benzoates, annatto and monosodium glutamate or MSG. My general rule of thumb is, "if I don't know what it is or can't pronounce it, I'd better find out what it's made of!"

High Cholesterol

In much the same way that we react to the word "fat", most of us have a tremendous aversion to the word "cholesterol". However, cholesterol, like fat, is essential for life. It is used by our body to construct cell membranes and protective sheaths for nerve fibers; to manufacture bile for the digestion of fats, as well as to produce stress-coping hormones such as adrenaline and all of our reproductive hormones including testosterone and estrogen. Animal products such as cheese, butter, meat and shellfish contain cholesterol, while foods that are high in saturated fats (solid at room temperature) like coconut and palm kernel oil tend to produce cholesterol in the body. However, 70 percent of us can process these foods without any significant problems - our bodies are efficient at eliminating the unneeded cholesterol. The other 30 percent of the population has a genetic tendency to create too much cholesterol and therefore do better on a reduced-cholesterol diet.

According to Western medical thought, cholesterol levels should be below 200. However, researchers are now saying that more important than our total cholesterol level is the ratio of our levels of LDL ("bad" cholesterol, known as low-density lipoprotein) to HDL (the "good" guy or high-density lipoprotein). If you are having problems with high cholesterol, below is a checklist to help you bring down those numbers!

Ned, a patient who inherited a tendency for high cholesterol from his father's side of the family, adopted some of the following suggestions - including the one about shiitake mushrooms - his count dropped 75 points (from an alarming 325 to 250) after only four weeks. By the end of eight weeks, his cholesterol had leveled out at 190.

Cholesterol Reduction Checklist

- Increase your consumption of **fresh foods** that help lower cholesterol: apples, grapefruit, bananas, carrots, leafy greens and cold-water fatty fish (such as salmon, sea bass, herring, anchovy, butterfish, mackerel, sardine, tuna and pilchard) non-fat or low-fat milk, yogurt and cottage cheese. Foods that are high in water-soluble dietary fiber help reduce serum cholesterol; these include oat and rice bran, barley, beans (like lentils, mung and black beans), fresh fruits, vegetables and whole grains (in moderation). Research has shown that by merely consuming two to three ounces of oat bran per day we can reduce LDL levels from 10 to 16 percent.
- Researchers from France, Italy and Ireland have confirmed that consuming 2 to 3 **apples** a day lowers cholesterol. **Apple pectin** can be purchased and taken as directed; it binds with fats and heavy metals, helping to eliminate them from the body. The great news is that fruits and vegetables are cholesterol-free!
- Purchase and consume only **unrefined cold-pressed oils** that are liquid at room temperature. Olive oil is excellent though

it is low in essential fatty acids; so be certain to supplement your diet with flaxseed or primrose or black currant seed oil. Omega-3 fatty acids (contained in flaxseed, fatty cold-water fish, or GLA's in evening primrose, borage seed and black currant seed oil) help eliminate cholesterol and fat deposits from the system; they also help reduce blood clotting and lower blood pressure. Israeli and Australian researchers have confirmed that olive oil, avocados and almonds (all rich in mono-unsaturated fats) assist in decreasing LDL levels. Several studies have demonstrated that grape seed oil helps lower cholesterol better than other oils. It is also extremely important to eliminate all hydrogenated fats from your diet - these include margarine and vegetable oils that are solid at room temperature.

- **Coffee**, in large amounts, doubles our risk of heart disease by elevating blood cholesterol levels. One study of 15,000 coffee drinkers, reported in *The New England Journal of Medicine*, revealed that blood cholesterol increases as coffee consumption rises - there is a direct correlation. Gradually reduce your coffee intake and try sipping on a cup of organic chamomile, mint or green tea in its place.
- **Non dairy coffee creamers** are very poor substitutes for dairy products. Most of these products contain overly-processed vegetable oils or tropical oils (such as coconut oil) with high-levels of saturated fat. Try soy, rice or almond milk instead.
- Studies conducted by Japanese researchers demonstrated that approximately **3 ounces of shiitake mushrooms** added to the diet on a daily basis lowers serum cholesterol by 12 percent in one week. Even when butter was added to the diet, the shiitake counteracted rises in cholesterol! *Note: Always cook shiitake mushrooms prior to consumption. Some individuals have shown allergic reactions to raw shiitake.*
- **Garlic** helps to reduce "bad" LDL cholesterol and triglycerides while raising "good" HDL cholesterol. Studies conducted by Dr. Benjamin Lau demonstrated a brief initial rise in LDL when garlic was added to the diet, followed by a considerable drop in serum cholesterol. Thirty-five percent of the persons in this study did not experience a drop in cholesterol; however, they drank heavily and consumed foods that are extremely high in fat. *(Ingest one to two cloves of garlic daily or garlic tablets as directed.)*

- **Artichoke** and it's cousin, **milk thistle**, can improve liver function and help lower blood cholesterol. American, Swiss and Japanese researchers have all confirmed that artichokes contain a cholesterol-lowering substance. One of my favorite herbs, milk thistle (a relative of artichokes), produces a beautiful lavender thistle flower whose seeds yield a remarkably healing oil known as silymarin. To date, many studies have been conducted on this substance that herbalists refer to as "virgin's milk" (because the constituents of this plant are so gentle). But don't let "gentle" fool you! - numerous European clinical studies on silymarin have shown that all subjects who ingested amanita mushrooms (containing one of the deadliest toxins in the world) survived even if they received silymarin up to 24 hours after ingesting the deadly poison. Other studies have shown that healthy liver cells are produced 3 times faster when silymarin is ingested. *Take 140 mg of a natural product standardized to contain 70 to 80% silymarin - 3 times per day - 6 days per week.*
- Research on **gugulipid** *(Commiphora mukul)*, an herbal extract made from an oleogum resin closely related to myrrh, confirms that it lowers cholesterol 14 to 27% and triglycerides 22 to 30% in four to twelve weeks; it helps to increase the liver's metabolism of LDL cholesterol as well. One of the three gifts given to the infant Jesus by the Three Magi, this healing substance has been used in the Middle East since biblical times to treat infected wounds and for digestive and bronchial disorders. In Ayurvedic herbal medicine it has long been used as a rejuvenative and Chinese medical texts from 600CE describe its medicinal properties. *Take 200 mg, four times daily, 6 days per week.*
- **Hawthorn berry tincture** is commonly prescribed in Europe to help reduce cholesterol levels as well as to treat angina pectoris, atherosclerosis, congestive heart failure and high blood pressure. Hawthorn is an extremely safe herbal food and medicine that has been used in the prevention and treatment of digestive and heart disorders for centuries. Hawthorn should be considered a long-term therapy, taking 4 to 8 weeks for its maximum effect to take hold. There are no known interactions of hawthorn with prescription drugs. Ingest 30 to 40 drops of tincture, two times daily, six days per week.
- **Stress** is probably one of the greatest contributors to high cholesterol and heart disease. Try to take a few moments each

day to check in with your body/mind/spirit to identify those stresses that tighten muscles, speed up breathing and send adrenaline coursing through your system to prepare you for the fight or flight mode. Those Wood/Warrior reactions helped keep our fleet-footed ancestors from being devoured by predators but do not serve us well when they are occurring throughout the day, especially when we are in a sedentary situation.

- **Exercise** is an excellent tool for reducing blood cholesterol and elevating HDL. A simple 30 minute walk, 5 times a week, will do wonders to bring your cholesterol levels back in line!

In **Ayurvedic** thought, high cholesterol is related to a *kapha* imbalance. In combating high cholesterol, persons should follow a *kapha*-pacifying diet (please see Chapter 10) eliminating fried foods, fatty dairy products, refined sweets and starches, as well as cold food and drinks. To start your day, Dr. Vasant Lad recommends drinking one cup of hot water into which is added one teaspoon of lime juice (or 10 drops of apple cider vinegar) and one teaspoon of raw, organic honey. In Ayurvedic thought, honey in its natural raw state is a great aid to help eliminate excess *kapha.* However, honey should never be cooked because it's properties change, making it toxic to the system.

One teaspoon of raw honey can be combined with 1/2 teaspoon of *trikatu* and taken two or three times daily to lower cholesterol and reduce *ama* (toxins in the system) and excess *kapha*.

Another effective Ayurvedic herb, *chitrak-adhivati* can be taken two times daily (ingest one 200 mg. tablet after lunch and dinner) to lower cholesterol levels.

An Ayurvedic herbal mixture to reduce cholesterol consists of 3 parts *kutki* to 3 parts *chitrak* and 1/4 part *shilajit.* Mix one teaspoon of raw honey with 1/2 teaspoon of herbs and take with hot water two times daily.

Bhastrika, is a breathing exercise which is also known as the Breath of Fire; it helps to reduce *kapha* as do the following yoga poses: Lotus, Spinal Twist, Cobra, Shoulder Stand and Sun Salutation.

Since cholesterol is a building block for the arteriosclerotic plaques that can clog our arteries, it has received considerable attention from scientific research. Studies have definitively demonstrated that reductions in total cholesterol, and specifically the LDL values (considered the "bad cholesterol"), significantly decreases the risk of coronary artery disease and strokes. Since these are the leading causes of death in the Western world, everyone needs to have a blood test that includes a lipid profile. A risk factor for heart disease can be calculated from the total cholesterol divided by the HDL (the "good cholesterol"). Exercise is known to raise this value, lowering the risk factor. If you have a strong family history or elevated cholesterol values on testing, taking appropriate dietary, herbal, or pharmaceutical measures is preventative medicine at its best.

Cholesterol is only found in animal products - meat, fish, eggs and dairy - so moving the diet in the vegetarian direction is a cornerstone of reducing cholesterol levels. When animal products are consumed, simple measures, such as trimming away fat, avoiding fried foods, eating egg whites instead of the yolk, and choosing non-fat dairy products makes a big difference. Rather than filling up on animal protein, this should be a limited part of the meal, supplemented by salads, vegetables, and whole grains. Consumption of high fiber foods holds dietary cholesterol in the intestines, so it can be eliminated instead of being absorbed into the bloodstream.

Diet is not the only source of cholesterol, as it is also produced in the liver, accounting for elevated values sometimes occurring in strict vegetarians. This is where genetic predispositions come into play. Consumption of foods high in saturated fats (even from vegetable sources) leads to an increase in cholesterol production, while polyunsaturated fats and fish oils have a lowering effect. Smoking and stress elevate LDL, contributing to the likelihood of heart disease. Niacin, which is vitamin B3 (also known as nicotinic acid or niacinamide), has been shown to lower cholesterol, especially at high doses of up to 3,000 mgm per day. In its simple form it may cause unpleasant symptoms of flushing, so use it as inositol hexaniacinate which is flush-free. Although diet and herbs ought to be the first-line of defense, if adequate reduction of cholesterol is not achieved, Western medicine has a lot to offer in this area. This is especially important for those with a family or personal history of heart disease or strokes. The "statin" drugs have a powerful cholesterol lowing effect and studies have repeatedly demonstrated their ability to significantly reduce the risk of the complications of arteriosclerosis. - *Dr. Gary*

Immune Disorders

The image of the Warrior is quite applicable when talking about our body's natural defense system and its ability to ward off foreign invaders that cause bacterial and viral diseases. Low immunity may be compared to an ineffective Warrior that is unable to defend the boundaries of the kingdom. Poor diet, combined with stress and lack of exercise contribute to an impaired immune system which sets the stage for a wide-range of dis-eases that can be associated with the Wood element - hepatitis, recurrent infections of any kind, and cancer. In Five Element thought, auto-immune disorders like rheumatoid arthritis, lupus and thyroiditis can also be linked to the Wood element. Here it is considered an excessive condition - it is as if our internal warrior becomes over vigilant and begins to attack the wrong enemy, waging war on our own organs. In these illnesses, laboratory measurement of antibodies that attack the body's tissues are used to confirm the diagnosis. - *Dr. Gary*

Wisdom from Around the World in Treating Imbalances Frequently Associated with the Fire Element

Anxiety

Every year in the U.S., over 5 billion doses of sleeping pills and tranquilizers are prescribed and ingested; an estimated 65 million Americans suffer from anxiety. According to the National Center for Health Statistics, pharmaceuticals to treat anxiety disorders are among the most often used medications.

A Few Folk Remedies from Around the World

Al-Samarqandi, a Muslim herbalist who lived during the 12th century, prescribed sniffing violets for patients suffering from migraine headaches due to anxiety. In the 20th century, due to aromatherapy research, we are beginning to understand the profound effects flavor and fragrance have on the emotions and moods.

For centuries, the French people have taken warm baths in lime flower (also known as Tilia, or linden flower) tea to lighten depression and ease anxiety. Add a cupful of loosely packed lime flowers to one quart of boiling spring water; reduce the heat to minimal; cover and simmer for fifteen minutes; remove from heat and let steep another 15 minutes; strain out the flowers and add the liquid to your next bath.

Favored for hundred of years throughout Europe and Russia, valerian root is still used to calm anxiety; you can find mention of valerian in novels by the famous Russian writer Tolstoy. Add ten to twenty drops of valerian tincture to your favorite herbal tea and drink before bedtime.

Basil has historically been been the herb of choice of people living in the Arabian Peninsula to fight off depression and anxiety. Fresh basil leaves can be added to salads or vegetable dishes, or simply make a tea by steeping one tablespoon of dried basil leaves in a cup of boiling water for ten minutes; strain and drink to lift the spirits.

In **Ayurvedic** medicine, anxiety is viewed primarily as an imbalance of the *vata dosha* which is associated with the nervous system. A delicious drink made from almonds is frequently prescribed. Soak 10 to 12 raw, organic almonds in spring water overnight; remove the skins and place the almonds in the blender; add a cup of warm milk, a pinch of ginger powder, just a dash of nutmeg powder and a touch of saffron; blend well and enjoy. If insomnia is a problem, you might prefer to soak the almonds throughout the day and enjoy this drink before bedtime. *(Note: People of a kapha constitution should avoid consuming dairy products in the late afternoon and evening.)*

An Ayurvedic herbal tea used to calm anxiety consists of 1/4 teaspoon *tagar* (valerian root) and 1/4 teaspoon *musta (Cyperus rotundus)*; bring 1 cup of spring water to a boil; stir in the herbs, remove from heat, cover and let steep 5 to 10 minutes. Drink a couple of cups of this tea per day.

Gotu kola is considered a prime nervine tonic in Ayurvedic medicine and is used to treat many disorders of the nervous system including anxiety, insomnia and stress. This calming herb promotes mental clarity.

In Ayurvedic medicine, different types of oils are frequently applied therapeutically to sooth imbalances of the three doshas. If you are experiencing anxiety and have a *vata* constitution, give yourself a full body massage (just prior to your morning shower) with organic, untoasted sesame oil (including the head and feet); *pitta* predominant types can use coconut oil and *kapha* types corn or light olive oil. (To discover your Ayurvedic body type, please take the quiz in Chapter 10).

The yoga posture known as the Corpse Pose or *savasana*, can help you relax. Lie down on the floor on your back; arms along your sides. Using long, slow, deep abdominal breathes, visualize your body as a bag filled with sand; now imagine the sand slowly draining out the tips of your fingers and toes as all muscles relax and let go. Practicing this pose for 20 to 30 minutes daily can do wonders to ease anxiety.

In **Chinese** medical thought, anxiety is viewed as an imbalance of the "heart-mind" or *xin*. The Heart not only circulates the blood but houses the mind, and is responsible for consciousness, memory, and sleep. The Heart, together with the Kidney, relate to the brain and nervous system. The Heart relies on all of the other organ systems for its energy and nourishment, therefore, most Heart imbalances are treated through other organ systems. Taking a wholistic approach, practitioners of Chinese Traditional Medicine would prefer that their patients address root issues that may be responsible for feelings of anxiety.

In the Five Element system, the Heart official is part of the Fire element and is termed "the supreme controller". It brings calmness and peace to the body/mind/spirit in the same way that the emperor brings order to the entire kingdom. No wonder that imbalances in this energy are associated with anxiety, panic and insomnia - it is as if a person is operating without an "emperor on the throne". - *Dr. Gary*

When we draw too much energy from our Water element (the Western equivalent of the "human battery pack", relating to the Kidney/adrenal and reproductive organ complexes in Asian thought) during our Fire years, the result can be burn out, anxiety and insomnia. Are job stresses taking their toll? What about your relationships - are they meaningful, supportive and fulfilling? Do you eat balanced meals or simply survive on snacks, fast foods, coffee and other stimulants? Regular exercise is also essential to relax the body and calm the mind. Is there sufficient time and space to simply sit, enjoy and do nothing but *be*?

Twentieth century life accentuated the importance of mental activity. We have lived in the age of "information" - our minds race with excessive thought and worry. It is the nature of Fire or heat to rise, and it is typical for this active energy to concentrate in the head, creating headaches, insomnia, irritability, anxiety and other mental disturbances. Hopefully, as we enter the twenty-first century, we can stop, reassess our lives and begin to devote quality time and energy to the activities, goals, and dreams that would give value to other aspects of life and bring more balance.

Following are some substances used in Chinese herbal medicine that help soothe the mind:

- Jujube date seeds calm the heart and nourish the spirit in Asian thought. *Diana (a Fire Type patient) found that by simply chewing a teaspoon of jujube seeds two to three times a day, anxiety and insomnia were both greatly relieved.* Chia seed also has calming properties.
- Naturally mineral-rich, mushrooms are commonly used in Chinese herbal medicine to settle the nerves, calm the mind and nurture the heart. *Fu Ling*, also known as poria cocos, was used as a food by North American settlers; it reduces anxiety and regulates fluid metabolism. *Ling zhi*, also known as reishi, calms the mind and is a effective immune tonic.
- Pearl powder and oyster shell are both used to settle the heart; calcium made from oyster shells is available in most health food stores.
- Whole grains like brown rice, millet, whole wheat and oats help calm the mind.
- Schisandra berries are prescribed in Chinese herbology to calm the spirit, increase concentration and reduce insomnia. They are astringent in nature and are useful in treating excessive perspiration, diarrhea and frequent urination.
- Foods that are rich in silicon improve the metabolism of calcium, strengthening both heart and nerve tissue, these include celery, lettuce, cucumber, and teas made from oat straw or oat groats.

Western herbalism offers a number of excellent herbal helpers to reduce anxiety, known as nervines, including California poppy, chamomile, gotu kola, hops, kava-kava, lemon balm, oat straw, passionflower, skullcap and valerian. A very strong decoction of organic chamomile flowers works wonders for many patients: Bring 4 cups of spring water to boil in a glass or stainless steel pan; remove from heat and gently stir in 2 to 3 ounces of chamomile; cover and let steep over night; strain and drink 1/4 cup as needed.

A blend of the following herbs in dried or tincture form can also be quite effective: Equal parts of gotu kola, lemon balm, oat straw, skullcap, Siberian ginseng, and 1/2 part licorice root. *(Note: Passionflower should not be ingested for more than two weeks at a time. Valerian should be avoided if you are taking mood-altering medications such as anti-depressants and tranquilizers).*

Aphrodisiacs & Love Potions

Passionate love, "Fire within Fire" in Five Element thought, has been celebrated in poetry and song from time immemorial. In its grips, we mere mortals can soar to great heights or plunge into depths of despair and confusion. Unfortunately, there is no known herbal cure for love itself (that's why this topic is included in the chapter on "chronic disorders")! The flames of love's powerful force drive us to seek union - and in the merging, both partners are both transformed - never to be the same. There is no greater aphrodisiac than genuine love for another individual, marked by care and concern for their well-being. The poet always says it best:

Love has no other desire but to fulfill itself.
But if you love and must needs have desires,
let these be your desires:
To melt and be like a running brook
that sings its melody to the night.
To know the pain of too much tenderness.
To be wounded by your own understanding of love;
And to bleed willingly and joyfully.

KAHLIL GIBRAN FROM *THE PROPHET*

A Few Folk Remedies from Around the World

Whether you wish to fan the flames of a mature relationship, enhance romance or spark the interest of a potential lover, here are tips from cultures around the globe.

Ever wonder where the term "honeymoon" comes from? In antiquity, Celtic brides drank honey-beer for a month after the wedding ceremony to stimulate sexual desire. Both honey and hops in the beer contain traces of hormones. To prepare your own brew, add 2 ounces of organic hops to 2 pints of boiling spring water; cover, remove from heat and let steep for 15 to 20 minutes; strain and refrigerate in a glass container. Simply add a teaspoon or so of raw honey to a glass of the brew and drink before each meal.

The English have also long used hops tea as an aphrodisiac specifically for women. There is a scientific basis for its success since hops contains small amounts of the female hormone estrogen. A bitter yellow extract found in the hops flowers known as lupulin appears to have a stimulating effect on members of the fair sex. Men beware, however, lupulin has a sedative and depressant effect on male physiology. Ever notice that you feel sleepy after sipping on a few beers? *Note: Alcohol, may loosen inhibitions, but, in general, has a sedative effect on the nervous system.*

Egyptian and Arabian men eat chaste berries to improve sexual prowess while in Africa, gum from the kino tree is used as an aphrodisiac.

French people believe the soft artichoke heart is a powerfully stimulating love enhancer. They serve sensuous steaming artichokes at intimate dinners; leaves are dipped in melted butter with a touch of Dijon mustard. French women have yet another secret in their repertoire d'amour; they sip on anisette or licorice water, a substance containing natural hormones.

In Mexico, leaves of the damiana shrub *(Turnera aphrodisiaca)* are used to make tea and added to liqueurs as a flavor enhancer. Commonly found growing in Mexico, California and the Antilles, damiana treats both impotence in men and frigidity in women. You can use damiana tincture (available at most health food stores) as a tonic - take 20 drops three times daily, six days per week. After a month, take a rest from the tincture for one week. Take 20 to 30 drops of damiana tincture an hour before intimacy to experience its aphrodisiac effects.

To enhance their sexual energy and magnetism, Turkish men and women eat powdered fenugreek seeds mixed with honey. Side benefits of fenugreek include its ability to sweeten the breath and perfume the body with a pleasant fragrance. It also helps eliminate perspiration. Gently crush 2 teaspoons of fenugreek seed; stir in to one cup of boiling water, cover and immediately remove from the heat; steep 5 minutes; strain and add a touch of lemon and/or honey to taste. Drink a cup a day. Or, you can make your own fenugreek romance enhancer by simply blending raw organic honey with fenugreek seed powder.

Why not sprinkle some fresh rose petals on your bed and in your bath? For eons, roses have been the flower of choice to carry our message of love to dear ones. The Romans heaped enormous quantities of rose petals on streets, in festive arenas and in bedrooms to stimulate feelings of romance.

It's rumored that Anthony and Cleopatra, to increase stamina during lovemaking, snacked on halvah during their cruises down the Nile. Halvah, a special Middle Eastern treat, is easy to make! Grind one cup of fresh organic sesame seeds and mix in just enough raw honey to create a dough-like texture. Break off chunks and enjoy as much as you dare.

Theobroma cacao comes from the Greek language - translated, it means "food of the gods." Rumor has it that Montezuma II, the famous ruler of the Aztecs (1480 to 1520), drank at least 50 cups of chocolate daily in order to keep up with his 600 wives. Then there was Casanova, the legendary lover, who always drank chocolate before bedtime. Western science has begun to unravel the mystery motivating us to give a box of chocolates for Valentine's Day. Chocolate contains a special phytocompound known as phenylethylamine (PEA for short); it triggers the release of certain brain chemicals which give us feelings of pleasure and euphoria. The neurotransmitters epinephrine and norepinephrine energize while dopamine regulates motor control and sex drive.

The scent used in India to enhance romance is jasmine; lovers are traditionally seen to bathe in moonlit gardens filled with fragrant flowering jasmine plants.

Ayurvedic medicine offers helpful advice and remedies for low libido. As a wholistic medicine, this system prefers to view the symptom in relationship to the whole person. It is possible that reduced sexual energy is the result of emotional and/or physical factors - high stress on the job; physical exhaustion; poor diet; and/or weakness in the male or female reproductive system. Reduced sexual desire could actually be a response by our body as it tries to heal itself from an exhaustive life-style.

Men can strengthen their reproductive systems with a rejuvenative Ayurvedic herb known as *ashwagandha (Withania somnifera)*. Mix 1 teaspoon of *ashwagandha* and 1/2 teaspoon of *vidari (Ipomea paniculata)* in to a cup of milk; warm the milk to infuse it with the essence of the herbs; drink before bed. Women can follow exactly the same directions but will substitute *shatavari* herb *(Asparagus racemosus)* for the *ashwagandha. ("Shatavari" in Hindi translates as "she who possesses 100 husbands." Need we say more?)*

Another interesting Ayurvedic remedy reputed to have aphrodisiac qualities is garlic milk. Stir one clove of peeled, minced garlic into 1 cup of milk and 1/4 cup spring water; simmer on low heat until the liquid has evaporated down to 1 cup. Drink at bedtime.

Here's a delicious almond milk drink to share with your loved one to enhance desire: Soak 10 raw, organic almonds in spring water overnight (double the recipe if you want to share it with your better half); peel off the skins of the almonds the next morning; in the blender add 1 cup of warm milk to the almonds plus: 1 teaspoon of ghee (clarified butter); 1 teaspoon of raw cane sugar or maple syrup; a pinch of nutmeg and of saffron. Blend and enjoy!

To restore sexual energy, figs, honey and *lassi* are recommended by Ayurvedic practitioners. After breakfast, eat 3 figs that have been drizzled with a teaspoon or so of raw, organic honey. An hour later, drink a cup of *lassi* made by blending one tablespoon of fresh yogurt into one cup of water with a pinch of cumin powder.

While jasmine is the blossom of romance in India, magnolia flowers are the choice of the **Chinese**. Lovers, in China, indulge in a special fragrant tea made of beautiful, large magnolia blossoms; it can be found in most health food stores or supermarkets.

In Traditional Chinese Medicine, herbal formulas tailored to the specific needs of your unique constitution are available through licensed acupuncturists/herbalists. Do to our frenetic lifestyle, Americans frequently suffer from adrenal exhaustion with such symptoms as fatigue, low back and knee pain, low sexual drive, and ringing in the ears. Often, Asian herbal treatment is aimed at tonifying the Water element by strengthening the kidney/adrenal and reproductive organ complex which such herbs as cuscuta, epimedium, eucommia, fenugreek seed, American ginseng, dendrobium or lily bulb. *Ch'i* and blood tonifying herbs may be added to the formula including astragalus, atractylodes, codonopsis, dioscorea, ginseng, jujube dates, licorice, *dang gui*, long berries, lycii fruit, white peony root, polygonum or cooked rehmannia.

In Asian thought, maintenance of a healthy Water element (the element that contains the seed for new possibilities while controlling and balancing our Fire element) is of great importance to fertility and longevity. **Kidney *Yang* Deficiency** is characterized by coldness, low energy, low sexual drive, impotence, infertility, premature ejaculation, edema, diarrhea, low back and knee weakness and/or pain, pale tongue and face, ringing in the ears and a general feeling that "the fire in your life is going out." If you suffer from these symptoms, it is important to consume warming foods like lean fish, chicken, eggs, black beans, sesame seeds, walnuts, chives, scallions, lentils, ginger and cinnamon bark tea. Avoid cold and raw foods.

Mildly spicy foods like chive, scallions, garlic and onion can tonify weak sexual functions by warming coldness and removing dampness. Following is a special nutritive recipe if you suffer from symptoms of Kidney *Yang* Deficiency: Soak 1/2 cup of organic black beans for twenty-four hours; strain and prepare as follows: add 4 cups spring water, 1/2 cup chopped chives (check frequently and add more water during cooking time if necessary; simmer on low heat for two to three hours or until the beans are soft and most of the water has evaporated). Remove from heat and let cool; blend 2 tablespoons of black sesame seeds, 1/4 cup of walnut pieces with one umeboshi plum (or one teaspoon sour plum paste) and 2 teaspoons of raw organic honey; add this to the black bean paste, and mix thoroughly. Eat one tablespoon of this tasteful, rejuvenating blend 3 to 5 times daily.

If you suffer from a Water element deficiency (known as **Kidney *Yin* Deficiency**) you may experience heat symptoms because there is not enough "water" to cool down the fire in your body. Symptoms include - insomnia, night sweats, irritability, low back pain, blurry vision, damp palms and soles of the feet, ringing in the ears, low fever in the afternoon, seminal emissions, dry mouth and a red, shiny tongue. Avoid eating hot, spicy foods, alcohol, stress and smoking. Consume cooling foods such as tofu, soybeans, mung beans, seaweed, millet, barley, water chestnuts, black sesame seeds, plenty of fresh organic fruits and vegetables and small amounts of animal protein - crab, clam, lean pork, eggs, cheese. You can purchase an excellent Chinese patent medicine formula specifically for this condition which is known as Liu Wei Di Huang Wan, Rehmannia-Six or "Six Flavor Tea Pills;" it is available at most health food or herb stores or Chinese pharmacies.

Saw palmetto berries were consumed by members of a number of **Native American** tribes to stimulate sexuality. The recommended dosage was four to five berries on a daily basis. Today, saw palmetto berries are used to treat enlargement of the prostate gland as well as atrophy of the testes. Some tribes recommended women eat the berries to firm up breasts. For lactating moms, the saponins contained in saw palmetto increase milk production.

Aging Navajo men and women of the American Southwest drank dayflower tea to enhance their potency; the same mixture was also given to animals used for breeding purposes. The Navajos used lupine as a remedy for sterility and believed that drinking lupine tea for several days prior to conceiving a baby would insure the birth of a daughter.

The Meskwakis, of Wisconsin, had a special love remedy that was given to an argumentative couple. The finely ground roots of both blue and red lobelias were secretly placed in the food of the feuding couple to rekindle the flame of love. Meskwakis women made a special love potion to find a mate; it was composed of mica, gelatin, snake meat and American ginseng root.

Pulverized seeds from wild columbine were used as an aphrodisiac by Ponca and Omaha tribesmen. The suitor rubbed columbine powder on the palms of his hands and contrived of a means to shake hands with the woman of his dreams; the unsuspecting maiden was supposed to be unable to resist his advances.

The Pawnee Native American people concocted a powerful love potion from American ginseng, carrot-leaved parsley, wild columbine and cardinal flower. A friend of the male suitor obtained hairs from the head of his beloved; once her hairs were added to the formula, she was completely captivated by his charms.

From Brazil comes *Pfaffia paniculata*, sometimes referred to as Brazilian Ginseng. Known for its tonifying and aphrodisiac properties, it is now becoming increasingly popular here in North America.

Insomnia

The National Sleep Foundation released findings of its 1999 survey revealing that 33 million American adults suffer from insomnia and another 100 million persons experience poor sleep on a regular basis. One out of every three Americans sleeps six or less hours per night.

It is a common belief in our culture that you need less sleep as you age. To the contrary, studies conducted by the University of Chicago suggest that sleeping less than eight hours each night can accelerate the aging process, hastening the onset of diabetes, hypertension, overweight and loss of memory. When men in the study cut back to only four hours sleep, their bodies responded with higher blood sugar levels while insulin secretion decreased by 30 percent - similar to persons who suffer from diabetes. The sleep-deprived men also experienced heightened levels of cortisol which is related to memory loss and insulin resistance.

Sleep researchers at Stanford University demonstrated in recent studies that lack of sleep can produce results similar to drinking too much alcohol. Persons who suffer from sleep apnea (a serious condition affecting an estimated 25 million Americans in which breathing can stop numerous times each hour) did more poorly on reaction time tests than did people who were actually drunk. The same subjects scored *worse* on three of the other seven components tested.

During the deepest stages of sound sleep, the human body completes some of its most important functions by rebuilding and restoring cells, tissues and organs, and replenishing enzymes, hormones and immune cells. Dreaming takes place during the REM (rapid eye movement) stage of sleep - without it, the human brain and psyche cannot function properly. Prolonged periods of REM sleep deprivation can result in serious emotional disorders. However, Eve Van Cauter, director of the University of Chicago study, says that the sleep deficit can be recuperated by resting longer than the normal eight hours per night.

Tension is a prime culprit keeping many of us awake at night. When you are under stress your body produces adrenaline which can overpower serotonin, a hormone the brain produces to promote feelings of relaxation and well-being. Serotonin is later converted into melatonin - the body's natural sleeping "pill".

Following are some helpful recommendations:

- Avoid caffeinated drinks and chocolate after lunchtime. Elimination of these stimulants alone can result in improved sleep.
- Avoid tobacco and alcohol. While a cigarette may seem to calm you down, nicotine is actually a neurostimulant and can disrupt sleep. While a little alcohol induces sleep at first, it disrupts deeper stages of sleep later.
- Avoid ingesting cold medications or nasal decongestants, such

as pseudoephedrine, late in the day. While antihistamines may cause drowsiness, the decongestant constituent acts as a stimulant to most people.

- Use your bedroom only for sleep and intimacy - not for watching TV, eating or working.
- Try taking a leisurely hot bath scented with lavender oil an hour or two before going to bed.
- If you are not sleepy, do not stay in bed. Get up, go to another room and do something until you do feel really sleepy.
- Try to set up a regular morning or afternoon exercise program - physical exertion can be very helpful in helping you relax. Avoid exercising in the evening before bed; it takes a while to wind down after exercise.
- Avoid consuming foods which contain tyramine at dinner time: bacon, cheese, chocolate, ham, sugar, sausage, spinach as well as members of the nightshade family including bell peppers, eggplant, potatoes and tomatoes. Tyramine increases the release of norepinephrine, a neurostimulant.
- At dinner, or in the evening, consume foods that are high in tryptophan (see page 315), a natural sleep inducer: bananas, chicken, dates, figs, milk, nut butters, turkey, whole grain crackers and yogurt.
- A balanced calcium/magnesium supplement relaxes muscles and can have calming effects. Magnesium is an important mineral naturally found in whole grains and fresh green vegetables. Unfortunately, it is not present in refined flour products since it is lost in the milling process. Without adequate magnesium, calcium does not function properly in the tissues of the heart and nerves. *Try supplementing your diet with 500 mg calcium citrate/250 mg magnesium tablets three times daily after meals, especially if you are interested in strengthening the bones and preventing osteoporosis in later life.*
- Inositol improves REM sleep. *Ingest 100 mg prior to bedtime.*

A Few Folk Remedies from Around the World

Polynesian people have long used a liquor made from kava-kava (a plant native to tropical forests) in religious ceremonies; it relaxes the mind and encourages restful sleep without side-effects. Kava-kava helps relieve anxiety and contains pain-relieving phytochemicals that are believed to be as effective as aspirin. Extensive studies now support the contention that this herb promotes higher quality sleep by decreasing muscle tension, promoting relaxation and encouraging a state of sleep within 30 minutes after ingestion.

If your ancestors were from Russia or Germany they probably drank the following mixture to relieve insomnia: Crush or grind 1/2 teaspoon of anise seed and mix into a cup of milk - warm over low heat; add a drizzle of raw organic honey and enjoy before bedtime.

Galen, the famous Greek physician, is said to have cured insomniacs by advising them to eat large quantities of lettuce at the evening meal. Interestingly, the Irish and English make a tea from chopped lettuce leaves as a remedy for insomnia. Irish people will add a sprig of mint to the decoction to promote digestion and improve the flavor.

In ages past, English and other European peoples made a strong infusion of hops tea to encourage sleep. Simply bring 1-1/4 cups spring water to a boil; remove from heat and stir in two tablespoons of hops; cover and let steep for 15 minutes; strain and flavor with a squeeze of lemon, add a touch of raw organic honey if desired.

Red clover blossom tea was used by American pioneers to calm the body and mind, promoting sleep. Red clover is naturally high in essential vitamins and minerals as well as blood-thinning coumarins. Follow the recipe immediately above, substituting two tablespoons of red clover blossoms for the hops - add a drizzle of honey.

Greek soldiers in Alexander the Great's army learned some Egyptian herbal medicine when they conquered that country and took these remedies back home to Greece. Before bed, mash two cloves of garlic with a few drops of olive oil; place the mixture on a piece of whole grain brain and enjoy. You can eliminate the garlic odor by chewing on a a sprig of parsley or a few fennel or anise seeds.

A popular Gypsy cure for insomnia entails drinking a mixture of hot water, honey and lemon or orange juice just before bedtime.

In East Indian **Ayurvedic** medicine, insomnia is viewed as a *vata dosha* imbalance affecting the mind or nervous system. A cup of warm milk is frequently prescribed. You can add a dash of nutmeg (no more than 1/16 teaspoon), and/or some almonds ground in a coffee grinder with a pinch of cardamom. Garlic milk is also prescribed: Simmer one clove of fresh crushed garlic in 1 cup of milk and 1/4 cup water on low heat for 10 minutes, ingest before retiring.

Following is an Ayurvedic herbal combination to help induce sleep: Combine equal parts of valerian root power and chamomile; ingest 1/4 teaspoon of the formula with warm water prior to bedtime.

Massaging warm sesame or *brahmi* oil into the scalp and soles of the feet just before going to bed helps soothe *vata dosha*, encouraging sound sleep.

A brief 20 to 30 minute period of meditation before going to bed can help still mental processes and resolve the stress and anxiety that keeps the mind active at night. Sit comfortably in your bed and follow your breath in and out. The mind might jump to other topics but bring it back to the breath. During the slow inhale think or hear the word *"So"* in your mind; gently exhale thinking *"Hum."* As you begin to relax, lay back in your bed, continuing to watch your breath, focusing on the third eye area between your eyebrows and repeating *So-Huṃ.*

Some everyday **Chinese** home remedies for insomnia include repeatedly yawning before retiring. Once in bed, place the tip of your tongue just behind the lower teeth; concentrate on keeping the tongue in this position until you fall asleep. If this fails, try inhaling the vapors of a crushed onion.

In Traditional Asian medicine, insomnia is frequently viewed as an imbalance of the Fire element and treatment is geared towards nourishing the heart and calming the mind and spirit. Mental hyperactivity, so prevalent in our modern age, sends the *yang* aspects of the heart (spirit, heat and *ch'i* energy) spiraling toward the head, leaving the heart impoverished. By enhancing Heart *yin*, the *yang* energies are restrained and superficial thinking will begin to cease. It is only then that we can begin to stay centered in the ever present "now".

Asian dietary and herbal recommendations for calming the mind include focusing on a simple diet with occasional light fasts. Rich, heavy meals, eating late at night, refined sugar, coffee and alcohol all contribute towards insomnia and excessive mental chatter. Foods and substances that help build the *yin* of the heart include:

- oyster shell (rich in calcium);
- whole grains and legumes like kamut, brown rice, rolled oats, lentils and mung beans;

- mushrooms that are naturally high in mineral salts which help settle the nerves *(please read about them in the preceding section on "Anxiety")*.
- foods rich in silicon improve the metabolism of calcium and help strengthen heart and nerve tissue, these include lettuce, celery, cucumber, barley and oats. Also try sipping on a cup of oat straw or horsetail rush tea.

Dill and basil are calming spices that can be added to food and teas. Most of the **Western** herbs already discussed in the preceding section on "Anxiety" are effectively used to treat insomnia, these include catnip, California poppy, chamomile, catnip, hops, kava-kava, passionflower, skullcap and valerian. It is best to try different herbal combinations and rotate the single herbs being ingested every two to three weeks. Always take a rest from herbs one day a week.

Native American Menominee people drank an infusion of partridge berry leaves as a remedy for insomnia. A very small quantity of black nightshade leaves (not to be confused with deadly nightshade, or belladonna) were steeped in a large amount of water to treat sleeplessness by the Comanche, Houma and Rappahannock natives of North America.

Wisdom From Around the World in Treating Imbalances Frequently Associated with the Earth Element

Bad Breath

There are many natural aides to freshen your breath - even if you are an onion and garlic lover! Most frequently, bad breath is due to poor dental hygiene or a diet that leads to weak or sluggish digestion. However, bad breath could be a sign of serious illness like ulcers, sinusitis, periodontal disease, kidney failure or liver trouble - so be alert and consult a professional health care practitioner if your problem persists.

A Few Folk Remedies from Around the World

Breath-sweetening licorice-flavored anise seeds were chewed by ancient Greeks to freshen their breath; after meals simply chew on five to ten seeds. A famous Greek historian named Theophrastus advocated eating grapefruit as a breath aid. Rich in natural vitamin C and bioflavonoids that support healthy gums, grapefruit as well as strawberries, red dates and persimmons were recommended to counteract garlic breath.

The people of Portugal use fresh basil to sweeten breath. Add a few sprigs to your salads or sprinkle them on other favorite recipes.

After meals try munching on a 1/4 teaspoon or so of whole fennel seeds like the East Indian people. Fennel's interesting flavor tends to grow on you and will soon become a palate pleaser; it is best described as a mixture of licorice, lemon and pine.

Fresh green foods with a high chlorophyll content are natural breath fresheners. The ancient Romans chewed on a sprig of parsley to cover up the odor of alcohol on their breaths.

Native Americans, Arabian and East Indian people rub sage leaves on their teeth to cleanse them as well as freshen breath.

Mint has been used world wide as a breath aide. Simply chew on a fresh mint leaf or brew up a cup of peppermint tea.

Cardamom, a fragrant spice commonly used in East Indian and Arabian cuisine to improve digestion, contains a potent antiseptic (cineole) which helps kill bacteria that can be responsible for bad breath. Simply purchase whole cardamom seeds and chew on a few to freshen your mouth.

Chinese cooks frequently add coriander (Chinese parsley) to meat dishes as a preventive measure to avoid bad breath. Chinese people will also chew on one to two pieces of clove spice to ease toothache pain and eliminate bad breath.

Still suffering from dragon's breath?

The coating (or lack of it) on your tongue reveals a lot about your health in both Ayurvedic and Chinese medicine. The basic idea here is that poor digestion and malabsorption leads to fermentation and putrefaction of the food in the gastrointestinal tract which is reflected in a thick coating on the back of the tongue. Basically, our whole system is affected by weak or sluggish digestion resulting in the retention of metabolic wastes in the fluid which surrounds each of our living cells.

Metabolic waste that clogs the extra cellular space in our

bodies is referred to as *ama* in Ayurvedic medicine and *tan* in Chinese medicine. Actually, most chronic dis-ease (in wholistic systems of healing) is viewed as an accumulation of toxins in this living matrix of our bodies. For example, once the fluid in our extra cellular space is loaded with toxins it is common to experience pain and stiffness as a result of the irritation created by the waste substances. Rheumatism or fibromyalgia, as it is currently called, is a good example of such a condition. Toxins pushed into the joints or sinuses become stagnant pools inviting various microbes to set up housekeeping.

But we were talking about bad breath! So let's start by taking a peek at your tongue in the mirror. In both Ayurvedic and Chinese systems of healing the whole body of the tongue and its different coatings can be analyzed to determine the health of various organ systems. However, let's keep it simple. Is the coating on the back of your tongue thick and white or yellow? If it is white, according to Chinese medical theory, you are too cold and probably consuming too many *yin* congesting foods like ice cream, cheese, sugary pastries, refined bread products and fruit juices (increase your consumption of fresh veggies and low fat protein like cold-water fish and lean poultry and meat). A yellow tongue coating indicates you are probably too warm and need to reduce the consumption of *yang* meats, eggs, and processed, fried and salty foods while significantly increasing your consumption of fresh fruits and vegetables.

Ayurvedic medicine, in order to address the root of the problem creating bad breath, emphasizes the need to rekindle the waning gastric fire *(agni)* which is responsible for poor digestion. Stay away from heavy cold and/or congesting meals that are difficult to digest. After eating, to improve digestion, chew one teaspoon of roasted fennel and cumin seeds (one to one ratio).

Aloe vera juice or gel will help restore freshness to the breath. Mix 1/8 teaspoon cumin powder in one tablespoon of gel or 1/3 cup aloe vera juice and ingest morning and evening (before breakfast and going to bed).

A digestive tea that can be ingested after each meal is composed of equal amounts of cumin, coriander and fennel seeds. Gently crush one teaspoon of the seeds and stir into one cup of boiling water; cover and remove from heat, letting the mixture steep for about five minutes; strain and drink.

Weight Problems

Every year, after January 1st, tens of thousands of Americans are afflicted with an unpleasant dis-ease called "post-holiday diet syndrome". With mixed feelings of remorse, resignation, regret, reluctance, repentance and resolution, we begin our annual pilgrimage to the multi-billion dollar diet industry's "magic mecca" of weight loss clinics. Armed with the latest low-fat, or low-carb or low-protein diet, with arduous consistency, over months and months, we heroically scale our personal Mt. Olympus . . . but sadly, like Sisyphus, the Greek mythological character forced to repeatedly push an enormous boulder up a steep mountainside, we finally reach the glorious summit (our target weight) only to watch in bewilderment as the boulder plummets down the mountain once again. You may have heard that 98% of all persons participating in weight loss programs have gained back MORE weight than they originally lost by the end of two years. A study published by the National Institutes of Health (NIH) in 1992 found that 99 percent of all dieters put back on all the weight they had lost within five years after completing a diet program. For all the dieting and deprivation, frustration, feelings of guilt and money spent, we Americans are heavier than ever.

There are many factors that can greatly influence our weight which will be discussed in the upcoming pages. Unfortunately, despite what advertisers try to lead us to believe, weight loss success does not boil down to the same simplistic calorie-reducing diet for everyone; or a special herbal brew that will enable us to burn fat; or a supplement that absorbs fat in the intestines. Dedicated researchers are gaining some valuable insights into the complex issues regarding weight control. Unfortunately, studies are conducted on one or two targeted hormones in one institution while across the country valuable information obtained by scientists studying other factors is never synthesized into a complete picture. Instead, we get book after book describing a single viewpoint and a new miracle diet cure that works great for some, for a while, and spells disaster for others. **Simplistic, reductionistic thought does not serve us well in the arena of weight control or chronic diseases where there may be many contributing factors.** While this book is not the place to go into great detail, I hope to briefly summarize various views to gain insight into the complex issues surrounding weight control. We will explore a number of contributing factors to overweight in the upcoming pages. *(Note: Most of the following problems are not limited only to persons with weight problems but can affect thin persons as well)*: 1) the "Famine Within" - malnutrition caused by low-calorie dieting or poor diets; 2) food addictions created by allergic reactions; 3) Omega 3 fatty acid deficiency, 4) fluctuating blood sugar levels due to carbohydrate sensitivity; 5) overwork, stress and anxiety; 6) adrenal exhaustion; 7) low thyroid function; 8) imbalances in our reproductive hormones related to PMS, menopause and andropause; 9) medications and prescription drugs; 10) yeast overgrowth; 11) food additives, MSG and artificial sweeteners, 12) lack of exercise; 13) genetics; 14) overeating; and 15) the beta endorphin and (16) serotonin connection to weight gain were discussed in the preceding section entitled "Healthful Carbohydrates Promote that Peaceful Feeling".

But first, a brief review of where we have been . . .

What Should We Count: Calories, Carbohydrates or Fat Grams?

In the 1950's and 60's we were told that food (calories) made you fat, so we went on the low calorie hard-boiled egg and grapefruit diet or drank meal replacers like Metrecal. By the 1970's and 80's we understood the importance of exercise, so we jogged and jazzercized while counting both carbohydrates and calories, ate three ounces of protein twice a day and guzzled diet sodas. Towards the middle of the 80's the lowly potato was on the comeback regaining respect as complex carbohydrates, more exercise and carbo-loading became the trend. In the 1990's we counted fat grams, ate complex carbohydrates and continued to exercise; though, towards the end of the decade, the high protein/low carbohydrate diet made an impressive come-back. Over the years, there have been hundreds of "miracle" diets or diet aids marketed. Many of us have tried a great number of them. For some of us, the sheer frustration of trying to live up to the Twiggy or Barbie image has prompted anorexia and bulimia. Believe me, after some of those diets, it seemed easier! Sadly, recent studies have confirmed that one out of every four college aged woman has an eating disorder.

America's War on Weight: Shapes and Sizes of Human Bodies — What's Perfect Anyway?

Greek humoric, Ayurvedic and Asian Medicine tells us that everyone inhabits a totally different, wonderful and unique bodyscape. The great diversity of humanity is broken down into four types in Greek humoral theory; three types in Ayurvedic thought and five elemental types in the Chinese Five Element model. What is the ideal weight? What is the ideal diet? For that matter, what is the ideal body?

Human heights range, more or less, from 3 1/2 to 7 1/2 ft. tall; but, fortunately, we never see a 7 foot person walking around with a 100 pound weight on their head to reduce their height. That, however, is the equivalent of what many women are trying to do in order to reach the "ideal" thin body with which our culture is so obsessed. Kelly Brownell, obesity expert at Yale University states that today's ideal body lies "beyond what many people can achieve with healthy and reasonable levels of dieting and exercise. The percent body fat required for the aesthetic ideal (in our culture) is probably less than half the normal level, so one has to question whether the individual meets biological resistance in pursuit of the ideal."

One of the major focuses of this book is to help you determine your unique bodyscape (its inherent strengths and weaknesses) and to assist you in finding a healthy lifestyle, herbs and nutrition that suit you best - something with which you can live. Interestingly, the 2% of dieters who manage to maintain weight loss are those who have devised their own programs. It should include a meal-plan (forget diets - they don't work!) filled with a great variety of delicious flavors derived from whole foods - basically, a plan for healthy living. It is important to remember that different flavors heal and balance different body types. And, one thing I can guarantee is that you probably will not look like Barbie - there are over three billion beautiful women on our planet who do not look like super models - there are only eight who do. One study found that three minutes spent looking at models in a fashion magazine caused 70% of the women to feel depressed, guilty and shameful. Probably the most frightening report of all was one published in *Newsweek* magazine in 1990 - 11% of parents surveyed said they would abort a child predisposed to obesity *(I would not be here, nor would Drs. Robert Atkins or Rachel Heller)*. Isn't something very wrong with this scenario? There are a great number of us walking around feeling pretty miserable about ourselves. In our society, excess weight is equated with gorging, laziness, ignorance, and slovenly habits - stereotyping and discrimination at its worst. Television and cinema have a heyday with their "humorous" portrayals of large persons. Let's try to get to the truth - to challenge and unmask the anti-fat messages with which we have grown up . . .

Dispelling the Myths

We have been told that 3,500 calories equals one pound of body weight. In one study, when identical twins were intentionally overfed, they gained weight at the same rate. Unrelated people on the same diet, with the same number of calories gained anywhere from 9.5 to 29 pounds.

> *"Fatness, in most cases," claim William Bennet, M.D., and Joel Gurin in* The Dieter's Dilemma, *"is not the result of deep-seated psychological conflicts or maladaptive eating behaviors; usually it is just a biological fact."*

One classic study was conducted at Middlesex Hospital in London forty years ago by Kekwick and Pawan. Various 1,000 calorie-per-day diets were compared, under hospital ward conditions, to assess their effect on weight loss. If weight was, indeed, dictated solely by caloric intake, then all patients should have experienced the same weight loss regardless of the type of calories ingested. Patients gained weight on 1,000 calorie-per-day diets consisting of 90 percent carbohydrates while losing weight on those diets that had a much lower carbohydrate content.

Set Point Theory and Other Factors That Determine Our Weight

Many years of scientific research and testing at major universities, such as Brigham Young and Cornell, have shown that low calorie diets just don't work and, in the long run, actually make you fatter. The body interprets a low-calorie diet as starvation. It reacts quickly by shedding mostly muscle tissue and water - this is the first weight loss you experience. While the first 20 pounds you lose may look great on the scale, as much as 10 pounds of that weight loss can be muscle tissue. And, unfortunately, you have just sabotaged your own ability to burn fat because fat can only be burned by lean muscle tissue. The more muscle tissue you lose, the less fat you burn.

A Rockefeller University study found that the body burns calories more slowly after weight is lost and faster than normal when weight is gained. "The body has an opinion about what it should weigh," states Richard E. Keesey, Ph.D., a researcher at University of Wisconsin. An individual's "weight range" is primarily determined by genetic and other physiological factors. The human body has a weight-regulating mechanism located under the brain in a gland known as the hypothalamus which is responsible for establishing your fat level or "set point." It signals you to take in more food when your supply of stored energy (fat) is threatened by a low-calorie diet and actually DECREASES your body's metabolic rate so that you burn less energy. Each time you undertake a low-calorie diet, you are diminishing your body's ability to burn fat and resetting your "fat thermostat" so the body struggles to retain more fat than before! Your body is intent on protecting you from the next cycle of "famine."

Obesity expert John Foreyt, Ph.D., who coauthored a book with G. Ken Goodrick, *Living Without Dieting*, explains:

> *We feel that losing weight by dieting is not unlike breath holding. The body will take over control after awhile, and it will cause breathing and eating even if the mind doesn't want to. After breath holding, a normal person will inhale a vast quantity of air to make up for the oxygen deficit. After a prolonged diet, the body will take in a large number of calories to make up for calorie deprivation.*

Susan Fried, Ph.D., speaking to members of NAASO in 1991, said the number of fat cells a person possesses stays constant (or increases with weight gains over 50 pounds). Once you have a fat cell, its yours for life, even with large weight loss. People tend to stop losing weight once fat cells reduce to "normal" size. People with excess numbers of fat cells will still be fat even though their cells are normal size. Dr. C. Wayne Callaway agreed, "If you have more fat cells than average, it will be difficult for you to achieve average weight." Fried added that maintaining a fat cell below its normal size appears to cause biological stress. At this same meeting, Robert Eckel, M.D., professor of medicine and biochemistry at the University of Colorado, concurred with Fried adding that reduced fat cells become "rebellious" by hanging on to their remaining fat and sucking in more outside fat. What can be done with this information in a society obsessed with a body size and proportion that only 5 to 7% of the population has the ability to ever achieve?

"If we learned to scorn obesity, we can unlearn it,"
says Carol A. Johnson,
author of Self-Esteem Comes in All Sizes.
"All it takes is an open mind and an open heart."

As you can see, the definitive answer regarding our nation's weight gain dilemma is not yet in. While keeping in mind that some people can be large *and healthy* due to genetics, let's briefly examine those fifteen factors that can greatly influence our ability to lose weight. Many overweight persons are contending with a combination of the complications discussed below:

(1) - Malnutrition Caused by Poor Nutrition or Low Calorie Dieting: The Famine Within

We Americans are surrounded by highly processed foods - foods high in salt, fat and caloric value, yet very low in nutritional value. The average American female ingests between 1,500 and 2,000 calories daily - the average male about 3,000. Of these, 30 to 40 percent come from poor quality fats (or 600 to 800 calories for the average female and 900 to 1,200 for the average male).

Compounding the problem, the average American consumes about 135 pounds of sugar per year (compared to 120 pounds in 1970 and 25 pounds in 1900) - amounting to well over 500 calories per day devoid of any nutritional value (meaning the calories contain virtually no protein, vitamins or minerals). If we take the lower figure for fat consumption for the average woman's daily diet based on 2000 calories - approximately 600 calories will be from fat, plus 500 calories from sugar, we get a total of 1,100 of relatively meaningless calories a person is consuming on a daily basis. This woman would have to get all of her essential nutrients from the remaining 900 calories. What can our human body and its millions of hungry cells interpret when confronted with empty calories other than there is a shortage of essential nutrients in the world. In response, it seems only logical that it would raise the body's set point and carefully guard its fat reserves.

Now, consider the fact that many weight-loss diets are based on the consumption of 900 to 1200 calories daily - prisoners at Treblinka, the dreaded Nazi camp were given 900 calories daily. In comparison, guidelines from the United States Department of Agriculture state that the minimum quantity of calories, recommended for a teenage girl or woman, is 2,500 per day. The World Health Organization (WHO), has established that starvation begins when less than 2,100 calories are consumed per day. This organization has many years of experience in dealing with worldwide starvation and uses this figure when calçulating emergency food rations. Many American women are barely existing on 900 meaningful calories per day while consuming another 1,100 calories in poor quality fats and sugar. Simply stated, we are not ingesting enough real food to subsist.

Research has shown that fat cells actually
increase in number and double in size
when children and adolescents
are subjected to low-calorie diets
- setting them up for a lifetime of dieting.

Do you have a tendency to skip meals and drink diet colas, cutting calories wherever possible while consuming too much fast food? Unless we have a thyroid dysfunction or other hormonal imbalance, the more whole food we consume, the faster we burn calories.

(2) - Food Addictions Created by Allergic Reactions

The very foods to which we have an allergic reaction are the ones that keep pulling us back for more of the same. Do you find yourself consuming the exact same food day after day? In response to a food allergy, the body releases hormone-like substances that give us a "lift", once the hormonal pick-me-up wears off the unpleasant allergy symptoms are back with a vengeance. We then unconsciously reach for the very food that caused the problem in the first place to recreate the "lift" experienced earlier. As an example, if you suffer from a wheat, corn, chocolate, or peanut allergy you might be tempted to snack all day long on high-calorie/low nutrient junk foods containing these ingredients. Unconsciously, you keep refueling the allergy cycle while being kept from eating healthful nutrients you would otherwise consume. Please read the section entitled "Allergies" page 325, where this topic is discussed in greater detail.

Amy, a forty-five year old professional woman and mother of two children, was afflicted with head-to-toe rashes and swollen, painful joints that had been bothering her for over six weeks. Due to side effects, she elected not to take the Prednisone prescribed by her medical doctor to help reduce the symptoms and sought alternative therapy instead. In questioning Amy, we discovered that she tended to snack all day on refined white flour products - cookies, pretzels, bread, muffins. I asked her to simply eliminate all wheat products from her diet for the next week while concentrating on eating more green vegetables, whole fruit and whole grains like brown rice. Improvement was immediate. By the end of the first week the rashes had disappeared; by the end of three weeks most of the joint swelling and pain was significantly reduced; by the end of six weeks Amy had lost 15 pounds that had plagued her for years and all symptoms were gone.

(3) - Omega 3 Fatty Acid Deficiency

Are you getting enough fat? As a nation our fat consumption is down to 35 percent of the calories we consume; however, many of those fat calories come from highly processed oils that contribute to ill-health.

If you find yourself overeating potato chips, French fries or other rich, creamy fatty foods it is possible that you are being driven by your body's inherent call for healthful fats. A number of my patients have found that by adding a constant supply of Omega 3 fatty acids to their diet that their fat cravings cease and their weight decreases (see page 301).

(4) - Carbohydrate Sensitivity and Addiction

Let's say it's 7:30 p.m., you just finished a good meal and your best friend drops off a plateful of delicious homemade chocolate chip or peanut butter cookies - still warm from the oven. Would you refuse taking a cookie because your appetite was well satisfied at dinner? Would you rather nonchalantly take one cookie, eat it now or perhaps save it for later? Or, would you immediately scarf down two or three cookies, possibly downing the whole plate of cookies once you got started? Persons suffering from severe carbohydrate addiction can only smile at that question - they know the answer. Most of the cookies would be gone within a short time.

Is it easier for you to skip breakfast and lunch and only eat dinner because you find yourself hungry all day once you start eating? For carbohydrate sensitive individuals, that one slice of toast and jam for breakfast can spell disaster and start the unbearable cravings associated with carbohydrate sensitivity throughout the rest of the day. Believe it or not, there is nothing wrong with your *will power* but you do suffer from a hormonal imbalance triggered by carbohydrate consumption.

In two to three days, all your cravings can be gone simply by eliminating foods that are high on the glycemic index from your diet while concentrating on eating healthful protein foods and vegetables *(Note: some orange colored vegetables, like carrots, are high on the glycemic index)*. Constructing a healthful diet that you can live with for a long time is much more difficult but there are a number of books on the subject (please see the Resource Section of this book for recommended reading). Using different methods to control insulin, Drs. Robert Atkins, Barry Sears and Richard and Rachel Heller have been studying and treating individuals with this imbalance for years.

According to Dr. Barry Sears, author of *The Zone*, about 25% of the population has a serious problem dealing with carbohydrates that rank high on what is known as the glycemic index. Regardless of the number of calories they ingest, weight loss is nearly impossible if certain carbohydrates, like those found in processed breads, pastries, cereals or even potatoes, certain whole grains like millet and cooked carrots are consumed in more than very minor quantities. These foods cause a rapid release of insulin in carbohydrate-sensitive individuals. Simply put, you can't burn fat with high levels of insulin in your blood stream no matter how severely calories are restricted - insulin is a fat-storing hormone. This was one of the answers to my lifelong problem (as I found myself gaining weight on an 800 calorie diet!) which forced me to discard much of today's dietary dogma.

For some, weight can *only* be held in check by controlling consumption of carbohydrates in order to manage excess insulin production. Sears' "block method" uses lean body mass and physical activity factors as a means of arriving at the quantity of food to be ingested daily. These calculations are to be used as a starting point for the minimum amount of protein and, therefore, calories to be consumed daily. I have found, however, unless someone has a very small frame, these calculations tend to be too conservative and consuming 2 to 6 more blocks per day than recommended by Sears still produces good results (as long as whole foods are eaten that do not rank high on the glycemic index). *A word of caution: watch out for convenience "balanced nutrition bars" - the highly refined sugars they contain hit the blood stream immediately and set off cravings for susceptible persons.* For those who can't bear the thought of calculating blocks, researchers Drs. Rachael and Richard Heller offer another approach to controlling insulin release in an informative book entitled, *The Carbohydrate Addict's Diet*. However, as your insulin levels come under control you may find yourself becoming more irritable, anxious and suffering from poor sleep. One reason for this could be that your body is not getting enough of the amino-acid tryptophan into the brain to manufacture sufficient quantities of serotonin (our natural mood enhancer) and melatonin (the hormone made from serotonin which promotes sleep) - please see page 315. Below you will find a chart showing various foods and their placement on the glycemic index:

Glycemic Index of Common Foods

Foods Ranking More Than 100% on the Glycemic Index

Very Rapid Insulin Inducers	
Tofu ice cream substitute	155
Maltose	152
Glucose	138
Rice cakes (puffed rice)	132
Wheat bread, French baguette	131
White rice, instant, boiled 6 minutes	121
Honey	126
Corn flakes	121
Potato, instant	120
Potato, baked russet	116
Bran flakes	104
Millet	103
Crackers, plain	100

Foods Ranking 80 to 100% on the Glycemic Index

Rapid Insulin Inducers	
Wheat (whole) bread	100
Wheat, white bread	100

Corn chips	99
Wheat, shredded	97
Parsnip	97
Muesli	96
Rye, crisp bread	95
Apricot	94
Raisins	93
Carrot	92
Banana, ripe	90
Oats, rolled	85
Rice, brown	81
Papaya, ripe	81
Corn, sweet	80

Foods Ranking 50 to 80% on the Glycemic Index

Moderate Insulin Inducers

Sucrose	78
Buckwheat	78
Kidney beans, canned	74
All bran	74
Spaghetti, white, boiled 15 minutes	67
Peas, green, frozen	65
Pinto beans, canned	64
Macaroni, white, boiled 5 minutes	64
Beets	64
Yam	62
Spaghetti, whole wheat, boiled 15 minutes	61
Chickpeas, canned	60
Sweet potato	59
Rice, white polished, boiled 5 minutes	58
Lactose	57
Custard	55
Orange, fresh fruit	54

Foods Ranking 30 to 50% on the Glycemic Index

Reduced Insulin Secretion

Oatmeal, long cooking	49
Apple, fresh	49
Rye kernels, steamed	47
Yogurt	44
Wheat, whole kernels, steamed	41
Applesauce, unsweetened	41

Milk, whole	41
Milk, skim	39
Yogurt, nonfat	39
Spaghetti, protein enriched	38
Barley, pearled	36
Lima beans	36
Pear, fresh	34
Rice bran	31

Foods Ranking Below 30% on the Glycemic Index

Low Insulin Response	
Peach, fresh	29
Grapefruit	26
Plums, fresh	25
Cherries, fresh	23
Soybeans, canned	22
Protein foods like fish, chicken, turkey	0*
Butter, olive oil, canola oil	0*
Whole nuts	0*

**Animal protein foods, butter and oils do not contain carbohydrates. Fresh whole nuts are primarily composed of fat with minimal quantities of carbohydrates.*

Not only over-weight persons suffer from carbohydrate sensitivity. Thin persons who do not produce excess insulin can also be carbohydrate addicted. This imbalance was discussed in the preceding section entitled, "Healthful Carbohydrates Promote that Peaceful Feeling."

(5) - Overwork, Stress and Anxiety

There's *good* stress like weddings, a new job, the birth of a baby, a new relationship, moving away from home to attend college - and then there's *bad* stress like overwork, financial difficulties, separation, divorce, illness and death. In response to either good or bad stress, your body releases hormones to help you cope. The adrenal glands secrete different hormones for short-term versus long-term stress, but both types of stress hormones stimulate the body's production of more insulin which can result in carbohydrate cravings and weight gain.

Do you find yourself reaching for "comfort" foods like cookies, candy bars or ice cream during or after a stressful event? These foods will make you feel better momentarily, but, ultimately, foods high in simple carbohydrates take their toll - creating even more physical stress. Start noticing your responses to stressful events in your life. What are your coping mechanisms? Can you talk about your feelings of anxiety, or do you keep smiling at all costs? Are you tempted to reach for a half-gallon of your favorite ice cream? Do you feel in control of your life - or helpless and unable to reduce the tension regardless of what you do? It's important to find ways to reduce the powerful impact modern-day stress has on your body. A good first step is to eat a balanced diet with adequate amounts of protein, healthful fats and complex carbohydrates that stabilizes blood sugar and helps reduce cravings.

If these issues are not addressed, after months or years of trying to cope, our body's delicate system of checks and balances begins to deteriorate and adrenal exhaustion sets in.

(6) - Adrenal Exhaustion

Sometimes referred to as "the human battery pack", the pyramid-shaped adrenal glands are situated on top of our kidneys. The outer layer of these glands produces steroid hormones responsible for regulating concentrations of water, salt and sugar in the body as well as secondary sexual characteristics. Throughout the day the adrenals are constantly responding to inner and outer stresses. The inner core of the adrenal glands produces adrenaline to prepare us for "fight or flight" in case of an emergency situation.

Maintaining stable blood sugar levels has become a complicated matter in 21st century life. Concentrated sugars found in highly refined sweet, starchy foods enter the bloodstream in seconds, rapidly spiking blood sugar levels. That donut or candy bar beckons; down it goes - you get a sugar high and feel positively wonderful! In response, the pancreas secretes insulin to reduce glucose levels - out it rushes, efficiently storing any excess sugar away as fat. You now suffer from hypoglycemia - a sugar crash, feeling irritable, anxious and/or depressed with cravings for more sweets. The human brain uses only glucose, or sugar, as fuel; if blood sugar drops too low for only a few minutes you will become comatose. When the starving brain calls out for more fuel, the adrenal glands must respond by secreting adrenaline to force the release of glycogen - a backup fuel source.

For many years, or even decades, the adrenal glands can manage to maintain blood sugar levels stable by releasing adrenaline to force that glycogen release. But it is hard work, and with too much overuse, the adrenals get overwhelmed. Diabetes can result when the pancreas is no longer able to keep up with the blood sugar rollercoaster. Prediabetic and diabetic people may find it very difficult to eat healthy foods because of constant carbohydrate cravings. It is not that they are self-indulgent, but that their back is up against a biochemical wall. It is essential that they seek professional care.

While adrenaline is produced to handle sudden emergencies, our adrenal cortex produces cortisol when we are under any kind of prolonged stress such as an illness, surgery, divorce, eating disorders, drug addiction, low-calorie dieting, financial pressures or even a job in which we feel miserable. Recent research has linked excess abdominal weight with chronic stress and excessive cortisol production. Until stress has been reduced, weight loss is next to impossible.

During the first stage of adrenal exhaustion other systems in our body attempt to compensate for the imbalance - the thyroid gland reduces its activity, slowing our metabolic rate, making us feel extremely tired. If we don't get a chance to rest and relax to repair the damage, during the second stage, immunity goes down and we might have difficulty sleeping; when cortisol levels are running low we feel drained, stressed and over-extended. In the third stage of adrenal exhaustion, we are running quite low on a number of important hormones including cortisol, thyroid, DHEA, progesterone, estrogen and testosterone. At this stage we feel exhausted all the time and just cannot cope with any stress.

A few of the more common symptoms of this disorder can include constant fatigue, depression or rapid mood swings; inability to tolerate exercise; lack of mental clarity; migraines; insomnia; edema; cravings for salt, sugar, alcohol or tobacco; low blood pressure; irritability; and recurrent chronic infections.

It is essential to look at lifestyle changes. There is a need to take time to rest, relax and recuperate; do not overexercise (that stresses your adrenals even more); consume at least three healthful meals of balanced whole foods daily. Get professional care to determine which natural herbs, hormones or medications can best help you recover.

(7) - Low Thyroid Function

Were you a very heavy child who preferred to play quietly rather than getting involved in physical activity? Was your weight gain associated with major "hormonal events" in your life like giving birth, or after a miscarriage or abortion? Or, did your weight gain begin after a low-calorie or starvation diet *(either can contribute to low thyroid function)*? Is there a history of thyroid problems in your family? Do you feel fatigued with a tendency to depression, require more than eight hours of sleep, have cold hands and feet, low blood pressure, constipation, heavy menses, brittle hair, low body temperature and are now unable to lose weight on the lowest calorie diets? It is possible you are suffering from low thyroid function. Other symptoms might include poor memory and concentration, headaches, high cholesterol, hoarseness, low sexual drive, water retention and difficulty swallowing (or sensation of a lump in the throat).

Your body requires a certain amount of heat, or *yang* energy to perform well. The thyroid gland (located behind the Adam's apple) regulates cell metabolism or the body's "burn rate" - it is our natural thermostat. Sometimes the thyroid does not produce enough hormones or, in thyroiditis, an over-reactive immune system attacks the thyroid gland, preventing hormone production. Other auto immune diseases that are also frequently associated with thyroiditis include: Addison's disease, allergies, candida, diabetes, lupus, multiple sclerosis, pernicious anemia and rheumatoid arthritis.

Studies have demonstrated that infants given soy-based milk formulas early in life have significantly higher rates of auto immune thyroid disease. Inadequate vegetarian diets that supply insufficient amounts of minerals like iron, zinc and selenium as well as the amino acid L-tyrosine can contribute to thyroid dysfunction. A number of pharmaceutical drugs inhibit thyroid function including (but not limited to) lithium, estrogen, antidiabetic and sulfa drugs - always check with your physician or pharmacist. Chlorine, fluoride and hydrocarbons found in our water supply can also suppress the thyroid gland.

Once thyroid function becomes sluggish, digestive fire diminishes and you are not able to extract nutrients from the foods and supplements ingested. Every cell and organ system in the body suffers - from head to toe. Your metabolic rate goes down and your weight goes up.

There is a simple test you can perform at home (studies show it is 77% accurate) to determine if you have a thyroid problem: In the morning, 30 minutes after awakening but before you arise, place a mercury thermometer under your armpit for 10 minutes. Do not use a digital thermometer - they are not as accurate. Take your temperature for three mornings; add the three numbers and divide by three to get your average temperature. If it is consistently less than 97.8 degrees, you are probably suffering from low thyroid function. (For women, your basal temperature can most accurately be measured during menses; temperatures normally rise during ovulation. Your basal temperature is not distorted by hot flashes.)

There are a number of standard medical tests that can be performed to examine your thyroid function. If you feel low thyroid function could be affecting you, talk to your healthcare professional. Be aware that many physicians, nutritionists and dietitians are not familiar with the multiple factors that can contribute to overweight - so seek additional opinions if necessary.

(8) - Changing Reproductive Hormonal Levels

For women, from the onset of menses through menopause, estrogen and progesterone levels are in continual flux. If estrogen levels drop too low, our mood plummets as well. This powerful female hormone stimulates important sites in the body that dictate moods - directly affecting production of *serotonin* (our built-in mood elevator), *endorphins* that act as endogenous painkillers and pleasure enhancers, and *norepinephrine* our body's natural stimulant that gives us a lift. Progesterone balances the effects of estrogen by increasing the levels of GABA in our systems; this brain chemical (our natural Valium) helps us relax. If it is deficient we can feel tense, anxious and suffer from poor sleep. Frequently, when we reach for that chocolate bar or pastry, we are unconsciously trying to self-medicate with food. Sweet, rich fatty foods indirectly increase serotonin levels as well as the levels of other mood enhancing hormones.

By the time we reach 35 to 40 years of age, our ovaries produce less estrogen and progesterone until, sometime during menopause, the levels run so low that only the adrenal glands produce these hormones. However, even healthy adrenals cannot adequately balance the hormonal deficit and too frequently we see middle-aged women afflicted with depression, anxiety, insomnia and weight gain. If we are suffering from adrenal exhaustion, as previously discussed, the situation is compounded and we may be living from one caffeine, nicotine or sugar fix to the next - just trying to get by.

Women who undergo complete hysterectomies, in which the ovaries are removed as well as the uterus and fallopian tubes, are plunged into immediate menopause. As mentioned above, the adrenal glands will only partially compensate for the hormonal imbalance created by the absence of the ovaries; hormone replacement therapy is almost essential in such cases.

For persons who are already carbohydrate sensitive (producing excess insulin with the consumption of refined carbohydrates leading to weight gain), the hormonal picture becomes extremely complicated.

(Note: Be certain to check out the recommendations for herbal helpers given under "Gynecological Disorders", "Menopause: Those Hormones Again!" and "Male Health: Tips for Maintaining a Healthy Reproductive System").

9) Medications and Prescription Drugs

Various medications as well as some herbal remedies can have a profound effect on insulin levels creating carbohydrate cravings and a tendency to gain weight. Sweetened cough drops, syrups, stool softeners, antacid tablets or liquids frequently contain ingredients that raise blood sugar levels. Other medications, such as drugs to lower cholesterol or blood pressure as well as hormone replacement drugs can increase insulin levels.

Corticosteroids (cortisones) frequently prescribed to reduce inflammation or to suppress immune reactions associated with auto-immune diseases can also take their toll. The adrenal glands shut down as a result of prolonged doses of pharmaceutical cortisone (such as Prednisone). Like its natural counterpart produced by the adrenal glands, cortisol, cortisone raises blood sugar and increases fat deposition.

If you find yourself craving more sweets after taking a medication, discuss these concerns with your physician so that you can jointly decide which medicines will best serve you. Never discontinue or reduce prescribed drugs without first consulting your healthcare professional.

(10) - Yeast Overgrowth

Candida or Monilia is one of the most well-known problematic yeasts found in the human body. However, there are actually many kinds of yeasts that live in harmony with us until something upsets the delicate balance and their overgrowth results in a problem. The most common places for yeast infections to occur include the mouth (thrush), vagina or intestines. In the digestive tract it causes symptoms of bloating, gas, indigestion, nausea, heartburn, foul-smelling diarrhea and/or constipation. There is a tendency to experience major cravings for the foods on which yeasts thrive - sugar, starch and alcohol found in bread, pastries, cookies, candies, chips, beer, soft drinks, etc. If you are already carbohydrate sensitive, the situation becomes even more difficult with the wildly fluctuating insulin levels created by the consumption of these foods.

According to Julia Ross, M.A., author of *The Diet Cure,* yeasts out of control are even more aggressive than viruses; they change into unfriendly fungi whose long roots penetrate the lining of the intestinal tract. These fungal forms then release toxins and undigested food into the bloodstream creating even further damage. Elson Haas, M.D., author of *Staying Healthy with Nutrition*, says that the chemicals released by yeasts into the blood stream also contribute to mood swings.

Since yeast is a normal inhabitant of the body, it is difficult to know when it is pathological. However, it is estimated that up to 25 to 35 percent of the population is afflicted with yeast or other fungal infections. There are a number of factors that can upset the delicate balance that give yeasts the upper hand in the human body, they include: 1) antibiotic therapy that kills friendly bacteria in our systems (such as lactobacilli acidophilus and bifidus) that would normally keep other microbes in check; 2) low immunity or steroid drugs, such as cortisone, which suppress the immune system, contributing to yeast overgrowth; 3) the excessive consumption of highly refined sugars and starches directly gives yeasts the food on which they thrive; 4) poor digestion and nutritional deficiencies help yeasts spread; 5) birth control pills increase glycogen (sugar) levels in vaginal secretions, helping yeasts to set up housekeeping; 6) nonoxynol 9, the active ingredient in spermicidal foams and creams destroys friendly bacteria while fostering the growth of candida and E.coli (a bacteria which causes cystitis).

If you suffer from frequent yeast infections or feel you might have a systemic yeast overgrowth, it is important to contact a health professional. Some things you can do immediately to help your immune system fight back include: 1) eliminate all breads, refined sugars, starches, alcohol and mushrooms from your diet; 2) daily, consume only one small portion of whole, gluten-free grains such as millet, corn, rice or quinoa; 3) consume adequate protein and vegetables; 4) avoid fermented foods such as vinegar, pickles and soy sauce; 5) in the beginning, you will find it necessary to avoid even fresh fruits and juices; 6) supplement your diet with unsweetened yogurt or a good source of acidophilus/bifidus culture.

In severe cases, anti-fungal medications (like Nystatin) can be prescribed. - *Dr. Gary*

(11) - Food Additives, MSG & Artificial Sweeteners

Commercially produced foods can contain one or more of over 3,000 different chemicals. Phosphates added to soft drinks, beer, ice cream, candy and pastries block our body's ability to absorb iron. At the same time, many food labels tell us that the contents are "fortified" with iron - unfortunately our body cannot assimilate the *ferric* iron used by many manufacturers - it requires *ferrous* iron. This book is not the place to go into great detail about chemicals used in food processing - but do try to become an informed consumer. In the meantime, one particular additive, MSG, could be a major contributor to our nation's collective weight gain.

Scientists feed MSG to laboratory animals used in research to make them fat *for experimental purposes.*

While the exact mechanism by which this chemical exerts its fattening effects is still being researched, MSG appears to influence the hunger and weight-control centers of the brain. Monosodium glutamate (MSG's scientific name) contains the neurotoxin "glutamate" that kills brain cells in laboratory animals. In the food industry, it is added to many processed foods to enhance flavor and is frequently found in canned soups, salad dressings, dips, sauces, luncheon meats, hot dogs, canned and frozen fish, fowl and meats; it is the main ingredient in most flavor enhancers. Listed on labels as *MSG, hydrolyzed food starch, monosodium glutamate, hydrolyzed plant protein, flavor enhancers or natural flavors*, this compound effects people in different ways. Some typical reactions might include leg swelling, severe headaches, irritability, fatigue, disorientation and strong cravings for carbohydrate-rich foods. While most of us believe that we can avoid consuming this chemical in Chinese restaurants by simply requesting, "no MSG," it is actually much more difficult than that - it is already present in many of the prepared sauces purchased by the restaurant (such as soy sauce and tamari, as well as in the bean curd). In fact, it is estimated that up to 30% of all foods we are served in *any* restaurant contains MSG.

Artificial Sweeteners

Sugar substitutes may reduce the total number of calories we are ingesting daily, but they do not fool our body's insulin response. Remember - insulin is our body's fat storing hormone and we can't burn calories when our system is filled with it. In response to the sweet flavor, no matter how "low-calorie" the food item, the body will release insulin if we are carbohydrate sensitive. Sugarless gums, candies, mints and sodas might be tempting but due to the extra insulin released as a result of their consumption, carbohydrate cravings increase - and we're hooked once again.

Before moving on, it is important to talk about Aspartame - the artificial sweetener that is marketed under different names but is present in many diet foods and drinks. When subjected to temperatures over 86 degrees Fahrenheit, the wood alcohol contained in Aspartame is converted into formaldehyde and then to formic acid. Grouped with the same class of drugs as arsenic and cyanide, formaldehyde is a deadly poison. Symptoms of methanol toxicity induced by Aspartame are similar to those of multiple sclerosis, systemic lupus and fibromyalgia and include joint pain, numbness or tingling in the arms or legs, shooting pains, cramps, spasms, dizziness, headaches, slurred speech, blurred vision, depression or memory loss.

Art, a 40 year old auto mechanic, came to me complaining of numbness alternating with shooting pains down both arms into his wrists and fingers. This condition had plagued him for four to five years and Xrays did not disclose any vertebral nerve impingement that could be responsible for the discomfort. In discussing diet, Art mentioned that he drank three to four diet colas daily. I asked him to eliminate the diet drinks and try to replace them with two to three pieces of fresh fruit. We did not follow-up with herbs or acupuncture, since both of us wanted to test the results of eliminating diet drinks. Art made this one simple change in his lifestyle and in two weeks there was some improvement. All numbness and pain was eliminated within three months.

(12) - Lack of Exercise

A sedentary lifestyle contributes to ill health. Every system in our body requires movement for fresh oxygen and nutrients to be carried to each cell with the circulating blood and lymph and for wastes and toxins to be taken away. Chinese medicine teaches that pain and discomfort is frequently an indication of stagnation - lack of motion. In other words, all of us need to keep active to stay healthy. However, the good news is that we do not need to be fitness fanatics to reap the health benefits of exercise.

A study conducted by Dr. Steven Blair and his colleagues at the Institute for Aerobics Research indicated that **simply walking 30 minutes a day reduced premature death almost as much as running 30 to 40 miles per week**. The eight year study tracked over 13,000 participants who were divided into 5 groups. The least fit, or sedentary group had a death rate more than three times greater than the active group (those that ran 30 to 40 miles weekly).

With that being said, let's talk about our society's perceptions regarding big people. Large persons are stereotyped as being lazy, undisciplined couch potatoes - this is not necessarily true. Many of their thin counterparts can be just an inactive - while, in contrast, many large persons exercise faithfully. Back in the 80's, I was a Covert Bailey, author of ***Fit or Fat***, exercise convert - jogging every lunch hour instead of eating, as well as faithfully attending dance aerobics classes 3 to 5 times weekly. Those were the days when I was following a low-calorie, low-fat macrobiotic diet impeccably (perfect by Drs. Ornish and MacDougall standards). The diet did not serve me well - I felt chronically cold, spacey, weak and fatigued - so all of that exercise was a real penance. Over that period of time my weight increased dramatically and my previously low cholesterol reading soared well over the 220 mark. And, I was particularly surprised because all that exercise did not seem to add up to more muscle mass. What could possibly be wrong if I was doing everything right? As discussed under the previous section entitled "Carbohydrate Sensitivity", even the carbohydrates found in whole grains turn some of us into fat storers instead of fat burners. I think about half of the population (probably mostly A, B, and AB Blood Types) function wonderfully using carbohydrates as fuel; however, for many O Blood Types or carbohydrate sensitive individuals, carbohydrate foods make us conserve energy by storing fat. Later, when I started the Sears' Zone Diet (which

I modified to be free of any refined carbohydrates with very few grains) I actually burned fat and protein quite efficiently as fuel and had boundless energy to exercise. I have to admit that I originally started the Sears' diet to disprove what I thought was a ridiculous theory. However, the weight began to drop off (without any exercise) at the steady rate of 6 to 7 pounds per month. By the end of ten weeks, the new energy I felt had me back on the exercise track - this time I began to build muscle. Needless to say, much research must be conducted in this area.

All too frequently, overweight people are chastised, sent home with a low calorie diet and told to "exercise". If their weight is due to any of the factors previously discussed, these people desperately need to make other lifestyle changes before being told to "hit the pavement". When dietary deficiencies, addictions and allergies are removed, fatigue begins to subside and there is natural energy to exercise. They are then getting the fuel that their body requires.

Most important - it is essential to start out slowly with any exercise program. That might mean walking only one block a day for the first week; two blocks a day for the second, etc. until you are walking a couple of miles or thirty minutes daily. Dr. John Shen, a very wise 86 year old Traditional Chinese healing master says that here in the West we have not learned the value of moderation, **"we rule our *limited* bodies with our *unlimited* minds."** Just because our mind wills something does not necessarily mean it is good for us. It is important to treat our body with love and respect, recognizing its uniqueness and limitations - any change that is going to remain a part of our lives must be gradual.

(13) - Genetics: Some People Can be Fit and Fat!

Many scientists are not so certain that it is unhealthy to be "overweight"; unfortunately, the public is largely left in the dark regarding their debate which is carried on in the scientific and academic circles. At a 1992 meeting of the National Institutes of Health, the benefits of weight loss were questioned. Several researchers announced they had reached the conclusion that weight loss, instead of prolonging life, was associated with earlier death. Francie Berg, respected publisher of a newsletter called *Healthy Weight Journal*, said the press was reluctant to report the findings of these studies, exclaiming, "We can't print that!" Researchers Susan Wooley and David Garner have extensively reviewed studies that attempt to link over-weight to disease and death. They state there are "conflicting opinions on the health risks associated with obesity; the conclusion that obesity is dangerous represents a selective review of the data." Unfortunately, in our "thin is in" society, data that supports a link between ill-health and obesity is considered newsworthy, while data contradicting this view is often withheld from the public.

At an American Heart Association meeting in March 1994, Steven Blair, an epidemiologist at the Cooper Institute for Aerobics Research in Dallas argued, "One of the fundamental tenets of the weight-loss industry is that if you get people to eat less, they'll lose weight. And if they lose weight, they'll be better off. And there is no evidence to support either one of those." Blair studied 12,025 Harvard University graduates. The study found that persons who kept a steady weight, even if they were overweight, had less risk of disease than persons whose weight fluctuated by as little as ten pounds. When questioned, "How often are you dieting?" Those who answered, "always" had a heart disease rate of 23.1% which is more than double the 10.6% heart disease rate of those who answered, "never."

Genes and Weight: Healthy Samoan Women Average 5'4" & Weigh 204 Pounds

In *The Dieter's Dilemma*, William Bennett, M.D., argues that human attributes follow the "bell curve." Weight is probably no different than height, I.Q. or other human qualities. For example, if you graph the I.Q.'s of an entire population, the majority of the people would fall into the average or middle range; however, a significant number of persons will have I.Q.'s much higher or much lower than average. Weight, like height or I.Q., is no different. Each person's ideal weight is determined by many factors including bone size and density, height and muscle mass.

Some people have naturally inherited greater numbers of fat cells from descendants who survived the ice ages thousands of years ago. These ancient ancestors were able to survive periods of famine, passing on their thrifty genes, thanks to an abundant store of reserved energy in fat cells. It is interesting to note that bodies of perfectly healthy Eskimo people may be composed of up to 75 percent body fat. Other species who live in cold climates are genetically equipped to gain large amounts of fat over a few months to hold them over through severe winter seasons. The polar bear puts on a walloping 400 to 500 pounds in just a few months! Could consumption of the carbohydrates found in maturing grains have served as an autumn trigger for the ice age body to start storing fat for long cold winters?

(14) - Overeating

If you read the preceding 13 factors which can contribute to overweight, you understand why "overeating" is next to last on my list.

C. Wayne Callaway of Mayo Clinic states that most of his big patients do not overeat, but are rather chronic dieters or persons who regularly skip meals. He believes that as many as 2/3 of the people with weight problems are not overeating. Studies indicate that at least 50% of people who enter formal weight-loss programs do not overeat. Dropout rates run as high as 85 percent for such programs because so many of us cannot lose weight by simply reducing calories.

As previously discussed, some persons may over consume certain types of foods due to hormonal imbalances or allergic reactions. Some large people may respond to stressful situations by eating - but so do their thin counterparts. **While it is true that some people (heavy or thin) may be "calorically overextended" it is often because they are "nutritionally bankrupt" and their body is searching for the real foods it desperately requires.**

(15) - Beta Endorphins & (16) Serotonin

Be certain to read about the beta endorphin and serotonin connection to weight gain which were discussed in in the preceding section entitled "Healthful Carbohydrates Promote that Peaceful Feeling", see page 314.

Wisdom From Around the World in Treating Imbalances Frequently Associated with the Metal Element

Asthma

Since the early 1980's, the number of Americans suffering from asthma has increased 61 percent.
Five mission children and
9.6 million adults are currently afflicted.
Asthma is on the increase.
Over the past 30 years hospitalization of children with asthma or asthma-related disorders has increased 500 percent.

Asthma is another one of those medical mysteries that is not yet completely understood by science. During an asthma attack the victim experiences difficulty breathing; the bronchial tubes become constricted and the sufferer begins to wheeze. Asthma is a potentially life-threatening disorder; in severe cases, trapped air cannot be exhaled and the victim feels like they are suffocating. Many different things can trigger an asthma attack - from cold, damp weather to allergic reactions, infections, pollution in the air, stress and even exercise. In my own practice, I have found that food and chemical allergies frequently play a major role in asthma attacks and many patients find great relief by simply removing certain trigger foods, drugs or other chemicals from their lives. *Please read the information given in the section on Allergies.*

While Western medicine most frequently relies on inhalants and other pharmaceutical drugs to relieve bronchial constriction and prevent asthma attacks, people from different cultures have dealt with asthma in many distinct ways.

(Note: Moderate to severe asthma ought to be treated by Western biomedicine. The following remedies should be used alone only in cases of mild asthma or alongside pharmaceutical regimens to enhance treatment and reduce dependence on drugs. Do not suddenly stop taking steroids or inhalants; when appropriate, their use can be gradually phased-out under your physician's guidance.) - Dr. Gary

A Few Folk Remedies from Around the World

You can probably find an unopened jar of fennel seed in the back of your spice cabinet. However, if you live in rural Greece you, more than likely, would be using this common household spice to help relieve asthma and other respiratory disorders. Simply crush two teaspoons of fennel seeds, stir it in to one cup of boiling water; cover and immediately remove from the heat; steep for 10 minutes; strain and drink.

Pungent foods like garlic, pepper and cinnamon were favored by ancient Greeks, Romans and Egyptians to help clear the nose and respiratory tract. Pliny, the early Roman historian, wrote that the ancient Egyptians used raw garlic and garlic juice to treat asthma-like coughs. For asthma prevention, various mineral-rich fruits were prescribed by ancient Egyptian physicians including grapes, figs and juniper.

Lemons and limes are used to relieve asthma by the residents of Amalfi, Italy, a beautiful port city that is also called "lemon land." Drink the juice of 1/2 organic lemon in one cup of cool water every morning as soon as you get up from bed. Between meals, it is recommended that the asthma sufferer ingest 1 teaspoon of undiluted organic lime juice. Italian physicians now commonly use motherwort and passionflower to treat asthma. These herbs help reduce anxiety and lessen the severity of lung spasms.

Musk mallow seeds, also known as Ambrette seeds *(Abelmoschus moschatus)*, are chewed by people living in Trinidad to relieve chest congestion and asthma. Before being chewed, these musky-smelling seeds are first steeped in rum or boiling water. The leaves and young shoots as well as the unripe pods (known as "musk okra") are eaten as a vegetable.

As a member of one of the nomadic Bedouin tribes, you would chew Ammi seeds *(Ammi visnaga)* to relieve asthma symptoms. In ancient Egypt this aromatic seed was used mainly to treat kidney stones. However, in 1946 an Egyptian pharmacologist discovered that extracts of this herb controlled asthmatic symptoms. His work lead to the production of sodium cromoglycate, a bichromone which halts the release of anti allergenic substances in the body that create the asthmatic response. Ammi is native to Syria, Arabia and West Africa. In the culinary arts, a close cousin, Ammi *(Ammi copticum)* seeds flavor curries, breads, pastries and other foods in Middle Eastern countries. Ayurvedic medicine uses Ammi seeds primarily to stimulate decongestion of the respiratory and digestive systems. Extracts of the seeds are currently added to commercially formulated cough medicines.

To stop asthma attacks, Russians from the Crimea deliberately inhale and exhale very slowly, taking a sip of water between breathes. A total of two glasses of lukewarm spring water is ingested over a 30-minute time span.

In **Ayurvedic** medicine, asthma is viewed as a *kapha* imbalance. Increased *kapha* lodges in the stomach and then moves into the upper respiratory tract blocking the smooth flow of oxygen. Avoid allergens like problematic foods, dust, mold, chemicals and refrain from dairy products including cheese. Avoid fermented and salty foods.

As an effective treatment for chronic bronchial asthma, it is recommended that seven pieces of clove (spice) be inserted into a peeled banana and left overnight. The next morning eat both the banana and the cloves. Do not ingest anything else for an hour, then drink a cup of hot water with one teaspoon of raw organic honey.

As an immediate aid to stop wheezing, boil one teaspoon of licorice root in one cup of spring water for 3 to 5 minutes; remove from heat and strain; add 1/2 teaspoon plain ghee (clarified butter) or 5 to 10 drops of *mahanarayan* oil; take a sip every five minutes. It is possible that the licorice tea may induce vomiting. In Ayurvedic thought this is beneficial since it helps to eliminate excess *kapha* and you will feel better immediately. Brew several cups and keep them refrigerated for up to 72 hours. *(Note: Persons suffering from hypertension should not drink licorice tea.)*

For a variation, you can follow the above recipe but use 1/2 teaspoon licorice root and 1/2 teaspoon ginger root per cup of tea.

To relieve congestion and for immediate asthma relief ingest 1/4 cup organic onion juice mixed with one teaspoon raw organic honey and 1/8 teaspoon black pepper.

A number of yoga postures aid in relieving asthma including the Cobra, Bow, Shoulder Stand and Plow poses as well as sitting in the *Vajrasana.*

Ideally, in traditional **Chinese** medicine the goal is to find the unique imbalance that is at the root of whatever condition is occurring. However, asthma can be subdivided into different categories - depending upon predominating factors: 1) Breathlessness due to Phlegm (mucus); 2) Asthma due to Wind-Heat; 3) Asthma due to Wind-Cold and Deficiency.

Breathlessness due to Phlegm is characterized by copious mucus production associated with chronic bronchitis. Breathing is extremely difficult when you are lying down and you are forced to breath with your mouth open; the tongue has a thick, greasy coating. Foods and herbs that could be helpful include organic lemon and lime juice, aduki beans, alfalfa sprouts, horseradish, fresh ginger tea and a little raw organic honey. This disorder can be permanently eliminated once the underlying cause has been addressed. *Hsiao Keh Chuan* is an excellent patent formula that eases breathing in 20 to 30 minutes and stops coughing; it comes in capsule or syrup form, and should be available at most health food stores that carry Chinese medicines. *Also see the following section on Bronchitis.*

If you suffer from asthma due to Wind-Heat, the dietary and herbal recommendations will be quite distinct from asthma due to Wind-Cold. This type of asthma is characterized by sensations of heat in the body; fast, heavy breathing; loud wheezing, headache; a barking cough; tightness of the chest; dry stools; scanty urine; yellow mucus and mental restlessness. Cooling detoxifying herbs and foods that are particularly helpful include the juice of sour fruits like lemons and limes in plenty of spring water, apricots, sprouts, tofu, daikon radish and horehound. There are a couple of excellent patent formulas for asthma due to Heat that can be found at health food stores: *Zhi Sou Ding Chuan Wan* (also known as Stopping Cough and Calming Breathlessness Pill); *Xiao Chuan Chong Ji* (Asthma Granules) is particularly good for asthma due to an acute viral infection since it contains isatis - an effective anti-viral/anti-microbial herb.

If you suffer from episodes of difficult breathing and wheezing associated with asthma and you frequently feel cold (cold hands and feet), tightness of the chest, tend to be pale and have clear or white foamy mucus, in Chinese thought you suffer from asthma due to Wind-Cold. Dietary recommendations would include cooking all food (including fruits and vegetables); and increasing your consumption of warming foods and spices such as onions, garlic, fresh ginger, mustard greens, basil. Small quantities of seeds and nuts eaten at regular intervals would be helpful including pumpkin, sunflower and flax seeds, almonds and especially walnuts. Other building food and herbs that could be helpful include Chinese or Korean Panax ginseng, black beans and warming soups or stews made with a few ounces of organic meat (particularly beef) and plenty of veggies and warming spices (leeks, onions, garlic and ginger). Be sure to enjoy two to three cups of ginger tea daily. Another patent formula specifically for Wind-Cold accompanied with sweating is *Qi Guan Yan Ke Sou Tan Chuan Wan* (Bronchial Cough, Phlegm and Dyspnoea Pill). A good formula for Wind-Cold without sweating is not available in patent form, it's known as *Ma Huang Tang* (Ephedra Decoction).

There are traditional Chinese herbal formulas that can be slightly adjusted to treat unique, individual constitutions and asthmatic conditions as they manifest in different persons. There are also many preventive formulas to help address the underlying weakness or deficiency that is the root cause of the problem (Kidney/Adrenal and Lung Qi Deficiency in Chinese thought). *(Note: Acupuncture can be effective in stopping an asthma attack. On numerous occasions I have treated patients undergoing an acute attack of asthma and within three to five minutes after needle insertion, normal breathing is restored.)*

Native Americans of the Dakota and Winnebago tribes used skunk cabbage *(Spathyema foetida)* to facilitate removal of phlegm due to asthma. Skunk cabbage, a stinky plant that thrives in swampy areas, was listed in the *U.S. Pharmacopoeia* from 1820 to 1882 as a treatment for respiratory and nervous disorders as well as for dropsy and rheumatism.

Indian tobacco *(Lobelia inflata),* a plant indigenous to central and eastern United States and Canada, was used by Native Americans for a number of ailments. In the late eighteenth century it became a popular remedy for asthma. Regarding its therapeutic attributes, the *Dispensatory of the United States* says: "Its most important use in medicine is as a nauseating expectorant in bronchitis . . . large doses will sometimes cause complete cessation of the asthmatic paroxysms." Alkaloids in the leaves of this species are currently under research. Lobelin, one of these alkaloid components, is a constituent in a number of anti smoking compounds.

Hyssop *(Hyssopus officinalis)* was used by Cherokee natives to stop asthma attacks and to treat respiratory ailments in general.

Yerba Santa was a favorite herbal ally of Natives living in Mendocino County, California. First the leaves were smoked and then chewed like tobacco to treat asthmatic conditions.

Mullein *(Verbascum thapsus)*, long used in Europe for respiratory problems, is a common weed found in abandoned pastures. Mullein was introduced to the Americas by the early settlers. Native Americans readily adopted this medicinal plant and used various preparations for a variety of ailments. Dried mullein leaves were used to relieve asthma by members of the Mohegan, Penobscott and Forest Potawatomi tribes. The Menominees smoked dried, pulverized mullein root for respiratory disorders. Native Americans of the Catawba tribe made cough syrup for their children by boiling the root and adding honey.

In South America the healing properties of the balsam tree were first discovered by natives of El Salvador. Peruvian Native Americans adopted the use of the reddish-brown syrupy sap from the Peruvian balsam tree to treat asthma. This tree produces valuable wood, fragrantly perfumed flowers and its healing sap relieves many respiratory disorders.

Parents living in South American countries will commonly give their asthmatic child a delicious tea made from lemon verbena *(Aloysia triphylla)* to ease wheezing. *(Don't sweeten with honey for young children; you can use a touch of stevia, organic maple syrup or blackstrap molasses.)*

Bronchitis

Bronchitis is an inflammation of the bronchial tubes and can be the result of infection, allergies or irritants. Symptoms frequently include a persistent cough (which produces yellow or green sputum only if there is infection). It is necessary to clear the lungs; therefore, any cough remedy should include an expectorant; a suppressant is appropriate only if there is a persistent, hacking cough that is creating more inflammation. Acute bronchitis due to infection usually lasts from 8 to 12 days. Since most cases are due to viruses, bed rest, a nourishing diet with plenty of liquids, and healing herbs is the order of the day. In more severe cases and possible pneumonia, or if there is an underlying medical condition that makes the infection more dangerous, antibiotics to fight bacteria may be needed. - *Dr. Gary.*

Chronic bronchitis can last two months, six months or a lifetime, leading to lung damage. Exacerbations of bronchitis need medical attention and require antibiotic therapy. If you have never used herbs before, this is not the time or place to start experimenting with them unless you are under the supervision of a licensed herbal practitioner. It is essential to get your health back on track with a nourishing vitamin and mineral-packed diet, adequate exercise and immune building herbs.

A Few Folk Remedies from Around the World

The old adage, "an apple a day keeps the doctor away," has been given new credence by Canadian researchers whose studies show that people who eat apples or drink apple juice daily have fewer colds and upper respiratory illnesses. In England, during Tudor times, bronchitis and coughs were treated with . . . yes, APPLES. Core an organic apple (leaving on the skin) and fill with a mixture of cinnamon, honey, and a few raisins and chopped walnuts (if desired); bake at 350 degrees 30 to 40 minutes (until done), then mash with a dash of ghee (clarified butter).

The Swedes use hot chili peppers to help break up the mucus congestion and ease the coughing that accompanies bronchitis. If you need to put out the fire after eating a chili pepper, eat a cracker or piece of bread, or have some yogurt or a little milk. Water will not help since the phytochemicals that make peppers fiery are oil based.

The Australians inhale eucalyptus leaf vapor to ease breathing and open obstructed airways. Bring two quarts of water to a boil; add four to five eucalyptus leaves; cover and simmer over low heat for five minutes; remove from burner and slowly remove lid so you are not scalded by the steam; cover pan and your head with a towel; slowly breathe in the healing vapors. Or, simply put two to three drops of eucalyptus essential oil on to a warm, wet washcloth; cover your face with the cloth (avoiding the eyes) and inhale the vapors for three to five minutes.

Throughout Europe á warm onion poultice is applied to the chest to ease breathing. Simmer a large onion in a cup of water until soft; strain the liquid; mash the onion and apply it to the chest once it has cooled down a bit; cover with a towel to help maintain the heat. Leave it on for 20 to 30 minutes, then gently cleanse the area with warm water and pat dry.

Herbalists in Spain and France prescribe warm chamomile tea for children suffering from bronchitis.

Irish moss is frequently recommended for persons who suffer from chronic bronchitis and other diseases of the lungs. Naturally high in mucilage, Irish moss soothes inflamed tissues in the respiratory tract. Bring one cup of spring water to a boil; remove from heat and add one teaspoon of the dried herb; cover and steep for five minutes, then sip. Drink two to three cups daily.

Following is an effective **Ayurvedic** home remedy for bronchitis: Mix one teaspoon of turmeric powder in one cup of warm milk and ingest on an empty stomach. One cup of turmeric milk can be taken two or three times daily.

Another popular remedy involves mixing equal quantities of dried ginger *(shunthi)*, long pepper *(pippali)* and black pepper *(maricha)*; this is an Ayurvedic formula known as *trikatu*. The dosage is 1/2 teaspoon three to four times daily. The powder can be added to tea, or mixed with a small amount of raw, organic honey and rolled into pea-sized herbal balls for easier ingestion.

The juice from the leaves of the Malabar Nut *(Adenanthera vasika)*, known as *vasa* in Sanskrit, is mixed in equal amounts with raw, organic honey and taken two teaspoonfuls three times daily for chronic bronchitis. This plant is native to India and thrives in most areas except the desert and high mountains.

Following is a **Chinese** herbal home remedy to relieve asthma and/or bronchitis; (however, for asthma due to heat, **omit** fennel and fenugreek seeds since they are warming): Combine equal parts of fennel seed *(Foeniculum officinalis)*, fenugreek seed *(Trigonella foenumgraecum)*, flaxseed *(Linum usitatissiumum)*, lobelia seed or leaf *(Lobelia inflata)*, mullein leaf or flower *(Verbascum thaspus)*, licorice root *(Glycyrrhiza glabra)*. Gently crush one tablespoon of this mixture and stir in to a rapidly boiling cup of water; cover and immediately remove from the heat; steep for 8 to 10 minutes; strain through muslin or cotton fabric (to remove the tiny hairs on the mullein leaves); ingest three to four cups daily.

For more Chinese formulas that help with bronchitis, see the preceding section on asthma.

In **Western herbalism**, echinacea and goldenseal extract may be recommended to help fight microbes and boost immunity. Every 2 to 3 hours, put 1/2 dropperful in your mouth and hold it there for 5 to 10 minutes, then swallow. *Do not use these herbs for more than one week at a time. Goldenseal should not be ingested during pregnancy.*

Popular herbal expectorants that loosen congestion, clear the lungs and boost immunity include elecampane, horehound, mullein and thyme. It is always best to combine them with soothing, anti-inflammatory herbs such as marshmallow, licorice or slippery elm. *Elecampane has an interesting history. The root was used by the English until about 1920 as a flavoring in sugar cakes. Asthma sufferers chewed on a piece of the root every morning and evening. When passing by a polluted waterway, people would chew on elecampane root as prevention against lung infections.* For quick and easy herbal relief, take the bottle of thyme off your spice rack; stir one teaspoon into one cup of boiling water; cover, remove from heat and steep for five to ten minutes; strain and drink.

There are a number of herbal cough syrups on the market that contain wild cherry bark, coltsfoot and slippery elm bark.

To treat bronchitis and other respiratory complaints, Omaha **Native Americans** chewed fresh pleurisy root while Natchez people ingested a tea made from the boiled roots to cure pneumonia.

In Mendocino County, California, Yokia people drank a tea made with the leaves of a local species of wormwood to treat bronchitis.

Wild bergamot can be found growing in thickets on dry hills in many eastern states from Maine to Minnesota and south to Florida, Louisiana and Kansas. To relieve bronchial problems, the Flambeau Ojibwa people boiled the dried root and extracted the oil which was then inhaled. The Koasati, Meskwaki and Menominee natives regularly used the plant when treating colds.

The Pillager Ojibwa people made a salve from the leaf buds of the balsam poplar mixed with bear or mutton fat. The ointment was rubbed into the nostrils and inhaled for relief of congestion due to bronchitis and colds.

South American Natives living in El Salvador and Peru treat bronchitis and asthma by ingesting the sap of balsam trees; it is an excellent expectorant which eases coughing and clears the lungs. You can ask for Peru balsam sap at most health food stores.

Pau d'arco is another natural antibiotic that comes to us from South America which can assist in treating bronchitis.

Constipation

Con stipati means "crammed together" in Latin. Liquid is removed from waste matter as it travels through the intestines, but excessive elimination of water results in dry, tightly packed stools that are extremely difficult to move. Constipation can result from a number of different factors: 1) Too little fluid or fiber intake; 2) lack of exercise or inactivity; 3) stress; 4) side-effects of medication; 5) not heeding your body's call to eliminate when it is ready resulting in suppression of natural contractions; 6) a tumor or some other type of intestinal obstruction; 7) hypothyroidism which slows colonic contractions; 8) hormonal changes associated with pregnancy or the second phase of the menstrual cycle.

There are many over-the-counter laxatives available, however, your body can become dependent upon them. Following are many natural remedies that help regulate the bowels and improve your health at the same time:

A Few Folk Remedies from Around the World

Ethiopians munch on pumpkin seeds to move the bowels - a natural laxative that's high in zinc. The African people have a special saying, "Small stool/big hospital; big stool/small hospital." This saying rings true to anyone interested in natural healthcare. Natural fiber that comes from eating plenty of fresh fibrous roots, vegetables, fruits, whole grains, seeds and nuts will bulk up the stool; help cleanse the colon; and promote health in general.

Canadians frequently consume one or two apples in the morning before breakfast to set the stage for proper elimination. Get organic apples, don't peel them - chew the skin thoroughly.

Muffins or biscuits made with barley flour are eaten by Israeli people to regulate bowels. Another favorite remedy of the Israeli's is honey; it was such an important commodity that the early Hebrews regulated who could own bees. First thing in the morning, dissolve a tablespoon of honey in 1/4 cup boiling water, then add *cold* water; drink on an empty stomach.

French people prefer to use oat bran in their muffins to maintain bowel health. Swedish researchers have confirmed that bran can help prevent constipation; 4 to 6 whole rye, wheat bran crackers or multi-grain cereals and breads can be a great aid.

German folks treat mild constipation by drinking dandelion tea; the bitterness of this herb moves stool along by stimulating colon contractions.

Ancient Greeks used licorice, known as "the grandfather of herbs," as a laxative. *(Note: Licorice is contraindicated for persons suffering from edema or high blood pressure).* In case of "obstinate" constipation, drink a cup of licorice root tea as a simple but effective aid. Another remedy is to simmer three to four prunes in 1-1/2 cups water with one tablespoon of licorice root for 25 to 30 minutes. Consume the prunes and drink the liquid before bedtime.

Figs, a fruit native to southwestern Asia, were also a favorite of Ancient Greeks; naturally high in fiber, the roughage provided by the seeds help move the bowels. Athenians had special laws prohibiting the export of figs from their city-state. *Suko phantai* (translated as fig informers) reported to Greek officials of anyone attempting to export the valuable commodity - that's where the English word "sycophant" comes from!

The laxative effect of figs was well known by the Egyptians - following is an ancient formula: *"Make a beverage for a patient suffering from constipation: figs; milk; notched sycamore figs; leave it overnight in sweet beer. Strain, give it to him to drink very often, and he will soon get well."*

A 19th century German cure for constipation involves drinking eight glasses of water daily plus herbal teas. Research conducted by Sebastian Kneipp of Bavaria, hydrotherapist and herbalist, showed that drinking one to two glasses of *cold* water first thing in the morning starts peristalsis - the movement that propels matter through the digestive tract.

My favorite formula for regulating bowels - the one I recommend for most patients - is known as *Triphala* (from Planetary Formulas); it is a renowned **Ayurvedic** internal purification formula. Composed of only three East Indian fruits, *Amla, Behada* and *Harada*, *Triphala* stimulates complete, yet gentle elimination while simultaneously toning and strengthening the digestive and elimination systems. *Amla* fruit (Indian gooseberry) contains one of the highest and most heat-stable sources of Vitamin C; it is second only to rosehips in Vitamin C content. *Triphala* is considered a bowel regulator; it effectively treats both diarrhea and constipation and helps to re-establish the normal bacterial flora necessary for a healthy colon. This simple, natural formula can be taken over a long period of time helping to avoid the dependency which often occurs with the use of harsh laxatives. *Take 2 Triphala tablets in the morning before breakfast and 2 tablets before retiring six days per week. After a month or so you may find that 1 to 3 tablets prior to bed is sufficient for desired bowel regulation.*

In **China** people eat fresh coconut before breakfast and bedtime; natural oils contained in coconut meat helps lubricate the intestines. Another Chinese folk remedy for constipation is sunflower seeds. Simply crush a tablespoon or two of shelled organic sunflower seeds; stir in a cup of boiling water with a little organic honey; enjoy a cup in the morning and in the evening. As a cure for chronic constipation, Chinese people consume a half cup or so of sweet potatoes just before bed.

Apricot and Linum Formula is a gentle Chinese herbal prescription from the Han dynasty relieves intense gastrointestinal heat and promotes evacuation - especially for the elderly. It is specific for dry stool, frequent urination, constipation, and dry skin. *Traditional Oriental herbal medicine offers a number of other effective formulas to treat constipation; these are geared towards treating the unique patterns of dis-ease as it manifests in your unique constitution.*

Again, Chinese medicine will tend to look at any problem in the broadest possible context. A person constipated on the physical level may also have a problem "letting go" on every level and be constipated in the mind as well, holding on to all sorts of negative patterns and unhelpful messages. We can see why depression and low self-esteem can also be associated with the Metal element. - *Dr. Gary*

Typical **Western** herbs used for stimulating evacuation include aloe vera, cascara sagrada, rhubarb root, senna leaves and yerba mate.

Depression

Every year in the U.S.:
More than $3 billion is spent on antidepressants;
approximately 17 million adults
experience a bout of serious depression.

According to Martin Seligman, author of *Learned Optimism* and psychology professor at the University of Pennsylvania, depression is ten times more common in persons born after World War II than for their parents and grandparents. Statistics show that women are twice as likely to suffer from depression than men.

A Few Folk Remedies from Around the World

A New and Complete American Medical Family Herbal, from 1814, offers a unique recipe for herbs steeped in Madeira wine to be used "in all debility, lowness of spirits, and dejection of mind." Bring two cups of spring water to a boil and add a handful of sage; cover, remove from heat and let steep for 30 minutes; strain. To the strained liquid add a pinch of each of the following herbal powders: cinnamon, ginger and cloves. Add a small piece of angelica root and pour in a bottle of port or Madeira wine. Steep for one hour then strain the liquid through muslin or a fine mesh strainer. Store in well-corked bottles in a cool cellar (in 1814) or your refrigerator. Drink three to four ounces every morning and before dinner.

As discussed in the preceding section on "Anxiety", French people traditionally took warm baths in lime flower (also known as Tilia, or Linden flower) tea to lighten depression and ease anxiety (see page 339).

Borage, a common pot herb, is called the "herb of gladness" by people living in Wales. They make a special drink by soaking borage leaves in water and sherry; the mixture is brought to a boil then covered and removed from the heat; let steep 20 to 30 minutes then strain; drink in the evening before going to bed.

Basil has historically been the herb of choice of people living in the Arabian Peninsula to fight off depression and anxiety. Fresh basil leaves can be added to salads or vegetable dishes, or simply make a tea by steeping one tablespoon of dried basil leaves in a cup of boiling water for ten minutes; strain and drink to lift the spirits.

In East Indian **Ayurveda**, depression is sometimes viewed as anger turned to the inside - associated with lost opportunities - of not being able to fully express ourselves in the world. Depression is considered to be of a *vata, pitta* or *kapha* nature and the following remedies for mild to moderate cases may prove helpful.

For *vata*-type depression (usually accompanied by nervousness, anxiety, fear and insomnia) a tea brewed from 1/2 teaspoon sage to 1/4 teaspoon holy basil *(tulsi)* per cup of hot water can be ingested twice daily. Organic, cold-pressed sesame oil is often used in the treatment of *vata* disorders. In the case of depression, use a dropper and apply 4 or 5 drops of warmed sesame oil into each nostril on an empty stomach both morning and evening. Rub the soles of the feet and top of the head with sesame oil each evening before bed. Loneliness is often one of the roots of *vata* depression so it becomes very important to reach out to people and to maintain healing, nurturing relationships.

Depression of the *pitta* type is accompanied by feelings of anger, or fear of making mistakes and failing or losing control. *Pitta* people tend to be addicted to succeeding in their endeavors and take it quite seriously when things don't work out the way they planned. *Pittas* can also suffer from seasonal affective disorders (SAD) that usually occurs in the darker fall and winter months. Suicidal thoughts are attributed to a *pitta* imbalance in Ayurvedic thought; please consult a health professional immediately. For mild to moderate *pitta* depression, a tea brewed from 1/2 teaspoon each gotu kola and/or ginkgo biloba per cup of hot water can be ingested two or three times daily. Ghee and coconut oil are the oils frequently used for *pitta* disorders. With a dropper, place 4 to 5 drops of warmed ghee in each nostril morning and evening on an empty stomach. Massage the bottoms of your feet and scalp with coconut oil prior to bedtime. Meditation is particularly beneficial in calming the *pitta* mind or a *pitta* imbalance.

Kapha depression is usually associated with weight gain, drowsiness, excess sleep and a general mental fogginess. A three to four day organic unfiltered apple juice fast can do wonders to lift a *kapha* depression; mix the juice half and half with spring water and sip throughout the day. You could also make a ginger tea with the spring water before mixing it with the apple juice. If not, drink two cups of ginger tea daily made with 1/2 to 1 teaspoon of ginger powder steeped in one cup of hot water. Exercise is essential to lifting *kapha* depression, so start walking. Yoga poses that will help include the Sun Salutation (12 repetitions daily); the Shoulder Stand and Plow pose; the breathing exercise known as *ujjayi pranayama* will also prove extremely helpful.

Ayurvedic medicine views depression as a potentially serious condition; treatment should be supervised by a qualified health practitioner.

One of the reasons why depression is related to the Metal element in **Chinese** thought is that this element is associated with the colon - our master organ of elimination. During our autumn years, we might need to eliminate or to let go of life's inevitable disappointments to live fully in the present - it is only by letting go of the past that we can step into the present moment that becomes a happy, fulfilled future.

The Metal element is also associated with the Lungs, the receiver of pure *ch'i* from the Heavens. The in-ability to take in the gifts that life has to offer can obviously result in the feeling of being cut-off, leading to the emotion of grief. - *Dr. Gary*

Depression is dealt with in great depth in Chinese Medical texts. Following is a brief summary of the Chinese view so readers and students of medical systems can become familiar with the thorough manner in which imbalances have been addressed over hundreds of years in Asian thought. This is only one example of the in-depth understanding and comprehensive description of dis-ease patterns which is so characteristic of Asian healing arts.

In 1271, Zhu Dan-xi wrote *Dan-xi's Insighted Method* describing six subdivisions of depression based on physiological symptoms:

- *Qi yu* refers to qi depression (lack of life force or fatigue);
- *Shi yu* refers to depression due to excess dampness (edema or water retention are good examples);
- *Re yu* or depression due to excessive heat (inflammation, infection or lack of body fluids);
- *Tan tu* or depression due to excess phlegm;
- *Xue yu* would be defined as blood depression (for example, anemia);
- *Shi yu* or depression due to poor diet.

Dr. Zhu created a special herbal formula to treat each of these six types of depression.

Approximately 350 years later, in *Jing Yue's Complete Compendium* written by Zhang Jiebin in 1624, five different types of depression are described based on organ system imbalances that are reflected in the patient's state of mind and predominant emotional tendencies:

- Depression that develops because of excessive anger *(nu yu)*;
- Depression due to excess thought *(students who are exhausted from too much study can develop si yu)*;
- Depression due to anxiety or excess worry *(you yu)*;
- Depression due to fright, known as *jing yu* (a sudden, terrible scare such as an auto accident, personal assault or robbery) and
- Depression due to fear or *kong yu* (different from fright in that this type of fear is more subtle and constant, for example, fear of the dark or the unknown).

Today, seven types of depression are recognized and treated based on the physical and mental imbalances described below. However, keep in mind that Chinese herbal medicine for depression can be tailored to each person's unique constitution and type of depression by a licensed practitioner of Chinese herbology. In cases of mild to moderate depression, the following traditional formulas are very effective:

- **Depression caused by *Heart and Kidney Yin Deficiency*** is distinguished by the following symptoms: Insomnia, night sweats, the person is running on empty, nervous energy. This calls for an herbal formula known as Celestial Emperor known or *tian wang bu xin dan;*
- ***Heart Fire Blazing*** with palpitations, nightmares, insomnia, flushed red face, dark urine, mouth & tongue ulcers calls for the use of *zhu sha an shen wan*, known as Cinnabar Calm the Spirit pill;
- **for *Liver Qi Depression*** resulting from restrained anger accompanied by chest oppression, costal discomfort, anxiety, bloating, acid regurgitation use *yue ju wan,* know as Overcome Depression Decoction;
- **for *Heart & Liver Blood Deficiency*** with insomnia, irritability, headache, palpitations, possible night sweats; dry mouth and throat use *suan zao ren tang* or Jujube Seed Decoction.
- **for depression characterized by what the Chinese refer to as "plum-pit throat",** *one feels a sensation of blockage in the throat* - perhaps there is a situation in one's life that "can't be swallowed", emotional upset (caused by depression of qi) use Pinellia & Magnolia Combination known as *ban xia hou po tang;*
- **for depression related to *Spleen & Heart Blood Deficiency*,** which is characterized by cloudy thinking, anxiety, possible palpitations, poor memory, fatigue of body & mind - use *gan mai dan zao tang* known as *gui pi tang* or Spleen Returning Decoction.
- **to treat a distinct type of depression that is frequently seen in women and children** with such symptoms as frequent sobbing, loss of emotional control, spaced out, possible palpitations (can be postpartum depression, menopause, colic, etc.) use *gan mai da zao tang* known as Licorice, Wheat & Jujube Decoction.

In **Western** herbalism, as early as 300 BCE (in the days of Hippocrates), depression was associated with an excess of the "melancholic" humor. There are a number of Western herbs that ward off bouts of anxiety (see page 339) and depression - these disorders are frequently linked, as it is common to experience symptoms of both simultaneously.

Used for centuries in Western herbalism, St. John's Wort has become the herb of choice in treating depression over the past few years. In Germany, doctors prescribe more St. John's Wort than all antidepressant drugs combined. It has been widely tested in Europe and in controlled studies in the U.S. and is now being taken by many persons across our country in the treatment of mild to moderate depression. In rare instances it may cause slight nausea as well as heightened photo-sensitivity, particularly in fair-skinned people. *To avoid any chance of nausea, take* ***one 300 MG tablet 4 times daily with meals and a snack*** *- for a total of 1200 MG daily. Be sure to ingest one tablet before bedtime with a snack.* Studies show most persons notice the affects of this herb in about four weeks. However some patients report feeling significantly better in only ten to fourteen days.

Wisdom from Around the World in Treating Imbalances Frequently Associated with the Water Element

Arthritis

It is estimated that over 250,000 children
and over 40 million adults in the U.S.
suffer from some form of arthritis.

Arthritis pain has been around since the beginning of time. Archaeologists found signs of arthritic joint inflammation in the skeletal remains of earth's most ancient civilizations. Osteoarthritis results when the cartilage that protects the ends of bones begins to wear away due to long time use - the final result is that the joints rub against each other. The bone can thicken and form painful spurs. Rheumatoid arthritis is an auto immune condition that causes all the signs of inflammation; the joints swell and become red, warm and painful. While these are the two major types of arthritis, over 100 other diseases can affect the joints; they include juvenile arthritis, lupus, fibromyalgia, polymyalgia, gout, ankylosing spondylitis (to mention a few).

A Few Folk Remedies from Around the World

Dioscorides, the famous Greek healer who lived during the first century, traveled widely with the Roman army, carefully observing and chronicling medical practices of his time. For arthritis-like pains, a substance called "oxymel" was prescribed. For centuries now, oxymel has been used for such diverse health problems as hay fever, nervousness and to help dissolve painful calcium deposits in the body. Oxymel is actually easy to make; simply combine 1 tablespoon of raw, pure organic honey and 1 tablespoon of apple cider vinegar in one cup (8 ounces) of spring water, mixing thoroughly. This is your oxymel base which should be kept in a glass container in the refrigerator. To ingest, remove a small portion and add 8 times the amount of water (for example - to 1/4 cup oxymel, add 2 cups of spring water). It will taste something like apple juice and can be sipped throughout the day.

For ages, buttercup poultices made from leaves and flowers of the plant have been used by French villagers to ease the pain that accompanies an acute attack of arthritis. Place 4 cups of buttercup flowers and leaves in a quart of water; bring to a boil; cover and remove from the heat; steep for 15 minutes; strain out the liquid; roll the buttercup mash in a soft cloth and apply to the affected area.

Poke roots are still used by Tennessee mountain folk to ease arthritis pain. *(Note: Poke root should not be ingested but applied externally).* Roast some poke roots in a fire; clean them by scraping the charred sections off with a knife; grind the remaining portions of the root into a fine powder; apply the powder directly to the bottoms of your feet. It doesn't matter where you are experiencing the discomfort, poke root powder should be applied to the soles of the feet. It reputedly draws pain out from anywhere it has lodged in the body.

If you were a member of an island culture, fresh pineapple would probably have been your cure of choice for arthritis pain. Bromelain, the enzyme in pineapple responsible for reducing pain of swelling the body's soft tissues, can be purchased in tablet form at most health food stores; adults can take 4 to 6 tabs daily. You could also enjoy several pieces of this refreshing fruit on a daily basis.

From South Africa's Kalahari Desert comes an anti-inflammatory herb known as devil's claw which helps reduce arthritis pain. Studies conducted in Germany and France have shown that one of its constituents, harpagoside, produces a therapeutic action similar to that of cortisone.

There are a number of age-old European remedies for arthritis pain. A hot bath in Epson salts helps the body rid itself of toxins through perspiration. Add 1 cup of Epson salts to your hot bath water; go straight to bed, and cover up to produce a heavy sweat. *(Note: Not recommended if you have heart trouble, high blood pressure, or are pregnant).* A cold water friction massage can help increase circulation to troubled joints. Keep the body covered; dip your massage mitt or washcloth into icy cold water; wring it out and briskly rub the exposed area; move from joint to joint - gently pat dry, cover, and move to the next area.

The 12th century German mystic Saint Hildegard recommended eating raw quince fruit to rid the body of toxins that create arthritic pain. For centuries, in Chinese medicine, dried quince has been considered one of the most effective herbs to reduce severe, cramping pain in the lower back and legs.

Ayurvedic medicine distinguishes arthritic symptoms according to their *vata, pitta,* or *kapha* nature. For example, joints that are cold or dry and pop when moved are due to a *vata* imbalance; movement aggravates joint pain which usually can be pinpointed to one particular spot. Strenuous exercise like jogging or jumping tends to aggravate this *vata*-type arthritis.

Inflammation characterizes *pitta-type* arthritis. The joints become red and swollen and are often hot to the touch with almost continuous pain - even without movement.

If you're suffering from *kapha-type* arthritis, the joints feel cold and clammy and are swollen and stiff. Usually, most pain is experienced early in the morning and once you start moving, it gradually diminishes.

In Ayurveda, treatment is unique for all three types, however, it always begins with colon cleansing. In this view, toxins from the colon are carried throughout the system and lodge in the joints causing pain and stiffness. For this reason, *Triphala,* an internal purification formula, is always prescribed. As mentioned in the previous section, *Triphala* (from Planetary Formulas) is my favorite formula for regulating bowels. *Take 3 to 4 Triphala tablets (or one teaspoon of the powder) before retiring each evening. After a month, reduce to 2 tablets nightly.*

For *vata*-type arthritis, follow the *vata*-pacifying diet in Chapter 10 being certain to eliminate all nightshades: bell pepper, tomato, potato and eggplant. All avoid cold foods and drinks. Rub *mahanarayan* oil on painful joints, then soak in very warm water. Take one tablet of *yogaraj guggulu* three times daily.

For *pitta*-type arthritis, follow the *pitta*-pacifying diet and avoid hot, spicy or sour foods such as: chile peppers, salsa, tomatoes, pickles, vinegar. Take one tablet of *kiashore guggulu* (350 mg) three times daily as well as 1/2 teaspoon of *sudarshan* twice daily with warm water. Gently apply cool coconut oil, castor oil or sandalwood paste to the painful joint. Cold compresses will help ease the pain and inflammation.

For *kapha*-type arthritis, follow the *kapha*-pacifying diet and avoid all dairy products and cold foods and drinks. Take one tablet of *punarnava guggulu* (250 mg) three times daily. A paste of calamus root powder *(vacha)* can be applied to the joint to ease discomfort.

Similar to East Indian Ayurveda, **Chinese** medicine recognizes four types of arthritis: cold, heat, damp and wind type.

Wind type arthritis, associated with the Wood element, is characterized by migrating pains that shift locations as well as occasional bouts of dizziness. Avoid red meat, alcohol, sugar and cigarettes. Foods that help include most whole grains, plenty of green leafy veggies, grapes, black beans and scallions.

Heat type arthritis, associated with the Fire element, is characterized by its sudden onset as well as red, swollen, hot, painful joints. Avoid alcohol, spicy foods, green onion, cigarettes and stress. Dramatically increase your consumption of cooling fresh fruit and green leafy veggies, mung beans, cabbage, dandelion greens and soybean sprouts. Apply a poultice of crushed dandelion greens to the painful areas - change every two hours.

Damp type arthritis, associated with the Earth element, is characterized by stiffness, swelling, dull, aching pain and sluggishness. Avoid cold foods, sugar, highly refined foods made with white flour, cheese and other fatty foods. Foods that will help drain dampness include aduki beans, barley, coix, cornsilk tea, mung beans and mustard greens.

Cold type arthritis, associated with the Water element, is characterized by coldness in the joints that creates sharp, stabbing pain - heat brings relief. Avoid all cold raw foods as well as exposure to cold weather. Foods that help include black beans, chicken, garlic, ginger, grapes, green onions, mustard greens, sesame seeds (especially black), parsnip, turnip, pepper and spicy foods. Gently rub ginger root juice on the painful areas.

Based on your unique constitution, there are a number of Chinese herbal formulas that help eliminate arthritic pain; acupuncture is also quite effective.

In the **West**, the pain-relieving properties of white willow bark have proven to be as effective as aspirin - and this herbal aid does not cause stomach irritation. The natural salicylic acid found in willow bark is nearly identical to that in synthetic aspirin. Stir one teaspoon of the bark into a cup of boiling water; cover and remove from heat; steep for 15 to 20 minutes then strain. Drink a cup three times daily - as needed. As a patient of the ancient Greek physician Dioscorides, you would have been advised to simply chew on a piece of bark.

Feverfew is an effective western herb that eases arthritic pain by suppressing the release of histamines and prostaglandins - chemicals that create inflammation. As is true of most herbs, feverfew can be taken in capsule, extract or tea form.

Nettles has long been prescribed to ease arthritic pain and stiffness. A controlled German study has confirmed that arthritis sufferers were able to cut their dosages of prescription drugs in half when taking 1,340 mg of nettles powder. Their next study will examine stinging nettles' ability to ease the pain from acute attacks of arthritis without the use of drugs.

Similar to Ayurvedic thought, Western herbalists view the cause of arthritis as being the improper elimination of wastes from the body. Dandelion and burdock root are frequently used to stimulate the detoxifying functions of the liver and kidneys. Bring three cups of water to a boil; stir in 1 teaspoon each of dried burdock and dandelion root; cover and simmer for five minutes; remove from heat, strain and sip the mixture throughout the day.

Native American Winnebago and Dakota people ingested black cohosh tea to ease pain from rheumatism. Native Americans living in Mendocino County rubbed the juice from the bruised rhizome of the California polypody fern on joints to reduce rheumatic pain.

Natives living in the American Southwest made a drink of mashed yucca root and water to treat arthritis pain. Mashed root can also be applied topically to inflamed joints to bring relief.

Other Recommendations

Sulfur is required by the body to repair bones, cartilage and connective tissue - it also aides in the absorption of calcium. Consume more foods that are rich in sulfur such as onions, garlic, asparagus and eggs.

A glucosamine sulfate supplement, a substance naturally found in cartilage, can repair and heal arthritic joints. Take 500 mg three times daily with meals. Patients have reported reduced pain levels in two to four weeks.

Many persons suffering from arthritis have high levels of iron and/or copper in their bodies. Avoid taking iron supplements or multivitamins that contain iron - it is suspected of contributing to inflammation of the joints. If anemia is a problem, consume foods that are high in *naturally occurring* iron such as dulse (a sea vegie), blackstrap molasses, broccoli, cauliflower, fish, lima beans and peas. Whole grains that have high levels of the amino acid histidine (wheat, kamut, spelt, rice and rye) help remove excess metals from the body.

Backache

Eighty percent of all Americans will experience back pain at one point in their lives. Twenty five percent of all sick leave and over $20 billion annually is spent on the medical treatment of backaches in the U.S. While many factors can contribute to back pain, Western researchers believe that most cases are related to simple muscle strains. Chronic conditions that can create back pain include arthritis, rheumatism, osteoporosis, herniated disks and other types of degenerative bone disease. Other causes of back pain might include poor lifting techniques; poor posture when sitting, standing or walking; sleeping on a mattress that is too soft or wearing shoes that do not fit properly (the higher the heel, the greater the chance of producing backache); constipation, menstrual cramping, kidney, bladder or prostate problems.

Lack of exercise and subsequent poor muscle tone can contribute to backache. Swimming, cycling, gentle yoga stretches and walking are all exercises that improve muscle tone and flexibility and are back friendly.

If you have back pain following a sudden movement or injury, apply cold packs for the first 48 hours to reduce swelling and inflammation - thereafter, apply heat to relieve pain, increase circulation and speed healing. If the pain is severe, lasts for more than seventy-two hours or radiates down the legs, consult your health care provider.

A Few Folk Remedies from Around the World

A Swedish technique to help relieve and prevent back pain suggests that during your shower, slightly bend at the knees and support your back by placing your hands on your thighs - then let warm water run over the painful area for five to ten minutes.

A number of the herbs mentioned in the preceding section on "Arthritis", such as white willow bark and feverfew, can help ease back pain caused by strain or over-exertion.

Magnet therapy has been used for a number of years in Asian healing practices to reduce back pain.

Backache, in **Ayurvedic** thought, is often caused by excess *vata dosha*. Reduce your consumption of *vata* increasing foods such as lentils, garbanzo, black, pinto and aduki beans and cruciferous vegetables such as cabbage, broccoli and cauliflower. *However, you can change the vata producing qualities of the veggies by stir-frying them in healthful oil with a little fennel.*

Rubbing *mahanarayan* oil on the painful area will also help (deeper massage would be beneficial for *kapha* types). Adding 1/3 cup each of baking soda and ginger powder to your bath water two to three times a week relaxes tense muscles - soak in the tub for 15 to 20 minutes.

Pain relieving herbs recommended by Ayurvedic practitioners include cyperus *(musta)* or valerian root powder. Take 1/2 teaspoon of either of these herbs with warm water (2 to 3 times daily) to relax muscles and promote restful sleep.

Consult with a trained yoga instructor. Gentle yoga stretches help release tensions, stretch out ligaments and tendons, and tone and build muscle strength.

According to **Chinese** medicine, the Urinary Bladder acupuncture meridian runs up and down the back and legs; points along this channel are frequently used in acupuncture to relieve pain and promote healing. Acupuncture and herbal treatment is an effective healing modality in dealing with most backaches.

Oriental medicine offers a unique view of back pain when compared to other healing traditions. Some Chinese physicians feel that Kidney/Adrenal deficiency is the underlying causative factor for most back pain. *(Note: The yin Kidney channel is paired with the yang Urinary Bladder channel in Asian medicine - both are associated with the Water element).*

Six possible causes for back pain, in Asian medical thought, include: 1) excessive physical work, 2) excessive sexual activity, 3) pregnancy and childbirth, 4) overexposure to cold/damp conditions, 5) fatigue due to overwork, 6) lack of exercise. All of these factors take their toll on our general well being and can contribute to low Kidney/Adrenal energy.

In my practice, I frequently see patients who sit behind a desk and in front of a computer for hours on end. Due to inactivity, energy, lymph and blood do not flow as they should - cells do not receive oxygen and nutrients, and toxins are not carried away. This congested condition results in localized pain that is sharp, deep and colicky in nature. Obviously, getting up and stretching frequently (every 30 minutes is suggested) would be essential. There are a number of herbal formulas to help remedy this situation. Achyranthes root and eucommia bark are frequently paired to relieve weakness, low-back and knee pain due to stagnation. You can also obtain excellent Chinese topical ointments at most health food store, such as Tiger Balm, to help relieve pain.

Dietary changes can help tremendously in easing chronic back pain. Avoid cold and congesting, fatty refined foods like ice cream, cheese, rich desserts and fried foods. Most patients are surprised and pleased to find that two weeks off such fare can make a major difference in pain levels.

If you suffer from chronic backache, review the information given in Chapter 7 on Kidney *Yin* and *Yang* Deficiency.

In **Western** herbal thought, arnica ointment or gel is an excellent topical remedy to ease muscle strains. Other herbs frequently recommended include alfalfa, burdock, oat straw, white willow bark and horsetail rush.

Osteoporosis

In Latin, osteoporosis means "porous bones". Over fifty percent of all women between the ages of 45 and 75 show some degree of this progressive disease in which the bones gradually become less dense - one-third of those women suffer from serious bone damage. Osteoporosis affects more women than breast cancer, heart disease, diabetes, stroke or arthritis.

Two basic types of osteoporosis have been recognized by researchers: **Type I** which is associated with mid-life hormonal changes (particularly estrogen deficiency) and subsequent loss of minerals from the bones; and **Type II** which is linked to insufficient dietary calcium and vitamin D (which is required for proper calcium absorption). Results from recent research conducted by the National Institutes of Health revealed that fifty percent of all Americans are calcium deprived; daily, they are ingesting less than half of the required amount of calcium their bodies need to prevent osteoporosis. It is a common belief that osteoporosis affects women only after menopause has begun. Studies indicate that bone loss actually begins early in life and accelerates after menopause; therefore, prevention needs to start early on as well.

Research conducted in New Zealand demonstrated that post menopausal women taking 1000 mg of calcium per day reduced bone loss by fifty percent. Unfortunately, substantial nutritional differences exist between the various calcium supplements available on the market, making choices difficult for consumers. The label might specify "calcium lactate 600 milligrams" but this only indicates that the total weight of each tablet is 600 milligrams. Out of the 600 milligrams of calcium lactate contained in the tablet, only 60 milligrams of assimible calcium may actually be available. Be certain to check for the amount of *elemental* calcium contained in your supplement - this is the kind your body can use. The highest percentage of elemental calcium available for absorption is usually found in **calcium carbonate** as compared to other forms. Another problem is that some calcium tablets do not dissolve readily in the body. To check this out, simply place one tablet in a cup of vinegar; stir every few minutes. If the tablet doesn't dissolve within 30 minutes, it is probably not being digested in your stomach. The suggested dosage for post-menopausal women is 1000 to 1500 mg of elemental calcium derived from both diet and supplements. It is best that calcium supplements contain magnesium in a 2 to 1 ratio (i.e. 500 mg calcium carbonate to 250 mg magnesium) as well as Vitamin D to facilitate absorption into the bones. *Consult with a physician before taking calcium supplements if you have a history of kidney stones.*

From a naturalist's point of view, acquiring our calcium from whole foods is more desirable than simply ingesting chemically compounded calcium supplements. Following you will find a chart that indicates the amount of calcium available in various foods - notice that most sea veggies provide over ten times the quantity of calcium available in milk. *Please read about sea vegetables, a valuable natural source of balanced minerals, page 322.*

Calcium Available in Foods Based on 3-1/2 ounce (100 mg) portions

Food Source	Calcium in mgs
Hijiki	1400
Wakame	1300
Kelp	1099
Kombu	800
Sardines	443
Agar Agar	400
Nori	260
Amaranth (grain)	222
Parsley	203
Sunflower seeds	174
Garbanzo beans	150
Quinoa (grain)	141
Black beans	135
Pinto beans	135
Kale	134
Yogurt	121
Milk	119
Sesame seeds	110
Chinese cabbage	106
Tofu	100
Walnuts	99
Salmon	79
Cottage cheese	60
Eggs	56
Brown rice	33
Halibut	13
Chicken	11
Ground beef	10

Following is a list of factors that influence a person's risk of developing osteoporosis:

- The density of our bones depends upon how much regular weight-bearing exercise we get. Lack of exercise contributes to loss of bone mass. Simply walking 30 minutes five or six times per week will help protect against osteoporosis.

- Small women with fine bones are more susceptible to debilitating bone loss. Women of Asian or northern European ancestry are more likely to develop osteoporosis than those of African descent.
- Processed foods and sodas contain excessive quantities of phosphorus and magnesium - an excess of these minerals inhibits the body from absorbing calcium properly.
- Our body buffers the effects of highly acidic foods (animal protein, coffee, colas, salt and sugar) by stealing calcium from the bones. Smoking tobacco, alcohol and many pharmaceutical drugs (such as the long term usage of anticoagulants, corticosteroids and anti seizure medications) produce a similar effect.
- Other factors that increase the likelihood of developing osteoporosis include: hyperthyroidism, chronic kidney or liver disease, late puberty or early menopause and a family history of the disease.
- As mentioned in the preceding section on "Pure Water", sodium fluoride, the chemical added to city water supplies *(an extremely toxic by-product of the aluminum industry commonly used as rat poison)* was once believed to promote bone growth. Studies show that ingestion of this chemical increases bone density in the vertebral column, but it is of inferior quality. Findings from a study conducted at Mayo Clinic in Minnesota indicate that women who took sodium fluoride supplements were three times more likely to suffer from hip, arm or leg fractures than those who took the placebo. We need to get this chemical out of our nation's drinking water!

For herbs rich in natural plant estrogens and calcium, please see Chapter 5, "Menopause: Those Hormones Again", page 175.

Vitamin & Mineral Allies: Our Third Line of Defense

As previously discussed, according to naturalistic thought, whole foods along with exercise and a healthy lifestyle form the first line of defense in creating health and combating chronic disorders; herbal remedies are the second while vitamin and mineral supplements are our third line of defense. In our fast-paced pill-oriented society, this sequence frequently gets reversed. Many first-time patients tell me they "take their vitamins and minerals" on a daily basis - however, little thought is given to the foods they ingest day in and day out. While good quality supplements made from natural sources can greatly contribute to our overall health and make up for nutrients that have been depleted from the soil, they shouldn't be considered the primary way to maintain health.

Throughout this book, various vitamins and minerals have been suggested when deemed appropriate. Following is a brief summary of the properties of some supplements that I frequently recommend to patients:

Multiple Vitamin & Mineral Supplement: Find a high quality capsule or tablet that contains the RDA (not mega-doses) of these essential nutrients - your diet should be supplying most of your needs. It would be good to find two different brands and alternate - for example, both Source Naturals and Rainbow Light produce sound products. *Take the vitamin/mineral supplement 6 days per week with a meal. Give your body a rest from herbs as well as supplements one day per week; and after 3 months on any particular supplement, a one to two week rest period is appropriate.*

Vitamin C helps remove Lipoprotein (a), or Lp(a) out of your system. Lp(a), a small particle that helps damage artery walls, is a substantial contributor to heart disease. Vitamin C aids the body in detoxification by scavenging free radicals. This important vitamin helps eliminate depression by enhancing the brains's production of serotonin (it does this by helping to convert tryptophan - *found in protein foods we eat like chicken and turkey.* - into this important neurotransmitter). While there is a great deal of debate about the RDA of Vitamin C, many chronically ill persons can benefit greatly from increasing their daily intake. You can determine your "bowel tolerance" level for Vitamin C ingestion by starting with 500 mg increments and adding one more tablet daily. If you begin to experience such symptoms as gas, diarrhea, or stomach distress, simply back off by reducing your dosage 500 mg at a time until the symptoms subside. *To start off, take 500 to 2,000 mg with breakfast and dinner and another 500 to 2,000 mg prior to bedtime. (Purchase buffered, time-released, vegetarian tablets).*

Calcium/Magnesium, see page 404.

Selenium, is a trace mineral with antioxidant and anti cancer properties. Research has shown that our soils and food supply are seriously lacking in this essential nutrient. While Vitamin E facilitates selenium's absorption, Vitamin C may actually interfere with the absorption of some forms of selenium. Your multivitamin will supply part of what you need but usually not enough. *Ingest 200 to 300 mgs of selenium at lunch time and NOT at the same time you take Vitamin C. (Note: Doses above 400 micrograms daily may not be healthy - so be sure to check how much you are already getting in your multiple vitamin/mineral tablet).*

Natural Vitamin E (d-alpha-tocopherol) another invaluable antioxidant needs to be taken with food since it is fat-soluble. *Take 400 to 800 IUs of natural vitamin E at lunch time* ***with selenium.***

Coenzyme Q10 is considered by some researchers to be a "miracle nutrient". Studies have shown that when body levels of CoQ10 start dropping, so does the general level of health. To enhance immunity ingest 100 to 300 mg/day.

Zinc is an essential component in over 300 enzymes that boost immunity, repair wounds, synthesize protein, preserve vision, promote bone formation and protect against free radicals (to mention a few). If you feel as though you have lost your sense of taste or smell, zinc supplementation may help. **Recent studies have shown a direct link between zinc and anorexia, bulimia and obesity. Persons suffering from these disorders have a low level of zinc.** Once liquid zinc supplements are added to the diet the recovery rate is much higher than for those persons not receiving zinc treatments. Be certain to purchase a supplement that is balanced with copper since too much of one can result in a deficiency of the other. *Daily, ingest 30 mg of zinc with 3 mg of copper along with a meal. Note: Premarin leeches zinc out of the system.*

Chromium, one of the most important minerals to maintain blood sugar levels and promote proper insulin utilization, can be very helpful for persons suffering from hypoglycemia or diabetes. *Diabetics should not start chromium supplementation without first consulting with their physician since this mineral alters insulin requirements.* Chromium helps to increase lean muscle mass while promoting weight loss. Chromium deficiency can result in fatigue, anxiety, increased risk of arteriosclerosis and inadequate amino acid metabolism. Excessive intake can result in chromium toxicity with such symptoms as gastrointestinal ulcers, dermatitis and/or liver and kidney function impairment. However, our soils as well as the average American diet are deficient in chromium. *The recommended dosage is* ***200 mcg of Chromium GTF (as polynicotinate) two times daily with a meal*** *- do not exceed this amount.*

Tips to Enhance A Speedy Recovery Before and After Surgery

Prior to surgery it is important to make as many healthful lifestyle adjustments as possible to maximize recovery. Below are a few additional tips to ease discomfort and speed renewal:

- Start a **high quality vitamin and mineral supplement** as soon as possible before surgery - it is best to find one that you can *take at regular intervals, with meals, throughout the day.*
- **Arnica Montana** is a homeopathic remedy which helps to reduce pain and trauma while speeding recovery. *As soon as possible after surgery, dissolve four small tablets under the tongue every two to three hours for two or three days (not to be taken with food or drink).*
- **Bromelain** *(or pancreatin)* can speed healing by helping to reduce inflammation and swelling at the surgical site. *The recommended dosage is 500 mg three times daily.*
- Be certain to schedule as much **recovery time** as possible before returning to work. Is there anything more important than your health?
- Be prepared with plenty of **entertaining activities** for your "downtime" - such as books that you have always wanted to read, or videos that you haven't had time to watch.
- After surgery, eat four to six healthful **mini-meals** throughout the day with plenty of fresh, lightly steamed (to facilitate digestion) fruits and vegetables (8 to 12 - 1/2 cup servings daily). Cold-water fish (such as salmon, sea bass, tuna, cod, etc.) provide healthful omega 3 fats.
- As soon as possible (with your doctor's approval) begin **light exercise**. Movement improves circulation and cell oxygenation - speeding recovery. Don't overdo - be certain not to tire yourself.
- You may find it helpful to consult with a licensed practitioner of **Chinese medicine** prior to surgery. There are many Chinese formulas designed to support the system and build immunity during such a stressful time; these can be tailored

to meet the needs of the individual. Acupuncture can also be used to reconnect meridian pathways that are disrupted by the surgical incision.

- **Ginger or chamomile** tea helps relieve nausea (see page 179).
- Other herbal aides might include **garlic** (see pages 206 and 335); **astragalus** (page 202); **milk thistle** (page 336); **gotu kola** (page 205); an extract made from tonifying, immune-building **Reishi/Maitake/Shiitaki Mushrooms** - *30 to 60 drops, two times daily.*
- **Essiac,** a well-known herbal preparation that has long been used in the treatment of chronic ailments, boosts immunity while cleansing the liver and blood. The formula for Essiac was given to Rene Caisee, a Canadian nurse, by a Chippewa Native healer. It is composed of four herbs: Burdock, Slippery Elm, Sheep Sorrel and Turkey Rhubarb. *The usual recommended dosage is 1/2 dropperful of tincture three to four times daily - one hour before or two hours after eating. Ingest it six days a week for four weeks; rest from it for one week and repeat the cycle.*

Maximizing the Potential and Minimizing the Side-Effects of Chemotherapy

Glutamine helps limit the side-effects of chemotherapy by supporting the immune system, reducing fatigue and preventing the destruction of gastrointestinal cells. *5 grams of glutamine powder can be dissolved in cool spring water and sipped between meals - up to 3 times daily for a total of 10 to 15 grams. It is important to drink this between meals since protein inhibits its effectiveness.*

Milk Thistle Seeds (Silymarin): Milk thistle helps protect the liver from the accumulation of chemotherapy drugs - once they've done their job in the tumor cell, silymarin helps move them out of the body. *The recommended dosage is 140 mg of a natural product standardized to contain 70 to 80% silymarin - 3 times per day - 6 days per week between and after chemotherapy rounds. See page 336 for more information about milk thistle.*

Red Clover Blossoms have been used in European folk medicine for centuries and are helpful in recuperating from chronic degenerative dis-eases. The blossom contains great quantities of vitamins and minerals and is considered an excellent blood purifier. It aides digestion by stimulating liver and gall bladder action and contains coumarins which have a mild blood-thinning effect *(do not ingest if you are currently taking blood-thinning pharmaceutical drugs)*. Several studies have shown that this herb has antibiotic effects against several bacteria (including those of tuberculosis). Red clover blossoms contain genistein, an estrogenic compound that may block estrogen receptors, thwarting tumor development in estrogenically-driven tumors.

Support During Radiation Therapy

Whey powder increases tumor sensitivity to radiation therapy by selectively stealing antioxidants from the cancer cells. It can be purchased in bulk at most health food stores. *The recommended dosage is usually one teaspoon with each meal and snack for a total of 5 to 6 teaspoons daily.*

Alkylglycerols are made from shark liver oil - they enhance the effects of radiation therapy on cancer cells while protecting the body against lowered immunity (frequently a side effect of radiation therapy). This product has been purified of heavy metals, pesticides and excess vitamin A and D. *The recommended dosage is 100 mg two times daily (with breakfast and dinner) during radiation therapy.*

Vitamin C helps boost immunity and enhances the effects of radiation while protecting healthy cells. *Ingest 1,000 to 10,000 mgs daily (depending upon your tolerance as described on page 407).*

Read about **sea veggies** on page 322, 1/4 cup per day can assist the body in eliminating radioisotopes. (Kelp root tablets are available at most health food stores.)

Apply 100% pure Aloe vera gel to areas receiving radiation treatment - it helps protect against radiation burn. Apply **Vitamin E** topically to any mouth sores to ease discomfort and speed healing.

In Chinese medicine, radiation, though it may be necessary to combat a cancer, is considered an "external causative factor" of disease. Specific acupuncture treatments can be used to counter this effect. - *Dr. Gary*

14

A Return to Natural Patterns

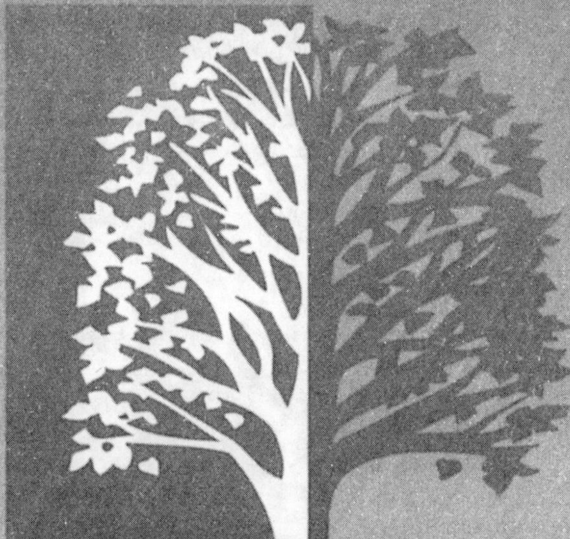

Conclusion

By Gary Dolowich, M.D., B.Ac.

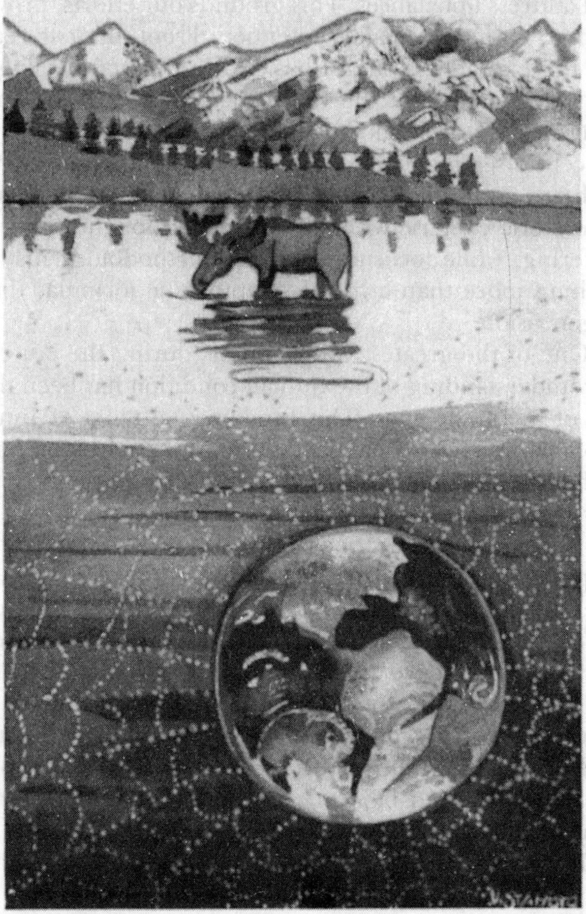

Whoever lets go in his fall,
dives into the source and is healed.

RILKE

It has been the intention in this book to hold a balance of *yin* and *yang* in our approach to illness. On the *yin* side we have Earth remedies, both herbal and dietary, to alleviate symptoms and address imbalances. This grounds our efforts, providing the form to express a healing intention. From the *yang* realm there are the energetic systems, basic to traditional healing, that offer a deeper insight into the processes involved. Through an awareness of these models there is a sense of meaning, as the concept of energy connects us to a spiritual dimension. Clearly, both are necessary, as purely energetic approaches can become an esoteric exercise without compassion for the need to relieve suffering, while focusing solely on methodology may result in nothing more than a list of symptomatic formulas that lacks a larger vision.

One of the greatest contributions during the last century to our understanding of the human condition has been the discovery of the archetypes. This fundamental tenet of Jungian psychology offers the view that there are basic underlying images within the unconscious which unfold during the progression of our lives. Bringing these potentials to expression is necessary for wholeness. Health then becomes more than the mere absence of pathology but, rather, an actualization of these archetypal energies. The process of *individuation* is the description of this journey of development, culminating in the mature man or woman. As we have seen, the images of depth psychology are not different from the energy models of traditional medicine that have been the focus of our exploration throughout this text. Indeed, the concept of the archetypes serves as a bridge between ancient and modern approaches to the patterns that lie beneath the mystery of life.

It is one of the main functions of traditional cultures to create the forms that enable these potentials to emerge in a healthy way. In the myths that are told, and in the rituals that are an enactment of these stories, we find the archetypes expressed in a balanced, complete way that supports the development of the individual in a direction that ensures enduring values. In addition, the connection to a higher source or Creator, inherent in mythology, links all undertakings to a greater purpose. Jung's concept of the collective unconscious points out that these images are universal, found in fairy tales, dreams, and art around the world. Thus, all humans share the same deep structures of the psyche and are truly brothers and sisters. Though we may live in a different time and place, the traditions of other cultures can become useful guides for our own maturation process.

Much of the suffering in our modern world can be understood to arise from a breakdown in traditional cultural forms, resulting in a failure to develop archetypal potentials in a life-affirming way. When the rituals that are so vital to individual growth are unavailable, these energies either remain dormant or are expressed in destructive forms, such as the shadow side of the Warrior leading to the increase of violence in the world. Without a viable myth, most people lack a sense of the sacred in their lives and find themselves cut off from meaning and purpose.

Often illness can serve as a catalyst for rediscovering this neglected archetypal realm. Especially when chronic in nature, the lack of an easy solution from conventional medicine forces us to change the questions that are asked. Instead of *how to fix it*, the inquiry extends to uncovering *what it is the condition may be asking from us*. This inevitably leads to digging deeper and exploring hidden parts of ourselves. Indeed, when symptoms are treated as inherently meaningful and looked at wholistically, they become the manure that enables the plant to grow. Jung compared the task presented by illness to the ancient science of alchemy. Through bringing the darkness into the light there is the opportunity to forge gold, which is the goal of the individuation process.

In seeking the answers to the problem of illness "across cultures and through time," there is an inevitable expansion of our worldview. Since, in general, medical practices are inseparable from the societies in which they have developed, by exploring ancient treatments we partake in the wisdom of traditions that have much to teach the Western world. Since these cultures are based on living in harmony with natural rhythms, this process can help us return to simplicity and find our own inner nature. One of the special gifts in studying traditional healing systems is to learn about various models for describing the energy that underlies life. This understanding opens up a side of existence that generally has been split off in the modern world, enabling us to reach beyond materialistic concerns to a more meaningful level.

The struggle with illness catapults us from a merely intellectual endeavor to a life-changing experience, while the medicine of traditional cultures brings the energetic potentials of the psyche into awareness. As we work with the healing systems of ancient peoples, we unlock undiscovered parts of ourselves and connect with natural patterns and the world of archetypal energies. These primal images literally vibrate with energy and are a rich source of vitality. Being in relationship with them allows us to lead the fullest, most satisfying life. It can be said that, ultimately, healing stems from contact with the numinous, that is, establishing a spiritual perspective to life. In uncovering the deeper meaning of the illness in terms of these traditional models, we indeed open to the Spirit and discover the truth behind Jung's statement that "if the archetypal meaning underlying the illness is expressed in the right way, the patient is cured."

Resource Guide

Ayurvedic Medicine

Organizations

American Institute of Vedic Studies
1701 Santa Fe River Road
Santa Fe, NM 87501

Ayurvedic Institute
P. O. Box 23445
Albuquerque, NM 87192-1445

Maharishi International University
1000 North 4th Street
D. B. 1155
Fairfield, IA 52557

Ayurvedic Herbal Products

Bazaar of India Imports
1810 University Avenue
Berkeley, CA 94703

Internatural
Dept. AR
P. O. Box 489
Twin Lakes, WI 53181 USA
800-643 4221 (toll free order line)
262-889 8581 (office phone)
262-889 8591 (fax)

E-mail: internatural@lotuspress.com
Website: http://www.internatural.com/
Retail mail order and Internet re-seller of Ayurvedic products, essential oils, herbs, spices, supplements, herbal remedies, incense, books, yoga mats, supplies and videos.

Lotus Light Enterprises
Dept. AR
P. O. Box 1008
Silver Lake, WI 53170 USA
800-548 3824 (toll free order line)
262-889 8501 (office phone)
262-889 8591 (fax)
E-mail: lotuslight@lotuspress.com
Website: http://www.lotuslight.com/
Wholesale distributor of essential oils, herbs, spices, supplements, herbal remedies, incense, books and other supplies. Must supply resale certificate number or practitioner license to obtain catalog of more than 10,000 items.

Planetary Formulas
P. Bo. Box 533
Soquel, CA 95073

Quantum Publications, Inc.
P. O. Box 598
South Lancaster, MA 01561
1-800-858-1808

Books

CHOPRA, Deepak, M.D. ***Perfect Health - The Complete Mind/ Body Guide***. New York, New York: Crown Publishers, Inc., 1991.

Frawley, David. ***Ayurvedic Healing: A Comprehensive Guide, 2nd Revised and En. Ed.*** Twin Lakes, WI: Lotus Press, 2000.

LAD, Vasant. ***Ayurveda - The Science of Self-Healing***. Twin Lakes, WI: Lotus Press, 1984.

Blood Types & Dietary Requirements

Books

D'ADAMO, Peter, Dr. with Whitney, Catherine. ***Eat Right for Your Type.*** New York, New York: G. P. Putnam's Sons, 1996.

GITTLEMAN, Ann Louise, M.S. ***Your Body Knows Best.*** New York, New York: Simon & Schuster, Inc., 1996.

Carbohydrate Sensitivity & Weight Loss

Books

HELLER, Rachael F., Ph.D., HELLER, Richard F., Ph.D. ***The Carbohydrate Addict's Diet.*** New York, New York: Penguin Books, 1993.

DesMAISONS, Kathleen, Ph.D. ***Are You Sugar Sensitive? Potatoes Not Prozac.*** New York, New York: Simon & Schuster, 1998.

SEARS, Barry, Ph.D. ***Enter the Zone.*** New York, New York: HarperCollins Publishers, 1995.

SEARS, Barry, Ph.D. ***Mastering the Zone.*** New York, New York: HarperCollins Publishers, 1997.

THOMPSON, Dr. Dennis ***Ayurvedic Zone Diet***. Twin Lakes, WI: Lotus Press, 1999

Fats in Our Diet

Books

ERASMUS, Udo. ***Fats that Heal - Fats that Kill.*** Burnaby BC, Canada: Alive Books, 1986.

Chinese Medicine

Books

BEINFIELD, Harriet, L.Ac. & KORNGOLD, Efrem, L.Ac., O.M.D. ***Between Heaven and Earth - A Guide To Chinese Medicine***. New York, New York: Ballantine Books, 1991.

FRATKIN, Jake. ***Chinese Herbal Patent Formulas - A Practical Guide.*** Boulder, Colorado: SHYA Publications, 1993.

L'ORANGE, Darlena, L.Ac. ***Herbal Healing Secrets of the Orient***. Paramus, New Jersey: Prentice Hall, 1998.

TIERRA, Dr's. Michael and Lesley ***Chinese Traditional Herbal Medicine***, Two Volume Set, Twin Lakes, WI: Lotus Press, 1998

Food Therapy

Note: Carbohydrate sensitive individuals can take advantage of the use of medicinal herbal soups and porridges given in the "Book of Jook;" however, substitute small amounts of whole barley, coix or oatmeal for rice (which is higher on the glycemic index). Consume your porridge with the appropriate amount of protein and fat as recommended by Sears in *The Zone.* If you follow the Heller & Heller method, simply consume a rice porridge during your daily "one hour Reward Meal."

FLAWS, Bob. ***The Book of Jook - Chinese Medicinal Porridges.*** Boulder, Colorado: Blue Poppy Press, 1995.

FLAWS, Bob & WOLFE, Honora. ***Prince Wen Hui's Cook - Chinese Dietary Therapy.*** Brookline, Massachusetts: Paradigm Publications, 1983.

HAAS, Elson M., M.D. ***Staying Healthy with Nutrition.*** Berkeley, California: Celestial Arts, 1992.

LU, Henry C. ***Chinese System of Food Cures - Prevention & Remedies.*** New York, New York: Sterling Publishing Company, 1986.

LU, Henry C. ***Chinese Foods for Longevity.*** New York, New York: Sterling Publishing Company, 1986.

PITCHFORD, Paul. ***Healing with Whole Foods - Oriental Traditions and Modern Nutrition.*** Berkeley, California: North Atlantic Books, 1993.

Chinese Herbs

The following companies sell Chinese herbs by mail order in the **United States:**

Spring Wind Herb Company
2325 Fourth Street Suite 6
Berkeley, CA 94710
Tel: (510) 849-1820
Fax: (510) 849-4886

Mayway Trading Corporation
1338 Mandela Parkway
Oakland, CA 94607
Tel: (510) 208-3123; (800) 262-9929

Nuherbs Company
3820 Penniman Avenue
Oakland, CA 94619
Tel: (415) 534-4372; (800) 233-4307

East West Herb Products
317 West 100th Street
New York, New York 10025
In New York: (212) 864-5508
Outside New York: (800) 542-6544

China Herb Company
6333 Wayne Avenue
Philadelphia, PA 19144
Tel: (215) 843-5864; (800) 221-4372
Fax: (215) 849-3338

Persons living in the **United Kingdom** can order most of the medicinals in this book from:

Acumedic Ltd.
101-105 Camden High Street
London NW1 7JN
Tel: 071-388-6704/5783
Fax: 071-387-5766

Harmony Acupuncture Supplies Center
629 High Road Leytonstone
London E11 4PA
Tel: 081-518-7337
Fax: 081-518-7338

Mayway Herbal Emporium
40 Sapcote Trading Estate, Dudden Hill Lane
London NW10 2DJ
Tel: 081-459-1812
Fax: 081-459-1727

Persons living in **Europe** can order most of the medicinals in this book from:

Tai Yang Chinese Herb Store
Elverdignsestr. 90A
8900 Ieper, Belgium
Tel: 057-21-86-69
Fax: 057-21-97-78

Apotheek Gouka
Goenelaan 111
3114 CE Schiedam, Netherlands
Tel: 010-426-46-33
Fax: 010-473-08-45

Persons living in **Australia** can order most of the medicinals in this book from:

Chinaherb
29A Albion Street

Surry Hills, NSW 2010
Tel: 02-281-2122

Egyptian Medicine

MANNICHE, Lise. ***An Ancient Egyptian Herbal***. Austin, Texas: University of Texas Press, 1989.

STETTER, Cornelius. ***The Secret Medicine of the Pharaohs.*** Carol Stream, Illinois: Quintessence Publishing Co., Inc., 1993.

Herbal Organizations

American Botanical Council
P. O. Box 201660W
Austin, TX 78720
Tel: (512) 331-8868
Write for a catalog. Publishes *Herbalgram*, which is available for a fee.

American Herbalists Association
P. O. Box 1673
Nevada City, CA 95959

American Herbalists Guild
P. O. Box 746555
Arvada, CO 8006-6555
Tel: (303) 423-8800
Fax: (303) 428-8828
The "AHG" is a professional body of herbalists dedicated to promoting and maintaining criteria for the practice of professional herbalism in America.

Herb Research Foundation
1007 Pearl Street, Suite 200F
Boulder, CO 80302

Institute for Wholistic Education
Dept. AR
33719 116th St.
Twin Lakes, WI 53181
Ph: 262-877-9396
Beginner and Advanced Correspondence Courses in Ayurveda.

International Herb Growers and Marketers Association
Box 77123
Baton Rouge, LA 70879

Herbal Studies

East West Herbal Correspondence School
by Michael & Lesley Tierra
P. O. Box 712, Santa Cruz, CA 95061

Live Herbs and Seeds

Shephards Garden Seeds
6116 Highway 9
Felton, CA 95018

Taylor's Garden, Inc.
1535 Lone Oak Road
Vista, CA 92083

Organic Herb Farms

Pacific Botanicals
360 Stephen Way
Williams, Oregon 97544

Trout Lake Herb Farm
Rt. 1, Box 355
Trout Lake, Washington 98650

Wildcrafters

Blessed Herbs
Michael Volchok
Rt. 5, Box 191A
Ava, Mo 85020

Mike and Debby Minear
Rt. 1, Box 60
Little Hocking, OH 45742

Reevis Mountain School of Survival
HC02 Box 1543
Roosevelt, AZ 85545

Bibliography

BAINES, John & MALEK, Jaromir. **Atlas of Ancient Egypt.** Cairo, Egypt: Les Livres de France, 1992.

BALCH, Phyllis, C.N.C., & BALCH, James, M.D. **Rx Prescription**

for Cooking. Greenfield, Indiana: PAB Books Publishing, Inc., 1991.

BASTIEN, Joseph W. **Drum and Stethoscope: Integrating Ethnomedicine and Biomedicine in Bolivia**. Salt Lake City, Utah: University of Utah Press, 1992.

BEIJING, SHANGHAI, & NANJING COLLEGES OF TRADITIONAL CHINESE MEDICINE & THE ACUPUNCTURE INSTITUTE OF THE ACADEMY OF TRADITIONAL CHINESE MEDICINE (Compiled by). **Essentials of Chinese Acupuncture**. Beijing, China: Foreign Languages Press, 1980.

BEINFIELD, Harriet, L.Ac. & KORNGOLD, Efrem, L.Ac., O.M.D. **Between Heaven and Earth - A Guide To Chinese Medicine**. New York, New York: Ballantine Books, 1991.

BENEDICT, Ruth. **Patterns of Culture.** Boston, Massachusetts: Houghton Mifflin Company, 1934.

BENSKY, Dan, & GAMBLE, Andrew (Translators). **Chinese Herbal Medicine Materia Medica**. Seattle, Washington: Eastland Press, 1993.

BENSKY, Dan, & BAROLET, Randall (Translators). **Chinese Herbal Medicine Formulas & Strategies**. Seattle, Washington: Eastland Press, 1990.

BERKOW, Robert, M.D. (Editor-in-Chief). **The Merck Manual of Diagnosis and Therapy.** Rathway, New Jersey: Merck Research Laboratories, 1992.

BHISHAGRATNA, Kaviraj Kunjalal. **An English Translation of the Sushruta Shamita Based on Original Sanskrit Text, Vol. 1.** Varanasi, India: Chowkhamba Sanskrit Series Office, 1996.

BHISHAGRATNA, Kaviraj Kunjalal. **An English Translation of the Sushruta Shamita Based on Original Sanskrit Text, Vol. 2.** Varanasi, India: Chowkhamba Sanskrit Series Office, 1996.

BHISHAGRATNA, Kaviraj Kunjalal. **An English Translation of the Sushruta Shamita Based on Original Sanskrit Text, Vol. 3.** Varanasi, India: Chowkhamba Sanskrit Series Office, 1996.

BINFORD, Lewis R. **In Pursuit of the Past.** New York, New York: Thames and Hudson, 1983.

BLY, Robert, editor. **News of the Universe.** San Francisco, California: Sierra Club Books, 1980.

BOWN, Deni. **The Herb Society of America Encyclopedia of Herbs & Their Uses.** New York, New York: Dorling Kindersley Publishing Inc., 1995.

CAMPBELL, Joseph. **The Mythic Image.** Princeton, New Jersey: Princeton University Press, 1974.

CARPER, Jean. **Total Nutrition Guide.** New York, New York: Bantam Books, 1987.

CHIN, Wee Yeow & KENG, Hsuan. **An Illustrated Dictionary of Chinese Medicinal Herbs.** Sebastopol, California: CRCS Publications, 1992.

CHOPRA, Deepak, M.D. **Perfect Health - The Complete Mind/Body Guide**. New York, New York: Crown Publishers, Inc., 1991.

CHOPRA, Deepak, M.D. **Quantum Healing - Exploring the Frontiers of Mind/Body Medicine**. New York, New York: Bantam Doubleday Dell Publishing Group, Inc., 1989.

CHOPRA, Deepak, M.D. **Unconditional Life**. New York, New York: Bantam Books, 1991.

CLAUDE-PIERRE, Peggy. **The Secret Language of Eating Disorders.** New York, New York: Random House, Inc., 1997.

COBO, Father Bernabe (1582-1657) translated by HAMILTON, Roland. **History of the Inca Empire.** Austin, Texas: University of Texas Press, 1998 ed.

COWAN, C. Wesley & WATSON, Patty Jo (Editors). **The Origins of Agriculture.** Washington, D.C.: Smithsonian Institution Press, 1992.

DASTUR, J. F. **Everybody's Guide to Ayurvedic Medicine.** Bombay, India: D. B. Taraporevala Sons & Co. Private Ltd., 1972.

D'ADAMO, Peter, Dr. with Whitney, Catherine. **Eat Right for Your Type.** New York, New York: G. P. Putnam's Sons, 1996.

DesMAISONS, Kathleen, Ph.D. **Are You Sugar Sensitive? Potatoes Not Prozac.** New York, New York: Simon & Schuster, 1998.

DUFTY, William. **Sugar Blues**. New York, New York: Warner Books, 1976.

ERASMUS, Udo. **Fats that Heal - Fats that Kill.** Burnaby BC, Canada: Alive Books, 1986.

ERICHSEN-BROWN, Charlotte. **Medicinal and Other Uses of North American Plants.** New York, New York: Dover Publications, Inc., 1989.

ESTES, J. Worth. **The Medical Skills of Ancient Egypt.** Caton, Massachusetts: Science History Publications/USA, 1993.

FLAWS, Bob. **The Book of Jook - Chinese Medicinal Porridges.** Boulder, Colorado: Blue Poppy Press, 1995.

FLAWS, Bob & WOLFE, Honora. **Prince Wen Hui's Cook - Chinese Dietary Therapy.** Brookline, Massachusetts: Paradigm Publications, 1983.

FOX, Stuart Ira. **Human Physiology**. Dubuque, Iowa: Wm. C. Brown Publishers, 1987.

FRATKIN, Jake. **Chinese Herbal Patent Formulas - A Practical Guide.** Boulder, Colorado: SHYA Publications, 1993.

GEERTZ, Clifford. **The Interpretation of Cultures**. New York, New York: Basic Books, 1973.

GITTLEMAN, Ann Louise, M.S. **Your Body Knows Best.** New York, New York: Simon & Schuster, Inc., 1996.

GLANZE, Walter D. (Managing Editor). **Mosby's Medical, Nursing, and Allied Health Dictionary**. St. Louis, Missouri: The D. V. Mosby Company, 1990.

HAAS, Elson M., M.D. **Staying Healthy with the Seasons**. Berkeley, California: Celestial Arts, 1981.

HAAS, Elson M., M.D. **Staying Healthy with Nutrition**. Berkeley, California: Celestial Arts, 1992.

Hammer, Leon, M.D. **Dragon Rises • Red Bird Flies (Psychology & Chinese Medicine)**. Barrytown, New York: Station Hill Press, 1990.

HAY, John. **Kernals of Energy, Bones of Earth**. New York, New York: Eastern Press, Inc., 1985.

HEATHERLEY, Ana Nez. **Healing Plants - A Medicinal Guide to Native North American Plants and Herbs.** New York, New York: The Lyons Press, 1998.

HEISER, Charles B. **Seed to Civilization (The Story of Food).** Cambridge, Massachusetts: Harvard University Press, 1973.

HELLER, Rachael F., Ph.D., HELLER, Richard F., Ph.D. **The Carbohydrate Addict's Diet.** New York, New York: Penguin Books, 1993.

HENDERSON, John S. **The World of the Ancient Maya.** Ithaca, New York: Cornell University Press, 1997.

HOBBS, Christopher. **The Ginsengs - A User's Guide.** Santa Cruz, CA: Botanica Press, 1996.

HOBBS, Christopher. **Handbook for Herbal Healing.** Santa Cruz, CA: Botanica Press, 1990.

HSU, Hong-Yen, PhD. & HSU, Chau-Shin, Ph.D. **Commonly Used Chinese Herb Formulas**. Long Beach, California: Oriental Healing Arts Institute, 1980.

JUNG, C. G. **The Archetypes and the Collective Unconscious.** Princeton, New Jersey: Princeton University Press, 1990.

JUNG, C. G. **Memories, Dreams, Reflections.** New York, New York: Vintage Books, 1961.

JUNG, C. G. **Symbols of Transformation.** Princeton, New Jersey: Princeton University Press, 1990.

JUNG, C. G. **Word and Image.** Princeton, New Jersey: Princeton University Press, 1979.

KAPTCHUK, Ted. **The Web That Has No Weaver.** New York, New York: Cogndon & Weded, 1983.

KUNZ, Jeffrey, M.D. & FINKEL, Asher, M.D. **The American Medical Association Family Medical Guide**. New York, New York: Random House, 1987.

KUSHI, Aveline. **Aveline Kushi's Complete Guide to Macrobiotic Cooking.** New York, New York: Warner Books, 1985.

KUSHI, Aveline & ESKO, Wendy. **The Changing Seasons Macrobiotic Cookbook.** Wayne, New Jersey: Avery Publishing Group, Inc., 1985.

KUSHI, Michio. **Book of Macrobiotics.** New York, New York: Japan Publications, 1977.

KUSHI, Michio. **Macrobiotic Home Remedies.** New York, New York: Japan Publications, 1985.

LAD, Dr. Vasant. **Ayurveda - The Science of Self-Healing**. Twin Lakes, Wisconsin: Lotus Press, 1984.

LAD, Dr. Vasant and FRAWLEY, Dr. David. **The Yoga of Herbs,** Second Revised and Enlarged Edition. Twin Lakes, Wisconsin: 2001.

LAO TZU (translated by John Wu). ***Tao Teh Ching.*** New York, New York: St. John's University Press, 1979.

LARRE, Claude. **Survey of Traditional Chinese Medicine.** Columbia, Maryland: Traditional Acupuncture Foundation, 1986.

LI, Cheng-Yu, C.M.D. (Editor). **Fundamentals of Chinese Medicine**. Brookline, Massachusetts: Paradigm Publications, 1985.

LONG, James W., M.D. **The Essential Guide to Prescription Drugs**. New York, New York: Harper Perennial, 1992.

LU, Henry C. **Chinese System of Food Cures - Prevention & Remedies.** New York, New York: Sterling Publishing Company, 1986.

LU, Henry C. **Chinese Foods for Longevity.** New York, New York: Sterling Publishing Company, 1986.

LUMBRERAS, Luis G. **The Peoples and Cultures of Ancient Peru.** Washington D. C.: Smithsonian Institution Press, 1989.

MACIOCIA, Giovanni. **The Foundations of Chinese Medicine.** New York, New York: Churchill Livingstone, 1989.

MACIOCIA, Giovanni. **Obstetrics & Gynecology in Chinese Medicine.** New York, New York: Churchill Livingstone, 1998.

MACIOCIA, Giovanni. **The Practice of Chinese Medicine.** New York, New York: Churchill Livingstone, 1994.

MANNICHE, Lise. **An Ancient Egyptian Herbal**. Austin, Texas: University of Texas Press, 1989.

McDOUGALL, John, M.D. **The McDougall Program.** New York, New York: Penguin Books, 1991.

McElroy, Ann & Townsend, Patricia K. **Medical Anthropology in Ecological Perspective**. Boulder, Colorado: Westview Press, Inc., 1985.

MERTON, Thomas. **The Way of *Chuang Tzu*.** New York, New York: New Directions, 1965.

MILLER, Mary and TAUBE, Karl. **An Illustrated Dictionary of The Gods and Symbols of Ancient Mexico and the Maya.** New York, New York: Thames and Hudson, 1997.

MOERMAN, Daniel E. **Native American Ethnobotany.** Portland, Oregon: Timber Press, Inc., 1998.

MONOD, Jacques. **Chance and Necessity**. New York, New York: Vantage Books, 1972.

MOORE, Robert & GILLETTE, Douglas. **King, Warrior, Magician, Lover.** San Francisco, California: Harper, 1980.

MOSELEY, Michael E. **The Incas and Their Ancestors.** New York, New York: Thames and Hudson, 1997.

MUNAKATA, Kiyohiko. **Sacred Mountains in Chinese Art.** Springfield, Illinois: University of Illinois Press, 1991.

MURAMOTO, Naboru. **Healing Ourselves.** New York, New York: Swan House Publishing Company, 1973.

MYERS, Isabel Briggs. **Gifts Differing - Understanding Personality Type.** Palo Alto, California: Davies-Black Publishing, 1995.

NI, Maoshing, Ph.D., CA, with McNEASE, Cathy. **The Tao of Nutrition.** Santa Monica, CA: Seven Star Communications Group, 1987.

NUNN, John F. **Ancient Egyptian Medicine.** Norman, Oklahoma: University of Oklahoma Press, 1996.

ODY, Penelope. **The Complete Medicinal Herbal.** New York, New York: DK Publishing, 1993.

ORNISH, Dean, M.D. **Dr. Dean Ornish's Program for Reversing Heart Disease**. New York, New York: Random House, 1990.

PEARMAN, Roger R. and ALBRITTON, Sarah C. **I'm Not Crazy - I'm Just Not You.** Palo Alto, California: Davies-Black Publishing, 1997.

PENNINGTON, Jean, Ph.D., R.D. (revised by). **Bowes and Church's Food Values of Portions Commonly Used.** New York, New York: HarperPerennial, 1989.

PITCHFORD, Paul. **Healing with Whole Foods - Oriental Traditions and Modern Nutrition.** Berkeley, California: North Atlantic Books, 1993.

Quenk, Naomi L. **Beside Ourselves - Our Hidden Personality in Everyday Life.** Palo Alto, California: Davies-Black Publishing, 1993.

RAVEN, Peter, EVERT, Ray & EICHHORN, Susan. **Biology of Plants.** New York, New York: Worth Publishers, Inc., 1987.

REA, Amadeo M.. **At the Desert's Green Edge - An Ethnobotany of the Gila River Pima.** Tucson, Arizona: The University of Arizona Press, 1997.

REQUENA, Yves, M.D. **Terrains and Pathology in Acupuncture**. Brookline, Massachusetts: Paradigm Publications, 1986.

RILKE (translated by Stephen Mitchell). **The Selected Poetry of Rilke.** New York, New York: Vintage Books, 1989.

ROBIN, Eugene D., M.D. **Matters of Life & Death: Risks vs. Benefits of Medical Care**. Stanford, California: Stanford Alumni Association, 1984.

ROBBINS, John. **Diet for a New America.** Walpole, New Hampshire: Stillpoint Publishing, 1987.

ROBBINS, John. **Reclaiming Our Health.** Tiburon, California: HJ Kramer, 1996.

ROSTWOROWSKI de DIEZ CANSECO, Maria, **History of the Inca Realm.** Cambridge, United Kingdom: Cambridge University Press, 1999.

RUMI (versions by John Moyne and Coleman Barks). **Open Secret.** Vermont: Threshold Books, 1984.

ST. BARBE BAKER, Richard. **My Life My Trees.** Scotland: The Findhorn Press, 1970.

SEARS, Barry, Ph.D. **Enter the Zone.** New York, New York: HarperCollins Publishers, 1995.

SEARS, Barry, Ph.D. **Mastering the Zone.** New York, New York: HarperCollins Publishers, 1997.

SOULIÉ DE MORANT, George. **Chinese Acupuncture.** Brookline Massachusetts: Paradigm Publications, 1994.

SMITH, Fritz Frederick, M.D. **Inner Bridges - A Guide to Energy Movement and Body Structure.** Atlanta, Georgia: Humanics Limited, 1986.

STETTER, Cornelius. **The Secret Medicine of the Pharaohs.** Carol Stream, Illinois: Quintessence Publishing Co., Inc., 1993.

THOMAS, Clayton, L., M.D. (Editor). **Taber's Cyclopedic Medical Dictionary**. Philadelphia, Pennsylvania: F. A. Davis Company, 1987.

THOMAS, David Hurst. **Archaeology - Down to Earth.** Orlando, Florida: Harcourt Brace Jovanovich College Publishers, 1991.

TIERRA, Lesley, L.Ac. **The Herbs of Life - Health & Healing Using Western & Chinese Techniques**. Freedom, California: The Crossing Press, 1992.

TIERRA, Lesley, L.Ac. **Healing With Chinese Herbs.** Freedom, California: The Crossing Press, 1997.

TIERRA, Michael, L.Ac., O.M.D. **Planetary Herbology**. Twin Lakes, Wisconsin: Lotus Press, 1988.

TIERRA, Michael, L.Ac., O.M.D. **The Way of Herbs.** New York, New York: 1983.

TURNER, Kristina. **The Self-Healing Cookbook.** Grass Valley, California: Earthtones Press, 1987.

VEITH, Ilza (translator). **The Yellow Emperor's Classic of Internal Medicine.** Berkeley, California: University of California - Berkeley, 1966.

VOGEL, Virgil J. **American Indian Medicine.** Norman, Oklahoma: University of Oklahoma Press, 1970.

VON HAGEN, Adriana and Morris, Craig. **The Cities of the Ancient Andes.** New York, New York: Thames & Hudson Ltd., 1998.

WEAVER, Jace. **Native American Religious Identity - Unforgotten Gods.** Maryknoll, New York: Orbis Books, 1998.

WEINER, Michael A. **Earth Medicine Earth Food.** New York, New York: Ballentine Books, 1980.

WERBACH, Melvyn R., M.D. **Nutritional Influences on Illness**. New Canaan, Connecticut: Keats Publishing, Inc., 1988.

WILHELM, Richard, translator. ***I Ching*.** Princeton, New Jersey: Princeton University Press, 1950.

WURTMAN, Judith J. **The Serotonin Solution.** New York, New York: Fawcett Columbine, 1997.

YEN, Kun-Ying, Ph.D. **The Illustrated Chinese Materia Medica.** Taiwan, Republic of China: SMC Publishing Inc., 1992.

ZHANG, Zhongjing (translated by Luo Xiwen, MA, Ph.D.). **Synopsis of Prescriptions of the Golden Chamber.** Beijing, China: New World Press, 1987.

ZIHLMAN, Adrienne L. **The Human Evolution Coloring Book.** New York, New York: HaperCollins Publishers, Inc., 1982.

To Learn About
the Five Elements,
the Real Teacher
is Nature.

Index

BOOKS OF RELATED INTEREST

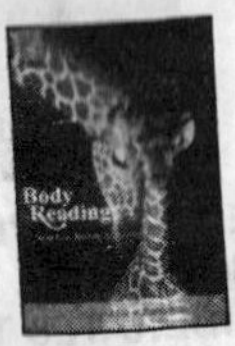

BODY READING
Your Body Reveals Your Personality

Gopesh Kumar Ojha
Ashutosh Ojha

81-7822-100-4

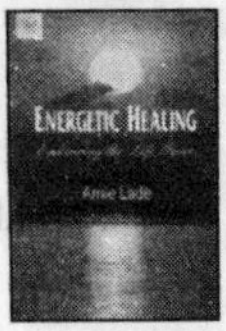

ENERGETIC HEALING
Embracing the Life Force

Arnie Lade

81-7822-005-9

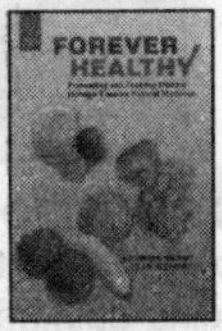

FOREVER HEALTHY
Preventing and Treating Disease through Timeless Natural Medicine

Kumuda Reddy
Stan Kendz

81-7822-171-3

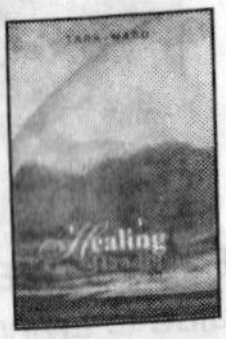

THE HEALING HANDBOOK
A Spiritual Guide to Healing Yourself and Others

Tara Ward

81-7822-034-2

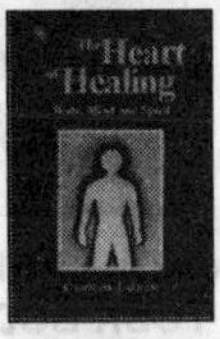

THE HEART OF HEALING
Body, Mind and Spirit

Caroline Latham

81-7822-019-9

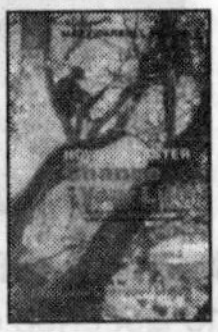

HOW TO MASTER CHANGE IN YOUR LIFE
Sixty-Seven Ways to Handle Life's Toughest Moments

Mary Carroll Moore

81-7822-036-9

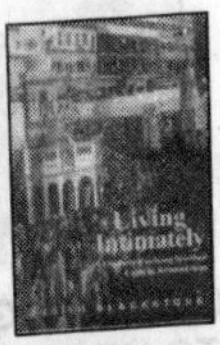

LIVING INTIMATELY
A Guide to Realizing Spiritual Unity in Relationships

Judith Blackstone

81-7822-143-8

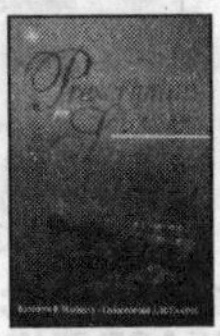

PRESCRIPTION FOR STRESS

Kenneth B. Matheny
Christopher J. McCarthy

81-7822-032-6

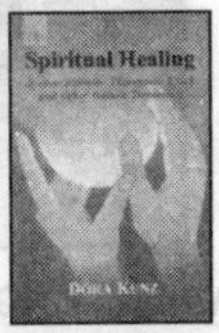

SPIRITUAL HEALING
Doctors Examine Therapeutic Touch and other Holistic Treatments

Dora Kunz

81-7822-011-3

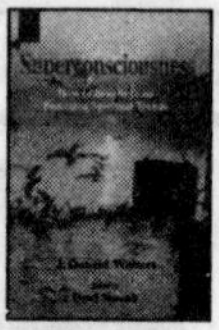

SUPERCONSCIOUSNESS
How to Benefit from Emerging Spiritual Trends

J. Donald Walters

81-7822-026-1

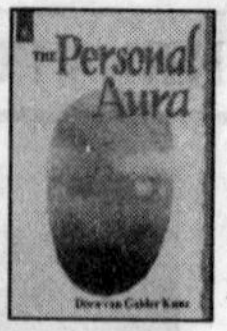

THE PERSONAL AURA

Dora Van Gelder Kunz

81-7822-073-3

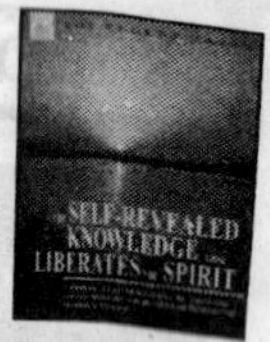

THE SELF-REVEALED KNOWLEDGE THAT LIBERATES THE SPIRIT

Roy Eugene Davis

81-7822-050-4

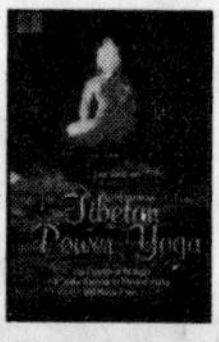

TIBETAN POWER YOGA
The Essence of All Yogas: A Tibetan Exercise for Physical Vitality and Mental Power

Jutta Mattausch

81-7822-006-7

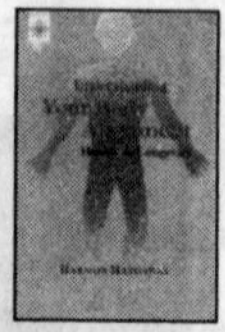

UNDERSTANDING YOUR BODY ALIGNMENT
Health and Longevity

Harmon Hathaway

81-7822-001-6

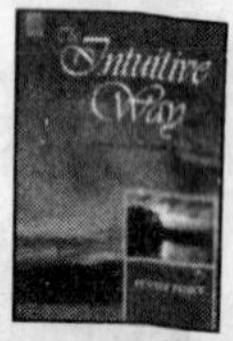

THE INTUITIVE WAY
A Guide to Living From Inner Wisdom

Penney Peirce

81-7822-008-3

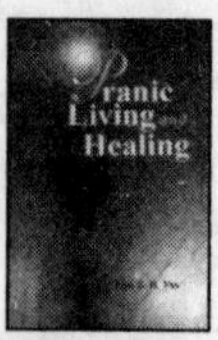

PRANIC LIVING AND HEALING

Luis S.R. Vas

81-7822-161-6

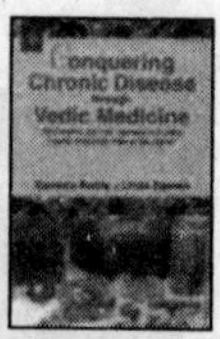

CONQUERING CHRONIC DISEASE THROUGH VEDIC MEDICINE
The Complete Ayurvedic Approach to Treating Chronic Complaints without Side Effects

Kumuda Reddy
Linda Egenes

81-7822-169-1

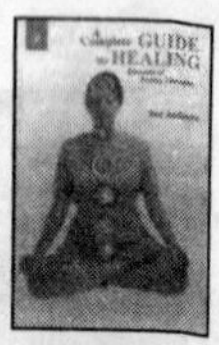

A COMPLETE GUIDE TO HEALING
Elements of Energy Therapies

Ted Andrews

81-7822-119-5